Comprehensive Gynecology and Obstetrics

Series Editors

Ikuo Konishi
National Kyoto Medical Center
Kyoto
Japan

Hidetaka Katabuchi
Department of Obstetrics and Gynecology
Kumamoto University
Kumamoto
Japan

This series presents the current and future perspectives of medical science in gynecology and obstetrics. The authors fully describe the current understanding of a disease including clinical features, imaging, pathology, and molecular biology, and also include the historical aspects and theories for exploring the etiology of the disease. Also, recent developments in diagnostic strategy, medical treatment, surgery, radiotherapy, prevention, and better health-care methods are clearly shown. Thus, each volume in the series focuses on the scientific basis for the pathogenesis of a disease and provides clinical applications that make it possible to offer personalized treatment for each patient. Over the past 20 years, physicians have been working to develop a standard treatment and publish clinical guidelines for a disease based on epidemiological evidence, mainly through the use of randomized clinical trials and meta-analyses. Recently, however, comprehensive genomic and genetic analyses have revealed the differences and variations in biological characteristics even among patients with the same diagnosis and have been focusing on personalized therapy. Now all physicians and patients are entering a new world of "precision medicine" through the use of genomic evidence. We are confident that readers will greatly benefit from the contents of the series with its purview of the exciting and promising future of gynecology and obstetrics.

More information about this series at http://www.springer.com/series/13621

Hideaki Masuzaki
Editor

Fetal Morph Functional Diagnosis

Springer

Editor
Hideaki Masuzaki
Nagasaki University
Nagasaki
Japan

ISSN 2364-1932 ISSN 2364-219X (electronic)
Comprehensive Gynecology and Obstetrics
ISBN 978-981-15-8170-0 ISBN 978-981-15-8171-7 (eBook)
https://doi.org/10.1007/978-981-15-8171-7

This Springer imprint is published by the registered company Springer Nature Singapore Pte Ltd.
The registered company address is: 152 Beach Road, #21-01/04 Gateway East, Singapore 189721, Singapore

Preface

The development of fetology has been dependent on advances in the field of prenatal diagnosis. There are numerous congenital abnormalities (structural, chromosomal, genetic, miscellaneous, etc.); the overall prevalence of disorders is approximately 2 per 100 of pregnancies. The early prenatal detection of congenital abnormality allows both parents and medical carers to plan the management for the pregnancy. Accurate provision of information regarding the incidence, likely outcome, screening, and diagnosis of congenital abnormalities is an essential part of pregnancy care. Without the ability to accurately evaluate the structure and the function of the fetus, it would not be possible to diagnose or treat the wide range of abnormalities that are now addressed by the special fetal medical care unit. This book shows new finding such as real-time 3D ultrasound, ultrafast fetal MRI, genetic counseling, fetal screening and diagnostic test, next-generation sequencing, and fetal therapy. Geneticists, obstetrician, pediatrician, genetic counselor, and nurses are interested in prenatal screening, genetic counseling, and prenatal diagnosis of the fetus. Numerous genetic syndromes exist, the majority of which are sporadic but some with established patterns of inheritance. The latter are relatively uncommon and are screened for only after the family has undergone genetic counseling regarding the disease, chance of recurrence, diagnostic tests, and possible therapeutic interventions. The distinction between screening and diagnosis of congenital abnormalities is often blurred in common usage. Screening tests (triple test, NT by ultrasound, NIPT, etc.) do not confer any risk to the pregnancy. Diagnostic tests on the other hand are carried out on pregnancies that have been identified as "high risk" by a prior screening test. They are usually invasive and have a risk of miscarriage. A number of different tests (amniocentesis, chorionic villus sampling, and cordocentesis) exist to detect sampling material of fetal origin. The sample obtained can be used for cytogenetic, biochemical, enzymatic, or DNA analysis to give a prenatal diagnosis. Generally, these tests are invasive and carry a risk of miscarriage.

This book covers both basic and clinical research. This book is very original, and all the authors are top scientists for prenatal screening, genetic counseling, and diagnosis. This book will be a good teacher for understanding recent findings in prenatal diagnosis.

Nagasaki, Japan Hideaki Masuzaki

Contents

Part VI Technical

Part I
Ultrasound Examination

Chapter 1
Ultrasonic Screening

Toshiyuki Hata, Mohamed Ahmed Mostafa AboEllail, Nobuhiro Mori, Aya Koyanagi, and Takahito Miyake

Abstract There have been several guidelines regarding antenatal ultrasonic screening of the fetus. These guidelines mostly focus on first- or mid-trimester fetal ultrasound scan. In Japan, the main target times are mid- and early third trimesters for fetal ultrasound scans. Recently, fetal sonographic screening has also been promoted in the first trimester in Japan. The main objective of fetal sonographic screening in Japan is the detection of fetal abnormalities and amniotic fluid volume abnormalities. In this chapter, we present Japanese standards of fetal sonographic screening in the late first, mid-, and early third trimesters.

Keywords Ultrasonic screening · First trimester · Second trimester · Third trimester · Normal fetus · Fetal abnormality · Amniotic fluid volume

1.1 Introduction

The fetus undergoes different stages of anatomical and physiological development throughout intrauterine life. This hidden life is no longer mysterious since the discovery and development of ultrasound technologies. They have enabled

T. Hata (✉) · T. Miyake
Department of Obstetrics and Gynecology, Miyake Clinic, Okayama, Japan

Department of Perinatology and Gynecology, Kagawa University Graduate School of Medicine, Miki, Kagawa, Japan
e-mail: toshi28@med.kagawa-u.ac.jp

M. A. M. AboEllail · N. Mori
Department of Perinatology and Gynecology, Kagawa University Graduate School of Medicine, Miki, Kagawa, Japan

A. Koyanagi
Department of Obstetrics and Gynecology, Miyake Clinic, Okayama, Japan

H. Masuzaki (ed.), *Fetal Morph Functional Diagnosis*, Comprehensive Gynecology and Obstetrics, https://doi.org/10.1007/978-981-15-8171-7_1

visualization of the fetus throughout different stages of growth and maturation. Such visualization opened the door for a better understanding of normal morphological development and differentiation between normal and abnormal fetal growth. In this chapter, we introduce the Japanese standards of fetal anatomical sonographic screening during different stages of intrauterine life.

1.2 Late First-Trimester Anomaly Scan (at 11–13 Weeks)

1.2.1 Aims of the First-Trimester Anomaly Scan

The first-trimester anomaly scan aims at: confirming fetal viability, accurately determining the gestational age, confirming the fetal numbers present inside the uterus, assessing fetal gross anatomy, and detecting signs of aneuploidy. The rationale of this scan is based upon the fact that embryogenesis is completed by 12 weeks of gestation so the detection rate can increase up to 51% in the first-trimester scan [1]; therefore, it is of marked value to perform first-trimester anomaly scan. Moreover, aneuploidy can show different markers after the first trimester, enhancing its predictability [2–6]. Identification of abnormal anatomical development of the fetus during intrauterine life enables prediction of lethal anomalies or permanent disabilities, which might become a physical and social burden on the parents. Therefore, an early decision regarding the continuation or termination of pregnancy with less morbidities and complications can be achieved with a first-trimester scan [7, 8].

1.2.2 Equipment Used

The minimal requirements for ultrasound equipment are not different from those in second- or late third-trimester scans. Real-time, grey scale two-dimensional (2D) sonography is used. The use of a transvaginal probe may be more beneficial than in second- and third-trimester scans, which mainly depend upon an abdominal approach [9–11]. A device that can provide freeze frames and zoom options, in addition to electronic calipers and cine loop, is essential.

1.2.3 Pre-examination Requirements

Clear, adequate counseling should be provided to the pregnant examinee and her family, aiming at clarifying the value of such a scan and resolving any concerns related to its safety. The shortest possible time of exposure is always advised as an ALARA (As Low As Reasonably Achievable) principle [12–14]. Having a regular

Table 1.1 Fetal anomaly scan checklist (11–13 weeks of gestation)

Head: regular hemisphere shape	Yes ☐	No ☐	Not visualized ☐
Thorax: symmetrical lung fields			
No effusions or masses	Yes ☐	No ☐	Not visualized ☐
Abdomen: stomach present on left side of the abdomen	Yes ☐	No ☐	Not visualized ☐
Extremities: four limbs	Yes ☐	No ☐	Not visualized ☐
Head, neck, thorax, abdomen: abnormal fluid collection	Yes ☐	No ☐	Not visualized ☐
Comments			

schematic strategy helps to avoid missing points in the scan. Therefore, using a checklist is advisable (Table 1.1). After confirming the viability and number of fetuses inside the uterus, the following items should be checked in the first-trimester (11–13 + 6 weeks) scan.

1.2.3.1 Head

The contour of the head should be examined carefully for any distortion or disruption. The shape should be regularly and uniformly rounded (Fig. 1.1a). The biparietal diameter (BPD) is used to determine the gestational age. The presence of a central interhemispheric fissure and a falx dividing the cerebral hemisphere equally should be assessed. The lateral ventricles predominantly appear in this view, filled with fluid, with the choroid plexuses in the posterior two thirds. This view might resemble a hydrocephalus [15]; therefore, meticulous examination is necessary.

1.2.3.2 Thorax

This involves assessment of the lung areas. They show homogenous echogenicity without any masses, cysts, or effusion. Exclusion of a diaphragmatic hernia is essential by ensuring the continuity of the diaphragm with all intrabdominal structures below it. A normal left-sided position of the heart (normal situs) should be confirmed. The four-chamber view of the heart should be checked (Fig. 1.1b). With high-quality devices, more detailed examination of the heart is possible; however, this is not part of the routine scan [16].

1.2.3.3 Abdomen

The integrity and continuation of the abdominal wall should be confirmed. Attachment of the umbilical cord to the abdominal wall should be checked closely. Care should be taken in order not to mistake the physiological umbilical hernia, which persists until 11 weeks of gestation, for anomalies like omphalocele or gastroschisis [17]. Visualization of the stomach in the left upper quadrant of the abdomen helps to confirm normal situs (Fig. 1.1c).

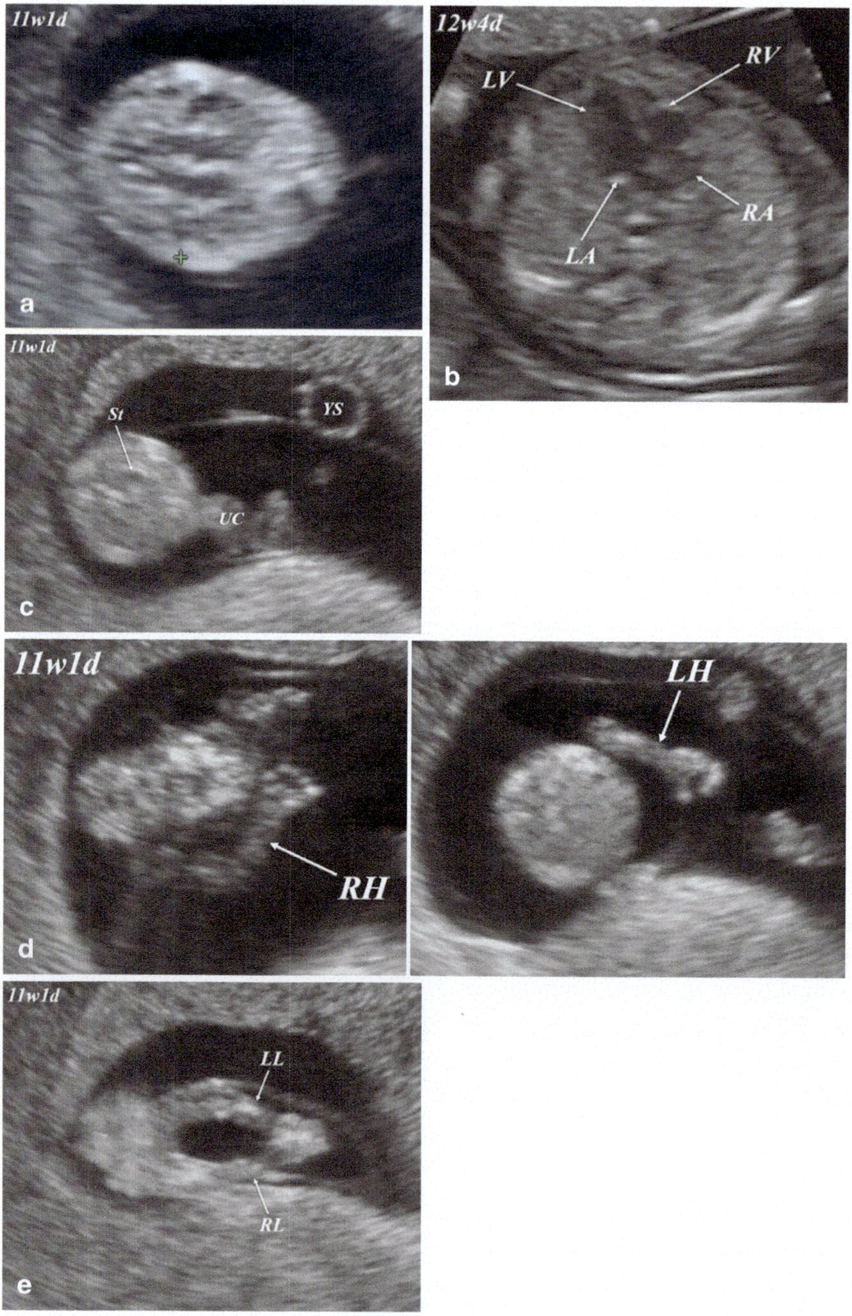

Fig. 1.1 Images of standard views of first-trimester fetal ultrasound examination. (**a**) Fetal head at the level of the biparietal plane. (**b**) Four-chamber view of the fetal heart. (**c**) Abdominal circumference plane showing the position of the stomach *(St)* on the left side, as well as attachment of the umbilical cord *(UC)* to the anterior abdominal wall. Yolk sac *(YS)* can also be visualized. (**d**) Right *(RH)* and left hands *(LH)* with fingers on two-dimensional (2D) sonography. (**e**) Right *(RL)* and left lower limbs *(LL)* demonstrated by 2D sonography

1.2.3.4 Extremities

The four extremities should be assessed regarding the bony parts. The normal orientation of the hands and feet should be confirmed. With high-resolution devices, the hand phalanges can be clearly visualized (Fig. 1.3d, e).

1.2.3.5 Abnormal Fluid Collection

Care should be taken not to overlook any abnormal fluid collection either in the nuchal area by detecting nuchal translucency or inside the body cavities as in the pleura, pericardium, and peritoneum to early identify any pathology or markers of aneuploidy [2, 4, 5].

1.3 Mid-trimester Anomaly Scan (at 18–20 Weeks)

It is the standard for fetal anatomical scanning [18]. The identification of some structures and anomalies like hypoplastic left heart syndrome and corpus callosum agenesis cannot be achieved in the first trimester [19]. Moreover, the first trimester requires more advanced machines and a higher level of education, which might not be possible in all facilities. The ultrasound requirements for the second-trimester scan do not differ from those mentioned in the first-trimester scan section. The following items should be checked during the mid-trimester anomaly scan (Table 1.2).

1.3.1 Head

The transthalamic view is one of the planes that should be used in the anomaly scan (Fig. 1.2a). Moreover, it is the standard view for BPD measurement for accurate gestational age and fetal weight calculation [20, 21]. The calipers should be placed at the outer edge of the near calvarial wall to the inner edge of the far calvarial wall. The head circumference can also be measured in the same plane, and it is more accurate in cases of dolicocephaly or brachycephaly [22]. Brain structures, including the lateral ventricles, choroid plexi, midline falx, cavum septi pellucidi, and thalami, should be assessed with this view. Abnormalities such as anencephaly, holoprosencephaly, encephalocele, and osteogenesis imperfecta are examples of abnormalities that can be diagnosed in this plane [23]. Measurement of the atria of the lateral ventricles should be less than 10 mm; otherwise, diagnosis of hydrocephalus should be considered [24–26]. The transcerebellar plane is obtained by moving the probe more caudally with slight posterior tilting. The

Table 1.2 Fetal anomaly scan checklist (18–20 weeks of gestation)

General	No edema	Yes ☐	No ☐	Not visualized ☐
Head	BPD consistent with gestational age	Yes ☐	No ☐	Not visualized ☐
	Abnormal fluid collection	Yes ☐	No ☐	Not visualized ☐
	Symmetry	Yes ☐	No ☐	Not visualized ☐
Face	Facial clefts	Yes ☐	No ☐	Not visualized ☐
Thorax	Normal thorax	Yes ☐	No ☐	Not visualized ☐
	Normal cardiac position	Yes ☐	No ☐	Not visualized ☐
Heart (four-chamber view)	Normal four-chamber view	Yes ☐	No ☐	Not visualized ☐
	Ventricular symmetry	Yes ☐	No ☐	Not visualized ☐
	Normal cardiac axis	Yes ☐	No ☐	Not visualized ☐
Heart (three-vessel view)	Three vessels alignment	Yes ☐	No ☐	Not visualized ☐
GIT	Left gastric position	Yes ☐	No ☐	Not visualized ☐
	Intestinal dilatation	Yes ☐	No ☐	Not visualized ☐
	Ascites	Yes ☐	No ☐	Not visualized ☐
	Omphalocele and gastroschisis	Yes ☐	No ☐	Not visualized ☐
	Renal abnormalities	Yes ☐	No ☐	Not visualized ☐
Spine	Abnormal spine	Yes ☐	No ☐	Not visualized ☐
Extremities	Short limbs	Yes ☐	No ☐	Not visualized ☐
Amniotic fluid	Polyhydramnios or oligohydramnios	Yes ☐	No ☐	Not visualized ☐
Comments				

BPD biparietal diameter, *GIT* gastrointestinal tract

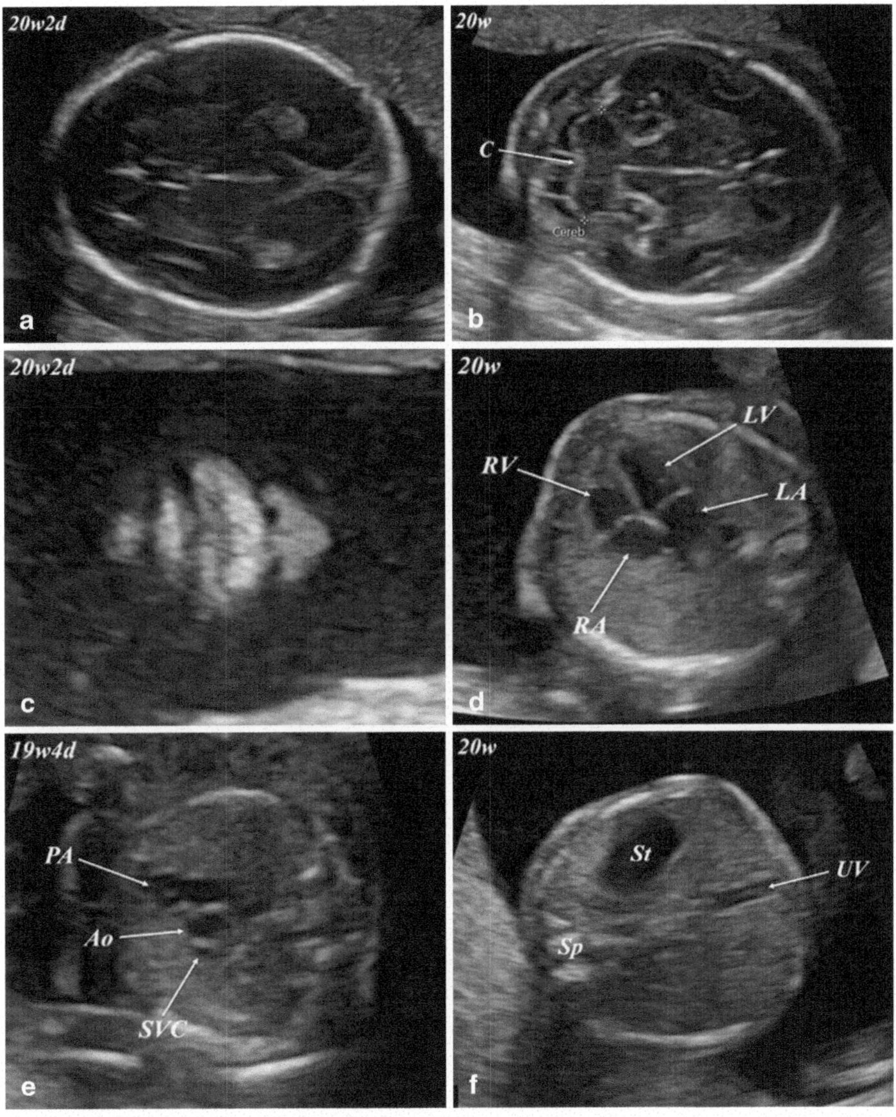

Fig. 1.2 Images of standard views on routine mid-trimester fetal ultrasound examination. (**a**) Biparietal diameter plane. (**b**) Cerebellum *(C)* and cisterna magna with calipers placed to measure the transcerebellar diameter. (**c**) Mouth, nose, and both nostrils. (**d**) Four-chamber view of the fetal heart, showing the right atrium *(RA)*, left atrium *(LA)*, right ventricle *(RV)*, and left ventricle *(LV)*. (**e**) Three-vessel view showing the main pulmonary artery *(PA)*, aorta *(Ao)*, and superior vena cava *(SVC)*. (**f**) Abdominal circumference plane demonstrating the spine *(Sp)*, stomach *(St)*, and umbilical vein *(UV)*. (**g**) Right *(RK)* and left *(LK)* kidneys (axial view) on both sides of the spine *(Sp)*. (**h**) Diaphragm *(D)* with the heart *(H)* above it and abdominal organs below it: liver *(L)*, stomach *(St)*, intestine *(I)*, and urinary bladder *(BL)*. (**i**) Spine (sagittal view). (**j**) Femur diaphysis length. (**k**) Hand with fingers by two-dimensional (2D) sonography. (**l**) Feet and toes demonstrated by 2D sonography. (**m**) Hand with fingers by three-dimensional (3D) ultrasound. (**n**) Feet and toes demonstrated by 3D ultrasound. (**o**) Single pocket vertical diameter measurement during amniotic fluid volume assessment

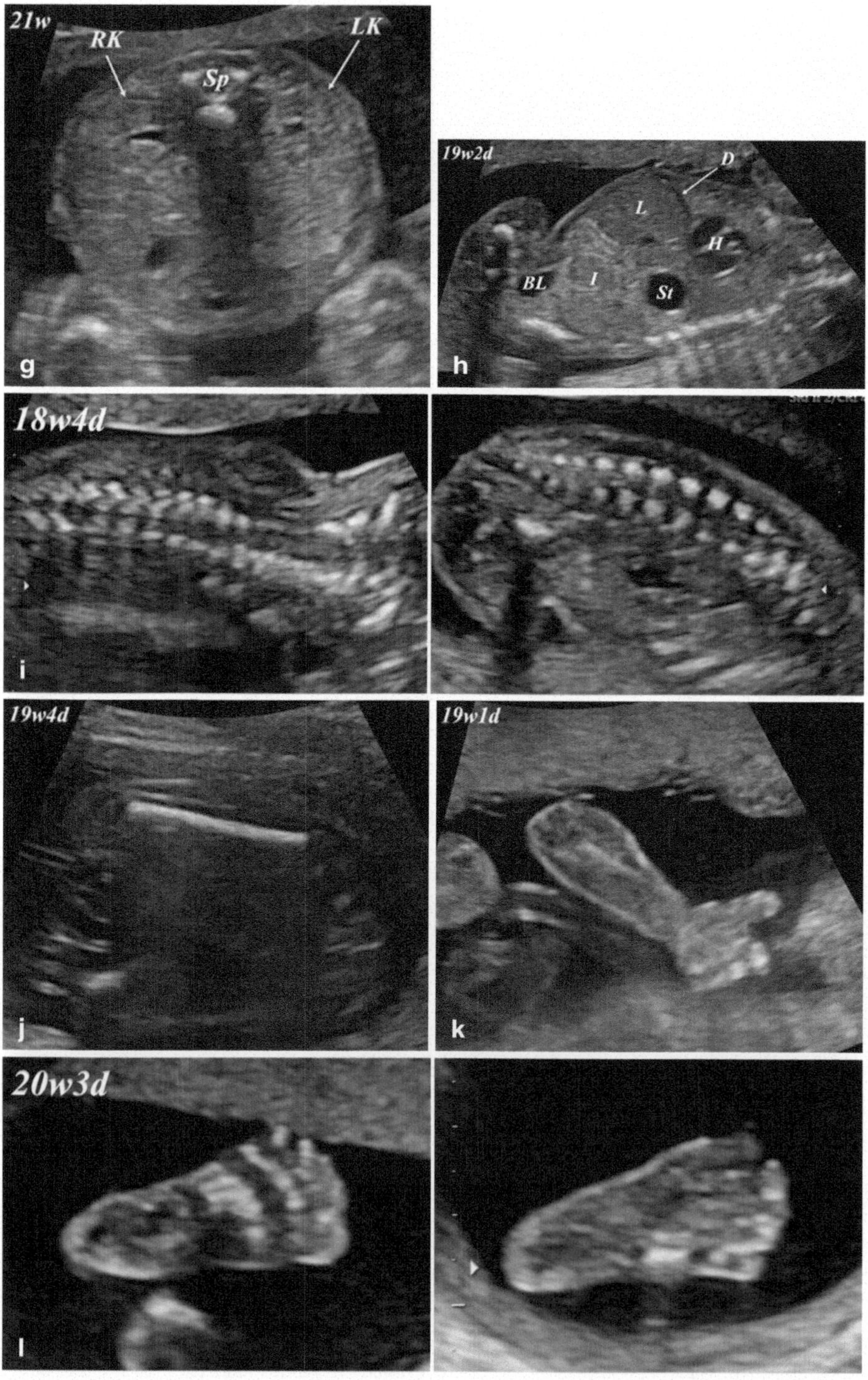

Fig. 1.2 (continued)

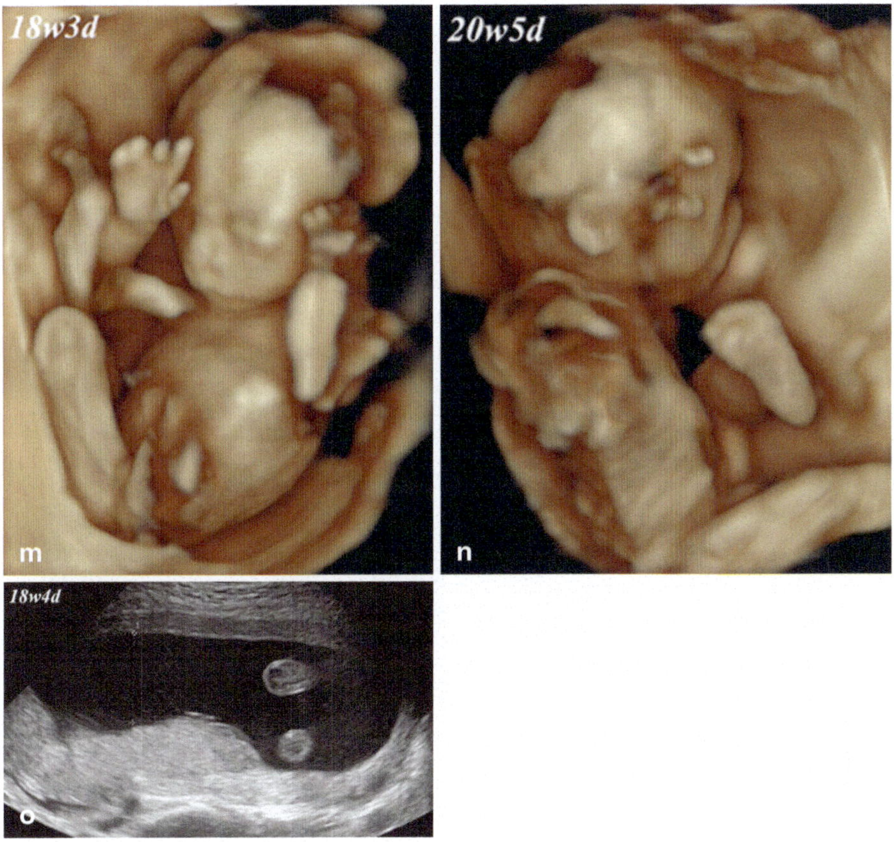

Fig. 1.2 (continued)

characteristic shape is a butterfly appearance showing two cerebellar hemispheres connected by the vermis, as the normal appearance (Fig. 1.2b). The transverse cerebellar diameter and cistern magna depth should be assessed. Abnormalities detected in this plane include a banana-shaped cerebellum in open spina bifida. Dandy Walker malformation, cystic hygroma, can also be diagnosed in this plane [27].

1.3.2 Face

A coronal view of the upper lip should be obtained to exclude cleft clip [28] (Fig. 1.2c). The nose, orbit, and nostrils should be evaluated whenever possible.

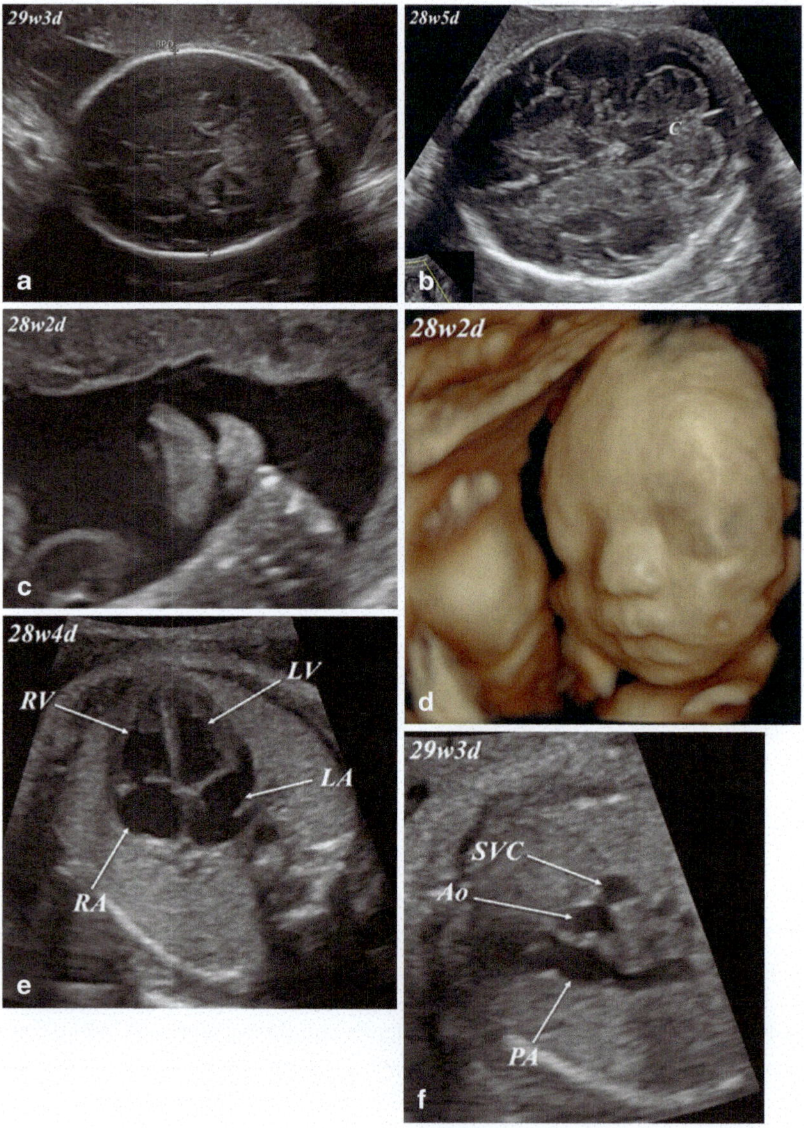

Fig. 1.3 Images of standard views for routine third-trimester fetal ultrasound examination. (**a**) Biparietal diameter plane with calipers placed to measure the biparietal diameter *(BPD)*. (**b**) Cerebellum *(C)* and cisterna magna. (**c**) Mouth, nose, and both nostrils by two-dimensional (2D) ultrasound. (**d**) Three-dimensional (3D) ultrasound view of the fetal face. (**e**) Four-chamber view of the fetal heart showing the right atrium *(RA)*, left atrium *(LA)*, right ventricle *(RV)*, and left ventricle *(LV)*. (**f**) Three-vessel view showing the main pulmonary artery *(PA)*, aorta *(Ao)*, and superior vena cava *(SVC)*. (**g**) Abdominal circumference plane demonstrating the spine *(Sp)*, stomach *(St)*, and umbilical vein *(UV)*. (**h**) Right *(RK)* and left *(LK)* kidneys (axial view) on both sides of the spine *(Sp)*. (**i**) Diaphragm *(D)* with the heart *(H)* above it and abdominal organs below as it: liver (*L*), stomach *(St)*, intestine *(I)*, and urinary bladder (*BL*). (**j**) Spine (sagittal view). (**k**) Femur diaphysis length. (**l**) Hand with fingers by 2D sonography. (**m**) Three-dimensional ultrasound view of a hand with fingers. (**n**) The feet and toes demonstrated by 2D sonography. (**o**) Feet and toes demonstrated by 3D ultrasound. (**p**) Single pocket vertical diameter measurement during amniotic fluid volume assessment

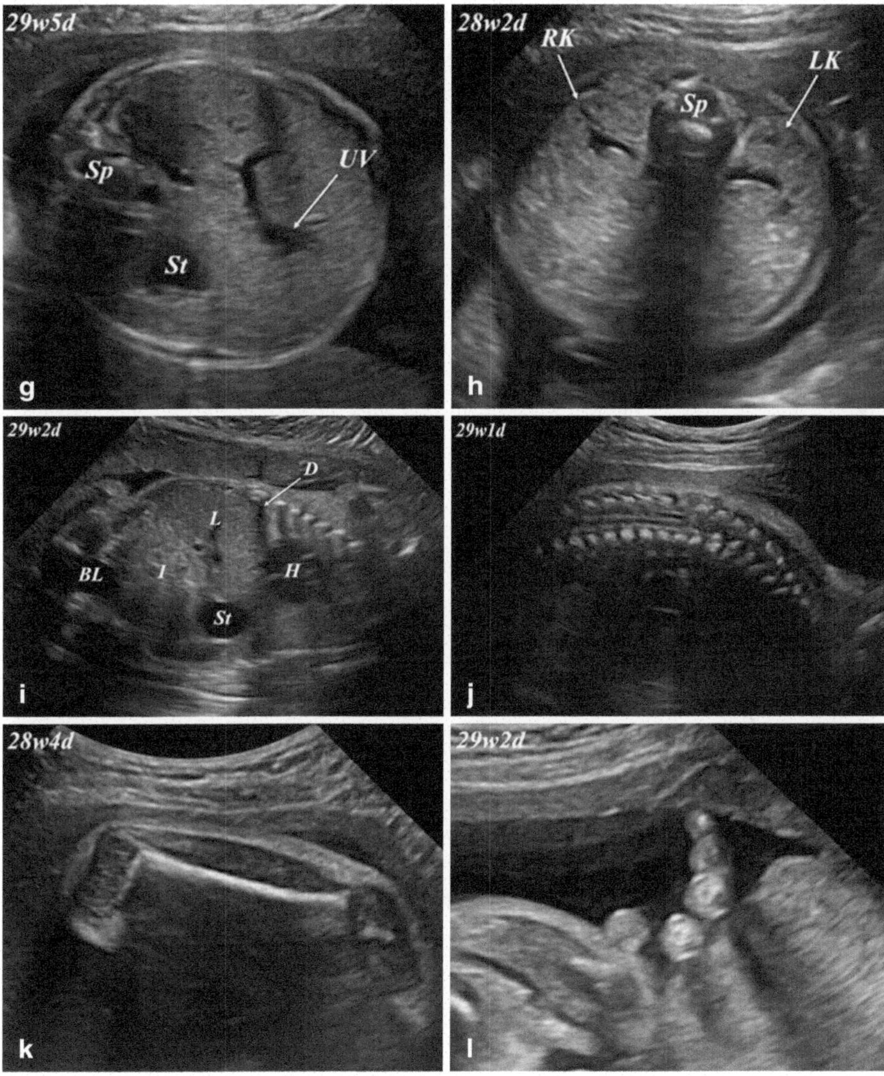

Fig. 1.3 (continued)

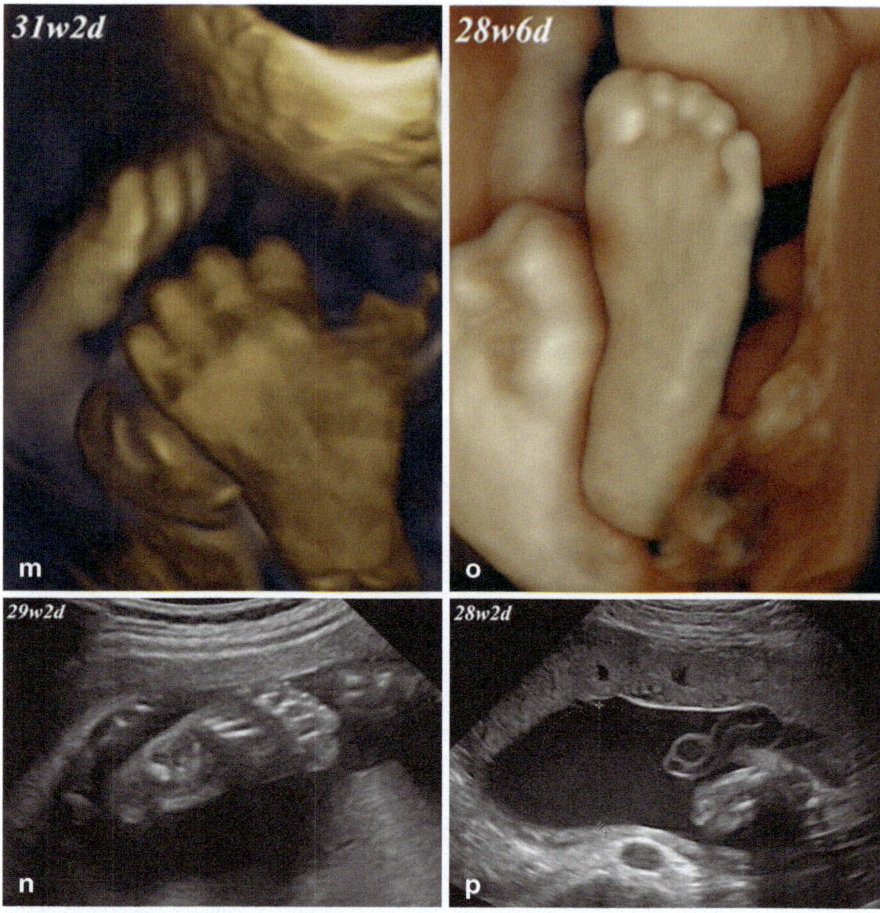

Fig. 1.3 (continued)

1.3.3 Chest and Heart

A mid-trimester scan is ideal for detailed cardiac examination. The heart should occupy about one third of the chest area with its axis pointing to the left at an angle of 45 ± 20° (Mean ± 2 SD) [29]. The standard four-chamber view (Fig. 1.2d) is necessary to evaluate the presence and symmetry of the two atria, two ventricles, and atrioventricular valves. The integrity of the interventricular septum and crux should also be confirmed. A rough evaluation of the fetal heart is advised to help diagnose arrhythmias [30]. The three-vessel view is a transverse view obtained at the upper mediastinum, with the pulmonary artery, aorta, and superior vena cava arranged in a straight line and aorta and pulmonary artery nearly equal in size (usually the pulmonary artery is a little bit larger than the aorta) (Fig. 1.2e). Adding this view to the cardiac examination (four-chamber view) improves the detection rate of fetal cardiac anomalies [31].

Elements in chest examinations are the same as those described in the first-trimester scan.

1.3.4 Abdomen

The presence of the stomach and its location on the left side should be confirmed during abdominal examination (Fig. 1.2f) [32]. This view is also used for measurement of the abdominal circumference to estimate the fetal weight [33]. The kidneys should be checked regarding their presence, echogenicity, and position (Fig. 1.2g). Anomalies such as ectopic kidney, dysplasia, and hydronephrosis can be detected. The intestinal loops should not be dilated, and their echogenicity should be less than the bone in normal cases. The urinary bladder should not be enlarged (Fig. 1.2h), and Doppler can be used to confirm the presence of umbilical arteries around it.

1.3.5 Spine

Transverse, longitudinal, and coronal views should be obtained to examine the whole spine from the cervical to sacral area to exclude anomalies such as spina bifida, vertebral anomalies, and sacral agenesis [27] (Fig. 1.2i).

1.3.6 Extremities

The femur length is measured as a factor in biometry and fetal weight estimation (Fig. 1.2j) [34]. Systematic evaluation of the extremities is essential, starting from the long bones ending at the hands (Fig. 1.2k)/feet (Fig. 1.2l). Checking the alignment of the bones and their densities can exclude anomalies as clubfoot and arthrogryposis [35]. Three-dimensional (3D) ultrasound can be used to count the fingers and toes to exclude anomalies (Fig. 1.2m, n) [36].

1.3.7 Amniotic Fluid

Amniotic fluid evaluation can be done roughly with a panoramic view of the uterus, or can be accurately estimated by measuring the deepest vertical pocket (Fig. 1.2o). Values of 2 cm or lower are considered to show oligohydramnios, while those of 8 cm or more show polyhydramnios. Another method is measuring the amniotic fluid index (AFI), where the four-quadrant technique is used. The deepest vertical length of each pocket of fluid not occupied by fetal parts or the umbilical cord is measured in each quadrant, and the total values are added together. Values of 5–25 cm are normal, those less than 5 cm show oligohydramnios, and those more than 25 cm show polyhydramnios [37–39].

1.4 Early Third-Trimester Anomaly Scan (28–30 Weeks)

The benefits of a third-trimester scan are numerous [40]:

(A) Confirmation of fetal size and exclusion of small- or large-for-gestational age fetus.
(B) Prediction of preeclampsia.
(C) Diagnosing previously (second-trimester scan) missed anomalies.
(D) Diagnosing anomalies that become more apparent after 20 weeks, such as cases of craniosynostosis, bowel atresia, and achondroplasia.
(E) Diagnosing anomalies that appear only in the third trimester, such as ventriculomegaly after fetal brain hemorrhage or maternal infection, or cases of ovarian cysts due to maternal estrogen stimulation.

The machine requirements and counseling are the same as for the mid-trimester scan. The checklist for this scan is shown in Table 1.3.

1.4.1 Head

The BPD is measured at the level of the transthalamic plane (Fig. 1.3a), the same as in the second trimester. Follow-up charts can help to detect whether the fetal growth is within the normal range or abnormal [41]. The transcerebellar plane should be checked too (Fig. 1.3b). Maternal infections can manifest as brain anomalies in the third trimester.

1.4.2 Face

A coronal view of the upper lip and nose (Fig. 1.3c) should be checked in the third-trimester scan. Three-dimensional modes can generate a realistic picture of the fetal face (Fig. 1.3d). Such images are beneficial to prepare the parents psychologically to accept facial anomalies such as cleft lip [42].

Table 1.3 Fetal anomaly scan checklist (28–30 weeks of gestation)

General	No edema	Yes ☐	No ☐	Not visualized ☐
Head	BPD consistent with gestational age	Yes ☐	No ☐	Not visualized ☐
	Abnormal fluid collection	Yes ☐	No ☐	Not visualized ☐
	Symmetry	Yes ☐	No ☐	Not visualized ☐
Face	Facial clefts	Yes ☐	No ☐	Not visualized ☐
Thorax	Normal thorax	Yes ☐	No ☐	Not visualized ☐
	Normal cardiac position	Yes ☐	No ☐	Not visualized ☐
Heart (four-chamber view)	Normal four-chamber view	Yes ☐	No ☐	Not visualized ☐
	Ventricular symmetry	Yes ☐	No ☐	Not visualized ☐
	Normal cardiac axis	Yes ☐	No ☐	Not visualized ☐
Heart (three-vessel view)	Three vessels alignment	Yes ☐	No ☐	Not visualized ☐
GIT	Left gastric position	Yes ☐	No ☐	Not visualized ☐
	Intestinal dilatation	Yes ☐	No ☐	Not visualized ☐
	Ascites	Yes ☐	No ☐	Not visualized ☐
	Omphalocele and gastroschisis	Yes ☐	No ☐	Not visualized ☐
	Renal abnormalities	Yes ☐	No ☐	Not visualized ☐
Spine	Abnormal spine	Yes ☐	No ☐	Not visualized ☐
Extremities	Short limbs	Yes ☐	No ☐	Not visualized ☐
Amniotic fluid	Polyhydramnios or oligohydramnios	Yes ☐	No ☐	Not visualized ☐
Comments				

BPD biparietal diameter, *GIT* gastrointestinal tract

1.4.3 Chest and Heart

It might be difficult to examine the heart in the third trimester due to shadowing effects of the bone. A four-chamber view (Fig. 1.3e) and three-vessel view (Fig. 1.3f) should be obtained. Elements are the same as those in the second trimester.

1.4.4 Abdomen

The abdominal circumference is measured to help estimate the fetal weight (Fig. 1.3g), the same as mentioned in the second-trimester scan. An axial scan should be done at the level of the kidneys to confirm their presence and exclude renal anomalies (Fig. 1.3h). A coronal view can be obtained to confirm the position of the viscera in relation to the diaphragm, excluding possible diaphragmatic hernia and confirming organ situs (Fig. 1.3i).

1.4.5 Spine

The whole spine from the cervical region down to the sacrum should be thoroughly examined (Fig. 1.3j).

1.4.6 Extremities

Measurement of the femur length is essential for fetal weight calculation (Fig. 1.3k). Moreover, evaluation of long bones is essential to exclude possible shortening in cases of achondroplasia, which is usually diagnosed in the third trimester [43]. Checking the hands with finger counting as well as feet with toe counting is mandatory, and can be done in 2D or 3D modes (Fig. 1.3l–o).

1.4.7 Amniotic Fluid

Checking the amniotic fluid with the same measurements and technique as in the mid-trimester scan should be performed in the late third trimester (Fig. 1.3p).

1.5 Summary

Fetal anatomical ultrasound scanning performed in the first, second, and third trimesters is required to detect fetal anomalies. With each trimester having its peculiar diseases and syndromes, a systematic approach will help to avoid missing anything, and make follow-up easy. A learning curve is needed to master the scan in order to minimize the time for examination, especially when encountering difficulties such as an unfavorable fetal position or actively moving fetus. In conclusion, fetal anatomical scan helps to detect anomalies early with subsequent good perinatal management of the condition and appropriate decision-making.

Conflict of Interest The authors have no conflict of interest.

References

1. Rossi AC, Prefumo F. Accuracy of ultrasonography at 11–14 weeks of gestation for detection of fetal structural anomalies: a systematic review. Obstet Gynecol. 2013;122:1160–7.
2. Nicolaides KH. Screening for fetal aneuploidies at 11 to 13 weeks. Prenat Diagn. 2011;31:7–15.
3. Maiz N, Valencia C, Kagan KO, Wright D, Nicolaides KH. Ductus venosus Doppler in screening for trisomies 21, 18 and 13 and Turner syndrome at 11–13 weeks of gestation. Ultrasound Obstet Gynecol. 2009;33:512–7.
4. Nicolaides KH, Azar G, Byrne D, Mansur C, Marks K. Fetal nuchal translucency: ultrasound screening for chromosomal defects in first trimester of pregnancy. BMJ. 1992;301:867–9.
5. Snijders RJ, Noble P, Sebire N, Souka A, Nicolaides KH. UK multicentric project on assessment of risk of Trisomy 21 by maternal age and fetal nuchal translucency thickness at 10 – 14 weeks of gestation. Lancet. 1998;352:343–6.
6. Kagan KO, Cicero S, Staboulidou I, Wright D, Nicolaides KH. Fetal nasal bone in screening for trisomies 21, 18 and 13 and Turner syndrome at 11–13 weeks of gestation. Ultrasound Obstet Gynecol. 2009;33:259–64.
7. Haak MC, Twisk JW, van Vugt JM. How successful is fetal echocardiographic examination in the first trimester of pregnancy? Ultrasound Obstet Gynecol. 2002;20:9–13.
8. Farraposo S, Montenegro N, Matias A. Evaluation of the role of first-trimester obstetric ultrasound in the detection of major anomalies: a systematic review. J Perinat Med. 2014;42:141–9.
9. Achiron R, Tadmor O. Screening for fetal anomalies during the first trimester of pregnancy: transvaginal versus transabdominal sonography. Ultrasound Obstet Gynecol. 1991;1:186–91.
10. Braithwaite JM, Armstrong MA, Economides DL. Assessment of fetal anatomy at 12 to 13 weeks of gestation by transabdominal and transvaginal sonography. Br J Obstet Gynaecol. 1996;103:82–5.
11. Guariglia L, Rosati P. Transvaginal sonographic detection of embryonic–fetal abnormalities in early pregnancy. Obstet Gynecol. 2000;96:328–32.
12. Miller MW, Brayman AA, Abramowicz JS. Obstetric ultrasonography: a biophysical consideration of patient safety—the "rules" have changed. Am J Obstet Gynecol. 1998;179:241–54.
13. Barnett SB, Ter Haar GR, Ziskin MC, Rott HD, Duck FA, Maeda K. International recommendations and guidelines for the safe use of diagnostic ultrasound in medicine. Ultrasound Med Biol. 2000;26:355–66.
14. Sheiner E, Freeman J, Abramowicz JS. Acoustic output as measured by mechanical and thermal indices during routine obstetric ultrasound examinations. J Ultrasound Med. 2005;24:1665–70.
15. Salomon LJ, Alfirevic Z, Bilardo CM, Chalouhi GE, Ghi T, Kagan KO, Lau TK, Papageorghiou AT, Raine-Fenning NJ, Stirnemann J, Suresh S, Tabor A, Timor-Tritsch IE, Toi A, Yeo G. ISUOG practice guidelines: performance of first-trimester fetal ultrasound scan. Ultrasound Obstet Gynecol. 2013;41:102–13.
16. DeVore GR. First-trimester fetal echocardiography: is the future now? Ultrasound Obstet Gynecol. 2002;20:6–8.
17. van Zalen-Sprock RM, Vugt JM, van Geijn HP. First-trimester sonography of physiological midgut herniation and early diagnosis of omphalocele. Prenat Diagn. 1997;17:511–8.

18. Salomon LJ, Alfirevic Z, Berghella V, Bilardo C, Hernandez-Andrade E, Johnsen SL, Kalache K, Leung KY, Malinger G, Munoz H, Prefumo F, Toi A, Lee W. ISUOG Clinical Standards Committee. Practice guidelines for performance of the routine mid-trimester fetal ultrasound scan. Ultrasound Obstet Gynecol. 2011;37:116–26.
19. Grande M, Arigita M, Borobio V, Jimenez JM, Fernandez S, Borrell A. First-trimester detection of structural abnormalities and the role of aneuploidy markers. Ultrasound Obstet Gynecol. 2012;39:157–63.
20. Hadlock FP, Harrist RB, Shah YP, King DE, Park SK, Sharman RS. Estimating fetal age using multiple parameters: a prospective evaluation in a racially mixed population. Am J Obstet Gynecol. 1987;156:955–7.
21. Taipale P, Hiilesmaa V. Predicting delivery date by ultrasound and last menstrual period in early gestation. Obstet Gynecol. 2001;97:189–94.
22. Hadlock FP, Deter RL, Carpenter RJ, Park SK. Estimating fetal age: effect of head shape on BPD. Am J Roentgenol. 1981;137:83–5.
23. Leung KY, Poon CF, Teotico AR, Hata T, Won HS, Chen M, Chittacharoen A, Malhotra J, Shah PK, Salim A. Recommendations on routine mid-trimester anomaly scan. J Obstet Gynaecol Res. 2015;41:653–61.
24. Cardoza JD, Filly RA, Podrasky AE. The dangling choroid plexus: a sonographic observation of value in excluding ventriculomegaly. Am J Roentgenol. 1988;151:767–70.
25. Cardoza JD, Goldstein RB, Filly RA. Exclusion of fetal ventriculomegaly with a single measurement: the width of the lateral ventricular atrium. Radiology. 1988;169:711–4.
26. Mahony BS, Nyberg DA, Hirsch JH, Petty CN, Hendricks SK, Mack LA. Mild idiopathic lateral cerebral ventricular dilatation in utero: sonographic evaluation. Radiology. 1988;169:715–21.
27. International Society of Ultrasound in Obstetrics and Gynecology. Sonographic examination of the fetal central nervous system: guidelines for performing the 'basic examination' and the 'fetal neurosonogram. Ultrasound Obstet Gynecol. 2007;29:109–16.
28. Rotten D, Levaillant JM. Two- and three- dimensional sonographic assessment of the fetal face. 1. A systematic analysis of the normal face. Ultrasound Obstet Gynecol. 2004;23:224–31.
29. Comstock CH. Normal fetal heart axis and position. Obstet Gynecol. 1987;70:255–9.
30. International Society of Ultrasound in Obstetrics and Gynecology. Cardiac screening examination of the fetus: guidelines for performing the 'basic' and 'extended basic' cardiac scan. Ultrasound Obstet Gynecol. 2006;27:107–13.
31. Yoo S-J, Lee Y-H, Kim ES, Ryu HM, Kim MY, Choi H-K, Cho KS, Kim A. Three-vessel view of the fetal upper mediastinum: an easy means of detecting abnormalities of the ventricular outflow tracts and great arteries during obstetric screening. Ultrasound Obstet Gynecol. 1997;9:173–82.
32. Bronshtein M, Gover A, Zimmer EZ. Sonographic definition of the fetal situs. Obstet Gynecol. 2002;99:1129–30.
33. Hadlock FP, Harrist RB, Sharman RS, Deter RL, Park SK. Estimation of fetal weight with the use of head, body, and femur measurements – a prospective study. Am J Obstet Gynecol. 1985;151:333–7.
34. Lessoway VA, Schulzer M, Wittmann BK. Sonographic measurement of the fetal femur: factors affecting accuracy. J Clin Ultrasound. 1990;18:471–6.
35. Holder-Espinasse M, Devisme L, Thomas D, Boute O, Vaast P, Fron D, Herbaux B, Puech F, Manouvrier-Hanu S. Pre- and postnatal diagnosis of limb anomalies: a series of 107 cases. Am J Med Genet. 2004;124A:417–22.
36. Kos M, Hafner T, Funduk-Kurjak B, Bozek T, Kurjak A. Limb deformities and three-dimensional ultrasound. J Perinat Med. 2002;30:40–7.
37. Magann EF, Sanderson M, Martin JN, Chauhan S. The amniotic fluid index, single deepest pocket, and two-diameter pocket in normal human pregnancy. Am J Obstet Gynecol. 2000;182:1581–8.

38. Kehl S, Schelkle A, Thomas A, Puhl A, Meqdad K, Tuschy B, Berlit S, Weiss C, Bayer C, Heimrich J, Dammer U, Raabe E, Winkler M, Faschingbauer F, Beckmann MW, Sütterlin M. Single deepest vertical pocket or amniotic fluid index as evaluation test for predicting adverse pregnancy outcome (SAFE trial): a multicenter, open-label, randomized controlled trial. Ultrasound Obstet Gynecol. 2016;47:674–9.
39. Nabhan AF, Abdelmoula YA. Amniotic fluid index versus single deepest vertical pocket as a screening test for preventing adverse pregnancy outcome. Cochrane Database Syst Rev. 2008;3:CD006593.
40. Ficara A, Syngelaki A, Hammami A, Akolekar R, Nicolaides KH. Value of routine ultrasound examination at 35–37 weeks' gestation in diagnosis of fetal abnormalities. Ultrasound Obstet Gynecol. 2019; https://doi.org/10.1002/uog.20857.
41. Shinozuka N. Fetal biometry and fetal weight estimation: JSUM standardization. Ultrasound Rev Obstet Gynecol. 2002;2:156–61.
42. Sajapala S, AboEllail MAM, Kanenishi K, Hata T. Fetal face abnormalities: from 2D sonography to HDlive and HDlive silhouette mode. DSJUOG. 2016;10:313–20.
43. Baujat G, Legeai-Mallet L, Finidori G, Cormier-Daire V, Le Merrer M. Achondroplasia. Best Pract Res Clin Rheumatol. 2008;22:3–18.

Chapter 2
Abnormal Findings in Ultrasound Examination

Junichi Hasegawa

Abstract One of the purposes of fetal ultrasound examinations during pregnancy is detection of fetal malformation. Antenatal ultrasound screening for morphological abnormalities has now become an accepted routine in obstetric clinical setting. Obtained antenatal information of the fetal abnormalities allows obstetricians to improve the management of pregnancy and gives parents earlier reassurance about the fetus. With improvement in the resolution of ultrasound, major congenital abnormalities have come to be identified in the first trimester, instead of the second trimester. However, examiners should be aware of potential pitfalls in the first trimester ultrasound diagnosis of the fetal anomaly. The use of a combination of first and second trimester ultrasound scan for detecting fetal anomalies was effective. In this section, important fetal congenital abnormalities are explained. In particular, anomalies associated with chromosomal abnormalities and genetic disease are selected.

Keywords Ultrasound · Fetal anomaly · Second trimester screening · Chromosomal abnormality

2.1 Introduction

The purposes of fetal ultrasound examinations during pregnancy are detection of fetal malformation, screening of aneuploidies, and evaluation of fetal growth and well-being. Antenatal ultrasound screening for morphological abnormalities has now become an accepted routine in obstetric clinical setting. Obtained antenatal

J. Hasegawa (✉)
Department of Obstetrics and Gynecology, St. Marianna University School of Medicine, Kanagawa, Japan

H. Masuzaki (ed.), *Fetal Morph Functional Diagnosis*, Comprehensive Gynecology and Obstetrics, https://doi.org/10.1007/978-981-15-8171-7_2

information of the fetal abnormalities allows obstetricians to improve the management of pregnancy and gives parents earlier reassurance about the fetus [1]. Occasionally, decision of fetal therapy can be made.

Most countries offer at least one mid-trimester scan as a part of standard prenatal care, although obstetric practice varies widely around the world [2]. Fetal ultrasound scans serve as an important baseline against which later scans may be compared for the evaluation of growth and health. Besides, prenatal diagnosis of fetal morphological anomalies is considered as an important purpose of scan [3, 4]. A multicenter project examined the accuracy of routine mid-trimester ultrasonographic examination in unselected populations. 56% of them were detected and 55% of major anomalies were identified before 24 weeks of gestation [5]. The other large studies and systematic reviews report detection rates of 16–44% of anomalies prior to 24 weeks of gestation [5, 6]. Higher detection rates of major and lethal anomalies have been reported.

With improvement in the resolution of ultrasound, major congenital abnormalities have come to be identified in the first trimester, instead of the second trimester. Abnormalities involving virtually every organ system detected in the first trimester have been reported. Nevertheless, second trimester assessments are easy to carry out using a detailed scan; first trimester assessments might be suitable for evaluating the whole body of the fetus and detecting major structural abnormalities.

However, examiners should be aware of potential pitfalls in the first trimester ultrasound diagnosis of the fetal anomaly. In some of the fetal parts, structures may not have already been fully developed at an early gestational age, including herniation of the intestine and development of brain. Unless confident prenatal diagnosis of fetal abnormality can be made during earlier gestational age, follow-up examinations should be performed. Furthermore, especially in the first trimester, though prenatal ultrasonography appears to be safe for clinical practice, examiners should be following the ALARA principle (As Low As Reasonably Achievable) during scan. Fetal exposure times should be minimized, using the lowest possible power output needed to obtain diagnostic information [7].

Therefore, it is considered that the use of a combination of first and second trimester ultrasound scan for detecting fetal anomalies was effective. The provision of intensive and focused ultrasound assessments should be essential for achieving accurate ultrasound prenatal diagnosis [8]. However, as limitation of the ultrasound scan for fetal anomaly should be aware by the examiners, smaller anomalies are unlikely to be detected, especially earlier in pregnancy. Some abnormalities, such as duodenal atresia and achondroplasia, are not suspectable until late in the second trimester. There are a lot of false negatives in the ultrasound screening of the fetal anomalies.

In this section, important fetal congenital abnormalities are demonstrated. In particular, anomalies associated with chromosomal abnormalities and genetic disease are selected.

2.2 Head and Neck

2.2.1 Neural Tube Defects

Neural tube defects (NTD) occur when disruption in closure of the neural tube occurs early in embryogenesis from 4 weeks' conceptional age. NTD include open spina bifida (myelomeningocele) which is a typical NTD located in the caudal portion of the fetus, anencephaly when the cranial portion of the neural tube fails to close, and occipital encephalocele which is a herniation of neural tissue through a cranial defect [9] (Fig. 2.1a–c).

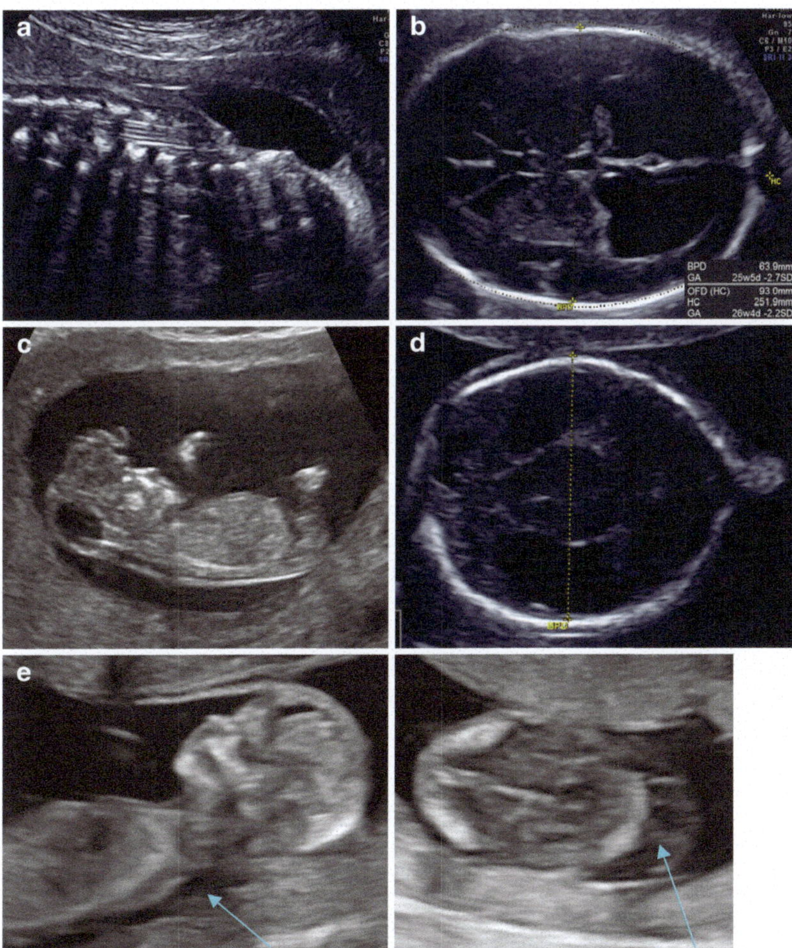

Fig. 2.1 Head and neck. (**a**) Myelomeningocele located in the caudal portion of the fetus. (**b**) Ventriculomegaly associated with myelomeningocele. (**c**) Anencephaly in the first trimester. (**d**) Holoprosencephaly: Incomplete cleavage of the forebrain with cyclopia. (**e**) Cystic hygroma in the first trimester

2.2.1.1 Anencephaly

Anencephaly can make diagnosis in the first trimester, because the cranial vault is possible to depict at 11 weeks [10]. Exencephaly is the finding of anencephaly when brain tissue is floating without cranial bone in the amniotic fluid.

Reduction in cerebrospinal fluid with corresponding reduction in the area of the cerebral ventricular system has been associated with myelomeningocele [11]. Imaging of the posterior fossa also can be helpful for ruling out and diagnosing NTDs in the first trimester. Intracranial translucency, which was first noted during nuchal translucency screening, is the normal fluid-filled area of the fourth ventricle seen in the midsagittal view (Fig. 2.1c).

2.2.2 Myelomeningocele

Spina bifida manifests in various forms. The most common form is myelomeningocele in a type of NTDs, which is the most clinically devastating form but is nonlethal. To diagnose spina bifida, complete ultrasound evaluation of the spine from cervical vertebrae to sacrum should be carried out in the second trimester. However, myelomeningocele is often found through identification of enlargement of the lateral ventricle (Fig. 2.1a, b).

2.2.3 Holoprosencephaly

Holoprosencephaly is a condition of incomplete cleavage of the forebrain. This malformation ranges from complete fusion (alobar), partial fusion with separation of the posterior cerebral hemispheres (semilobar), and partial fusion with separation of both the anterior and posterior cerebral hemispheres (lobar) [9]. Ventriculomegaly also often coexists in cases of holoprosencephaly [12]. Midface abnormalities include incomplete facial development such as cleft lip, single nostril or blind ended nose, iris coloboma, single maxillary incisor, or simply absent philtrum [13] (Fig. 2.1d).

2.2.4 Ventriculomegaly

Ventriculomegaly, which enlarged the lateral cerebral ventricles, is an ultrasound finding of abnormal brain development after the second trimester. Width of the atrium or posterior horn of the lateral ventricle is less than 10 mm throughout the second and third trimester in a normal fetus. Cases whose ventricular atrial width of more than 15 mm indicates severe ventriculomegaly are strongly associated with an intracranial malformation. Severe ventriculomegaly has an increased risk of perinatal death and long-term poor neurologic prognosis [14], though the outcomes depend on the underlying cause.

Mild ventriculomegaly with intermediate value, 10–15 mm of the atrial width, is less frequently associated with significant CNS anomalies [15], but is associated with chromosomal abnormalities. 10% of them might have neurodevelopmental abnormalities of variable types and magnitude. However, most fetuses with mild ventriculomegaly will have a normal outcome [15, 16] (Fig. 2.1b).

2.2.5 Cystic Hygroma and Lymphangioma

Increased nuchal translucency is well-known as a risk factor for aneuploidy. Besides, cystic hygroma is a condition of edema at the fetal neck associated with malformation of the lymphatic system. Early cystic hygromas should be considered associated with congenital syndromes and other malformations [17]. Cystic hygromas should also be distinguished from lymphangiomas which develop later in pregnancy. Cystic hygroma is defined as a septated hypoechoic area behind the fetal neck extending along the fetal back. Half of the cases that diagnosed cystic hygroma have chromosomal abnormalities, and among the chromosomally normal cases, one-third complicated a major structural anomaly, such as cardiac anomaly [18] (Fig. 2.1d).

2.3 Thorax

In the first trimester ultrasound, congenital pulmonary airway malformation (CPAM), bronchopulmonary sequestration (BPS), and congenital diaphragmatic may be diagnosable. However, detection of these malformations is usually performed in the second trimester [9].

2.3.1 CPAM and BPS

CPAMs are the most common lung lesions depicted by ultrasound. CPAMs have been described as hamartomatous malformations of the lung. These malformations are characterized by abnormal branching of immature bronchioles which communicate with the normal tracheobronchial tree and derive their blood supply from normal pulmonary circulation. On the other hand, BPS is a mass of nonfunctioning lung tissue and has aberrant systemic arterial blood supply (descending aorta) [19, 20].

CPAMs are often categorized into three types: Type 1: a lesion with a dominant cyst (3–10 cm); Type 2: multiple small cysts (0.5–2.0 cm); and Type 3: small micro-cyst or solid type of cyst [21]. Larger cyst has more prognostic importance because of shift in the location or axis of the fetal heart and esophageal compression and consequent polyhydramnios, but most of CPAM and BPS have little clinical significance [9].

2.3.2 Congenital Diaphragmatic Hernia

CDH results from absence or deficiency of a portion of the diaphragm owing to incomplete formation of the structure, with subsequent herniation of abdominal contents into the fetal chest.

CDH is most often a sporadic condition, and 85% of the defects are posterolateral and on the fetal left side. Right-sided defects are seen in approximately 10–15% of cases, and 2% of defects occur bilaterally or centrally [22].

The normal primitive diaphragm is formed by the end of the 8th week of gestation with development of the muscular diaphragm completed by the 14th week. Although the failure of fusion of the pleuroperitoneal canal occurs early in gestation, the herniation of intra-abdominal contents may not occur until later in fetal life, making small defects difficult to identify early in pregnancy. Most CDHs are detected at the time of second trimester fetal morphological assessment, with a median gestational age at diagnosis of 19 weeks.

An eventration of the diaphragm may appear as herniation of intra-abdominal contents into the fetal chest and can be mistaken for CDH. Eventration results from failure of muscularization of the otherwise intact primitive diaphragm and has a better prognosis.

In cases of left CDH, assessment of the location of the fetal liver is necessary for providing prognosis and patient counseling. Liver herniation is consistently associated with higher rate of postnatal mortality as well as morbidity, and increased liver herniation appears to predict outcome [23]. As mentioned, a portion of the left hepatic lobe is likely herniated into the thorax (liver up) if the fetal stomach is located posteriorly within the chest. This can also be suggested by deviation/distortion of the midhepatic portion of the umbilical vein toward the left [9, 22].

2.3.3 Cardiovascular Disease

Causes of cardiovascular disease are clearly considered as multifactorial. Cardiovascular disease can develop both inherently and sporadically. A large number of syndromic disorders are associated with congenital heart disease and genetic disorders have also been shown to be associated with isolated congenital heart disease [24]. Genetic disease with congenital heart disease coexisted with aneuploidies such as Down syndrome may result from chromosomal deletions such as 22q11.2

deletion, or may be secondary to a single DNA base mutation such as Alagille syndrome due to a JAG1 mutation [9]. However, cases with congenital heart disease in association with recognized genetic condition are not many. Cardiovascular diseases should be screened in all pregnant women by the ultrasound in the second trimester as a part of fetal assessment.

2.4 Abdomen

Abnormalities of the fetal abdomen include abdominal wall defects, gastrointestinal malformations, and the genitourinary system abnormalities.

2.4.1 Abdominal Wall Defects

Abdominal wall defects include gastroschisis and omphalocele. Gastroschisis is typically an isolated anomaly; however, omphaloceles are frequently associated with other structural anomalies or chromosome abnormalities. When abdominal wall defect is detected, additional anomalies should be ruled out. In cases with omphalocele prior to 14 weeks of gestation, more than half have chromosome abnormality, especially trisomy 18. Gastroschisis and omphalocele are mostly able to be distinguished; however, ultrasound confirmation after 12 weeks of gestation is required because of the midgut herniation [9] (Fig. 2.2a, b).

2.4.2 Gastrointestinal Malformations

2.4.2.1 Esophageal Atresia

The normal esophagus cannot be depicted. However, esophageal atresia is suspected when a persistently small or absent stomach exists accompanied with polyhydramnios [25]. Esophageal atresia is an interruption of the esophagus such that the upper esophagus ends in a blind pouch, most often at or above the tracheal bifurcation [9]. Most esophageal atresias have tracheoesophageal fistula which is connected from the trachea to the distal esophagus [1].

2.4.2.2 Duodenal Atresia

When obstruction occurs in upper gastrointestinal tract, polyhydramnios usually appeared after third trimester. Duodenal obstruction, including atresia and

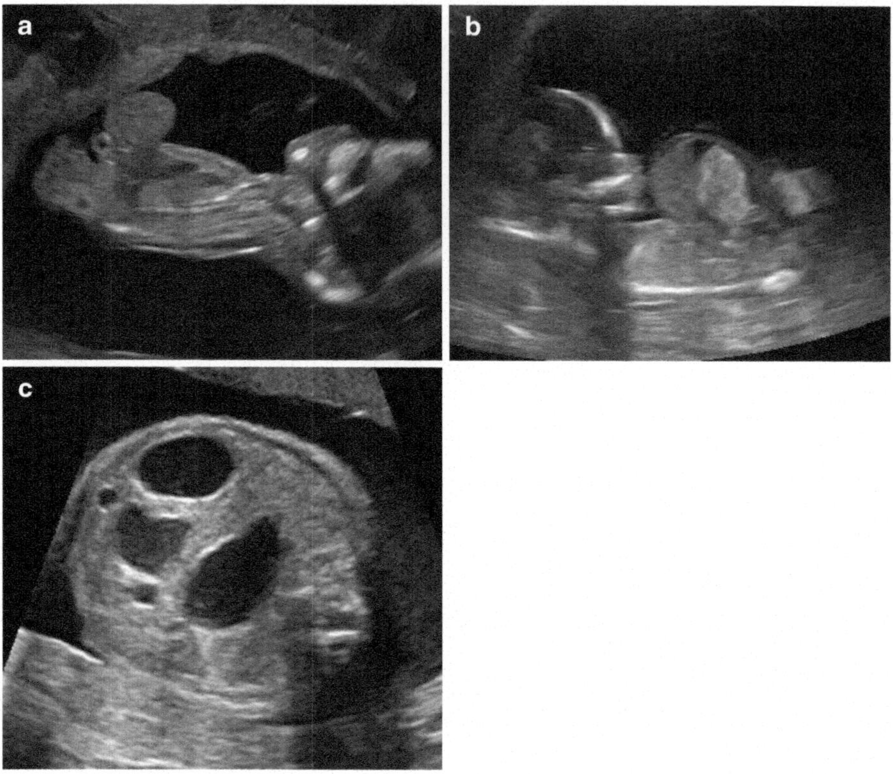

Fig. 2.2 Abdomen. (**a**) Gastroschisis. (**b**) Omphalocele. (**c**) Duodenal atresia

constriction due to annular pancreas, is also associated with polyhydramnios. However, in ultrasound screening at 20 weeks of gestation, the detection rate is only about 50% [26]. Diagnosis of obstruction in gastrointestinal tracts is more reliably made in the third trimester.

"Double cyst sign" is a characteristic ultrasonographic finding of duodenal obstruction. However, a more specific diagnosis requires demonstration of continuity of the dilated duodenum with fluid in the stomach, crossing the midline of the fetus. If such continuity cannot be established, other causes of an upper abdominal cyst, such as choledochal, mesenteric, hepatic, or enteric duplication cyst, should be considered [9, 26, 27].

Although survival rate is approximately 100%, most important thing associated with duodenal obstruction is the fact that up to a half of fetuses with duodenal obstruction have Down syndrome [26, 28] (Fig. 2.2c).

2.5 Kidney and Urinary Tract

2.5.1 *Urinary Tract Dilatation*

Urinary tract dilation is one of the most common sonographic prenatal diagnoses. This abnormality includes megacystis hydronephrosis, pyelectasis, pelviectasis, and pelvicaliectasis.

Megacystis is a ultrasonographic finding of lower urinary tract obstruction (LUTO), which is the most commonly detected genitourinary abnormality in the first trimester. LUTOs are caused by several abnormalities. The most common cause of severe bladder outlet obstruction is a posterior urethral valve (PUV). PUVs are membranes within the posterior aspect of the urethra [9]. The obstructive cause may resolve or progress throughout the pregnancy, thus when megacystis is diagnosed in the first trimester, outcome varies. Dysplastic nonfunctioning kidneys due to LUTO may involve anhydramnios and pulmonary hypoplasia resulting in perinatal death. Chromosomal abnormalities were found in 20% of the cases with megacystis in the first trimester [1] (Fig. 2.3a).

2.5.2 *Dysplastic Kidneys*

Renal dysplasia is a histologic diagnosis reflecting either abnormal early development or disturbed terminal maturation, while dysplasia expresses ultrasonically various findings, such as echogenic, cystic, abnormal sized, and structured kidney [9]. Obstruction of the urinary tract associated with multi-cystic dysplastic kidney (MCDK) involves antecedent of renal dysplasia. Bilateral dysplasia is likely to result in anhydramnios [1] (Fig. 2.3b).

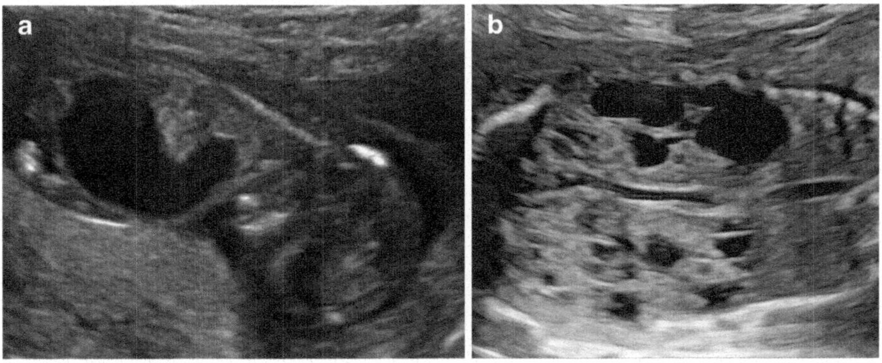

Fig. 2.3 Genitourinary abnormalities. (**a**) Pyelectasis due to lower urinary tract obstruction. (**b**) Multi-cystic dysplastic kidney (MCDK)

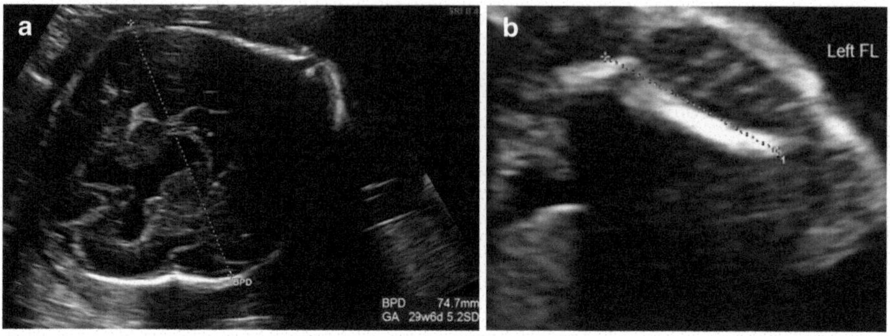

Fig. 2.4 Extremities thanatophoric dysplasia: (**a**) Enlarged BPD, (**b**) short femoral length

Nonobstructive dysplasia may be involved by heritable [autosomal recessive polycystic kidney disease (ARPKD) and autosomal dominant polycystic kidney disease (ADPKD)], or sporadic conditions, or genetic syndromes, etc [29]. Ultrasound findings of ARPKD are bilaterally enlarged, hyperechoic kidneys consisting of numerous microcysts which are undepictable using ultrasound and lack of corticomedullary differentiation [29].

2.6 Skeleton

The most common skeletal abnormalities detected in the first trimester are osteochondrodysplasias followed by limb-reduction defects and arthrogryposis [30]. Skeletal dysplasia characterized by severe rhizomelia, small thorax, normal trunk length, normal bone mineralization, no fractures, thickened redundant skin, and platyspondyly is also diagnosed antenatally during fetal biometry [9]. Minor skeletal abnormalities such as clubfoot, syndactyly, and polydactyly become to make diagnosis with advancing gestation, but low antenatal detection rate [9, 30] (Fig. 2.4a, b).

2.7 Ultrasound Features of Chromosomal Abnormalities

2.7.1 Trisomy 21

Characteristic phenotypes in trisomy 21 including distinctive facial features including midface hypoplasia and upslanting palpebral fissures, short stature, brachycephaly, a short neck with redundant skin on the nape, short broad hands with a single transverse palmar crease, and hypotonia are unrealistic for screening of fetal morphological assessment. Usually, this anomaly is screened ultrasonically using nuchal translucency, nasal bone, flow of ductus venosus, etc. in the first trimester.

Congenital heart defects are reported in a half of newborns with trisomy 21 [31]. Hydronephrosis and duodenal atresia are also associated with trisomy 21. Up to one half of fetuses with duodenal obstruction have Down syndrome [28].

2.7.2 *Trisomy 18*

Postnatal survival is poor resulting in neonatal death because of major structural abnormalities. However, recently, some of infants with trisomy 18 can survive for more months, but it depends on phenotype without severe abnormalities. Characteristic ultrasound findings include cardiac malformations, growth restriction, a prominent occiput, dolicocephaly, small mandible, short sternum, clenched hands with overlapping fingers, and rocker-bottom feet [9].

2.7.3 *Trisomy 13*

There is a high stillbirth and perinatal mortality rate because of multiple severe structural abnormalities. Ultrasound findings include growth restriction, midline defects including severe central nervous system malformations such as holoprosencephaly, cleft lip and palate, and microphthalmia, omphalocele, polydactyly, clenched hands with overlapping fingers, heart abnormalitis, and renal abnormalities such as polycystic kidneys [9].

2.7.4 *Turner Syndrome*

Fetuses with Turner syndrome often have an increased nuchal translucency or cystic hygroma, lymphangiectasia, structural renal abnormalities, and congenital heart diseases such as coarctation of the aorta. However, specific ultrasound findings are not present.

Conflict of Interest There are no conflicts of interest to declare.

References

1. Luchi C, Schifano M, Sacchini C, Nanini C, Sceusa F, Capriello P, Genazzani AR. Detailed fetal anatomy assessment in the first trimester at 11, 12 and 13 weeks of gestation. J Matern Fetal Neonatal Med. 2012;25:675–8. https://doi.org/10.3109/14767058.2011.587058.
2. Salomon LJ, Alfirevic Z, Berghella V, Bilardo C, Hernandez-Andrade E, Johnsen SL, Kalache K, Leung KY, Malinger G, Munoz H, Prefumo F, Toi A, Lee W, Committee ICS. Practice

guidelines for performance of the routine mid-trimester fetal ultrasound scan. Ultrasound Obstet Gynecol. 2011;37:116–26. https://doi.org/10.1002/uog.8831.

3. Saltvedt S, Almstrom H, Kublickas M, Valentin L, Grunewald C. Detection of malformations in chromosomally normal fetuses by routine ultrasound at 12 or 18 weeks of gestation-a randomised controlled trial in 39,572 pregnancies. BJOG. 2006;113:664–74. https://doi.org/10.1111/j.1471-0528.2006.00953.x.
4. Tegnander E, Williams W, Johansen OJ, Blaas HG, Eik-Nes SH. Prenatal detection of heart defects in a non-selected population of 30,149 fetuses--detection rates and outcome. Ultrasound Obstet Gynecol. 2006;27:252–65. https://doi.org/10.1002/uog.2710.
5. Grandjean H, Larroque D, Levi S. The performance of routine ultrasonographic screening of pregnancies in the Eurofetus Study. Am J Obstet Gynecol. 1999;181:446–54. https://doi.org/10.1016/s0002-9378(99)70577-6.
6. Whitworth M, Bricker L, Neilson JP, Dowswell T. Ultrasound for fetal assessment in early pregnancy. Cochrane Database Syst Rev. 2010:CD007058. https://doi.org/10.1002/14651858.CD007058.pub2.
7. Abramowicz JS, Kossoff G, Marsal K, Ter Haar G, International Society of Ultrasound in O., Gynecology B., Safety Committee. Executive Board of the International Society of Ultrasound in O. and Gynecology. Safety Statement, 2000 (reconfirmed 2003). International Society of Ultrasound in Obstetrics and Gynecology (ISUOG). Ultrasound Obstet Gynecol. 2003;21:100. https://doi.org/10.1002/uog.36.
8. Takita H, Hasegawa J, Arakaki T, Nakamura M, Hamada S, Tokunaka M, Oba T, Matsuoka R, Sekizawa A. Usefulness of antenatal ultrasound fetal morphological assessments in the first and second trimester: a study at a single Japanese university hospital. J Med Ultrason (2001). 2016;43:57–62. https://doi.org/10.1007/s10396-015-0653-1.
9. Norton M. Callen's ultrasonography in obstetrics and gynecology. Elsevier: City, 2017.
10. Chatzipapas IK, Whitlow BJ, Economides DL. The 'Mickey Mouse' sign and the diagnosis of anencephaly in early pregnancy. Ultrasound Obstet Gynecol. 1999;13:196–9. https://doi.org/10.1046/j.1469-0705.1999.13030196.x.
11. Loureiro T, Ushakov F, Montenegro N, Gielchinsky Y, Nicolaides KH. Cerebral ventricular system in fetuses with open spina bifida at 11-13 weeks' gestation. Ultrasound Obstet Gynecol. 2012;39:620–4. https://doi.org/10.1002/uog.11079.
12. Chervenak FA, Isaacson G, Hobbins JC, Chitkara U, Tortora M, Berkowitz RL. Diagnosis and management of fetal holoprosencephaly. Obstet Gynecol. 1985;66:322–6.
13. Peebles DM. Holoprosencephaly. Prenatal Diagn. 1998;18:477–80.
14. Patel MD, Goldstein RB, Tung S, Filly RA. Fetal cerebral ventricular atrium: difference in size according to sex. Radiology. 1995;194:713–5. https://doi.org/10.1148/radiology.194.3.7862967.
15. Melchiorre K, Bhide A, Gika AD, Pilu G, Papageorghiou AT. Counseling in isolated mild fetal ventriculomegaly. Ultrasound Obstet Gynecol. 2009;34:212–24. https://doi.org/10.1002/uog.7307.
16. Gupta JK, Bryce FC, Lilford RJ. Management of apparently isolated fetal ventriculomegaly. Obstet Gynecol Surv. 1994;49:716–21. https://doi.org/10.1097/00006254-199410000-00027.
17. Malone FD, Ball RH, Nyberg DA, Comstock CH, Saade GR, Berkowitz RL, Gross SJ, Dugoff L, Craigo SD, Timor-Tritsch IE, Carr SR, Wolfe HM, Dukes K, Canick JA, Bianchi DW, D'Alton ME, Consortium FTR. First-trimester septated cystic hygroma: prevalence, natural history, and pediatric outcome. Obstet Gynecol. 2005;106:288–94. https://doi.org/10.1097/01.AOG.0000173318.54978.1f.
18. Molina FS, Avgidou K, Kagan KO, Poggi S, Nicolaides KH. Cystic hygromas, nuchal edema, and nuchal translucency at 11-14 weeks of gestation. Obstet Gynecol. 2006;107:678–83. https://doi.org/10.1097/01.AOG.0000201979.23031.32.
19. Achiron R, Hegesh J, Yagel S. Fetal lung lesions: a spectrum of disease. New classification based on pathogenesis, two-dimensional and color Doppler ultrasound. Ultrasound Obstet Gynecol. 2004;24:107–14. https://doi.org/10.1002/uog.1110.

20. Alamo L, Gudinchet F, Reinberg O, Vial Y, Francini K, Osterheld MC, Meuli R. Prenatal diagnosis of congenital lung malformations. Pediatr Radiol. 2012;42:273–83. https://doi.org/10.1007/s00247-011-2303-0.
21. Stocker JT, Madewell JE, Drake RM. Congenital cystic adenomatoid malformation of the lung. Classification and morphologic spectrum. Human Pathol. 1977;8:155–71. https://doi.org/10.1016/s0046-8177(77)80078-6.
22. Richards DS, Kays DM. Fetal umbilical vein deviation in congenital diaphragmatic hernia. J Ultrasound Med. 2013;32:263–8. https://doi.org/10.7863/jum.2013.32.2.263.
23. Lusk LA, Wai KC, Moon-Grady AJ, Basta AM, Filly R, Keller RL. Fetal ultrasound markers of severity predict resolution of pulmonary hypertension in congenital diaphragmatic hernia. Am J Obstet Gynecol. 2015;213:216 e211–8. https://doi.org/10.1016/j.ajog.2015.03.036.
24. Fahed AC, Gelb BD, Seidman JG, Seidman CE. Genetics of congenital heart disease: the glass half empty. Circ Res. 2013;112:707–20. https://doi.org/10.1161/CIRCRESAHA.112.300853.
25. McKelvey A, Stanwell J, Smeulders N, Nasr R, Curry J, Pandya P. Persistent non-visualisation of the fetal stomach: diagnostic and prognostic implications. Arch Dis Child Fetal Neonatal Ed. 2010;95:F439–42. https://doi.org/10.1136/adc.2009.179341.
26. Choudhry MS, Rahman N, Boyd P, Lakhoo K. Duodenal atresia: associated anomalies, prenatal diagnosis and outcome. Pediatr Surg Int. 2009;25:727–30. https://doi.org/10.1007/s00383-009-2406-y.
27. Malone FD, Crombleholme TM, Nores JA, Athanassiou A, D'Alton ME. Pitfalls of the 'double bubble' sign: a case of congenital duodenal duplication. Fetal Diagn Ther. 1997;12:298–300. https://doi.org/10.1159/000264490.
28. Cohen-Overbeek TE, Grijseels EW, Niemeijer ND, Hop WC, Wladimiroff JW, Tibboel D. Isolated or non-isolated duodenal obstruction: perinatal outcome following prenatal or postnatal diagnosis. Ultrasound Obstet Gynecol. 2008;32:784–92. https://doi.org/10.1002/uog.6135.
29. Winyard P, Chitty L. Dysplastic and polycystic kidneys: diagnosis, associations and management. Prenatal Diagn. 2001;21:924–35. https://doi.org/10.1002/pd.208.
30. Grande M, Arigita M, Borobio V, Jimenez JM, Fernandez S, Borrell A. First-trimester detection of structural abnormalities and the role of aneuploidy markers. Ultrasound Obstet Gynecol. 2012;39:157–63. https://doi.org/10.1002/uog.10070.
31. Freeman SB, Bean LH, Allen EG, Tinker SW, Locke AE, Druschel C, Hobbs CA, Romitti PA, Royle MH, Torfs CP, Dooley KJ, Sherman SL. Ethnicity, sex, and the incidence of congenital heart defects: a report from the National Down Syndrome Project. Genet Med. 2008;10:173–80. https://doi.org/10.1097/GIM.0b013e3181634867.

Chapter 3
Fetal MRI

Keiko Segawa

Abstract Magnetic resonance imaging (MRI) is used in conjunction with ultrasound (US) to provide additional information for prenatal diagnosis. US is the imaging method of choice during the first trimester for the diagnosis of cardiovascular abnormalities and for screening. The main indication for fetal MRI is further evaluation of inconclusive US findings. It is also useful for evaluation prior to fetal and/or perinatal surgery and for specific information necessary for a fetal delivery plan. Knowledge about MRI sequences is useful for creating adequate scan protocol and accurate diagnosis.

Keywords Magnetic resonance imaging · Sequences · Prenatal diagnosis · Fetus

3.1 Introduction

3.1.1 The Advantages of MRI

MRI has the advantage of objectively demonstrating the pathology of the brain, lungs, and complex syndromes. In contrast to US, MRI is not affected in conditions associated with a reduction of amniotic fluid (Fig. 3.1). On MRI, the use of multiple planes for reconstruction and the large field of view facilitate the visualization of complicated anomalies.

The original version of this chapter was revised. A correction to this chapter can be found at https://doi.org/10.1007/978-981-15-8171-7_28

K. Segawa (✉)
Department of Radiology, Nagasaki University Hospital, Nagasaki, Japan
e-mail: segawamiyata@nagasaki-u.ac.jp

H. Masuzaki (ed.), *Fetal Morph Functional Diagnosis*, Comprehensive Gynecology and Obstetrics, https://doi.org/10.1007/978-981-15-8171-7_3

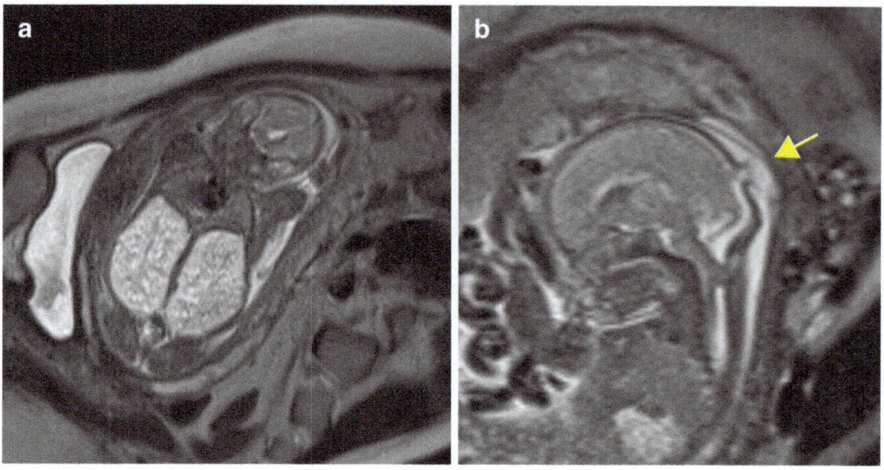

Fig. 3.1 (**a**) Coronal MRI of the fetus at 20 weeks shows severe oligohydramnios. The kidneys are grossly enlarged with abnormal hyperintense parenchyma. (**b**) Sagittal MRI of the brain in the same fetus shows an occipital calvarial defect and posterior encephalocele (arrow). These findings are classic features in Meckel-Gruber syndrome

3.1.2 The Disadvantages of MRI

MRI is not suitable for scanning in real-time observation of fetal movements. Usually, MRI is performed without IV contrast; therefore, it cannot evaluate vascularity of organs or tumors. In addition, various artifacts, especially fetal motion, degrade the quality of the images.

3.2 MRI Sequences

3.2.1 T2-Weighted Sequences

T2-weighted sequences are the major initial indication for fetal MRI, as they provide excellent soft-tissue contrast and the best anatomic detail imaging. T2-weighted images (T2WI) enhance contrast and allow visualization of cystic lesions. Most fetal body cavities, such as the nasal and oral cavities, the middle and inner ear, trachea, stomach, gallbladder, the renal pelvis, and urinary bladder, are fluid-filled; therefore, these cavities are hyperintense on T2WI.

The signal intensity of the fetal lungs on T2WI increases during gestation, which is used for the assessment of lung growth.

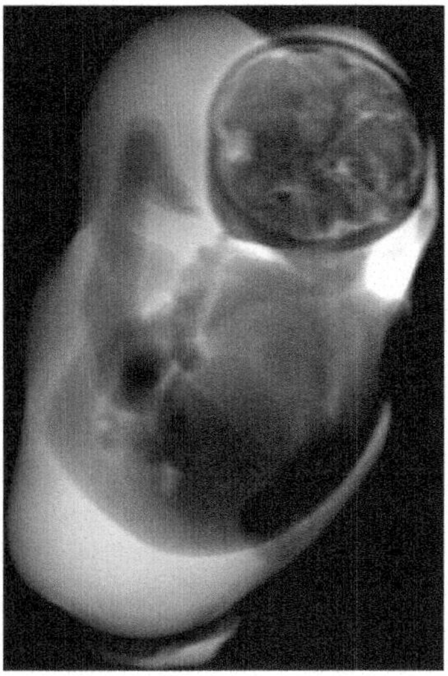

Fig. 3.2 Coronal thick-Slab imaging of the fetus with limb contracture. Limb positions are twisted

3.2.2 *Thick-Slab Imaging*

Thick-slab acquisitions with a slice thickness of 30–50 mm of the fetus provide a three-dimensional impression of the fetus and its surroundings. Acquisition of one image takes less than 1 sec. These images are useful for the assessment of the whole fetus, fetal proportions, surface structures, and extremities. Furthermore, this kind of imaging is useful for parents and those who are not familiar with sectional anatomy understand any abnormality (Fig. 3.2).

3.2.3 *Steady-State Free-Precession Sequences*

Using SSFP sequences, cavities and vessels show hyperintensity. The hepatic vein and intrahepatic portal vein that surrounded the liver parenchyma hypointense on T2WI and have better contrast on SSFP than T2WI. In addition, SSFP are the only sequences that demonstrate the morphological features of the cardiovascular system.

3.2.4 *T1-Weighted Sequences*

T1-weighted sequences are excellent for the detection of hemorrhage. The meconium in the large bowel is characteristically hyperintense on T1-weighted images (T1WI). The fetal pituitary, thyroid, and liver also show hyperintensity. T1-weighted fat-suppressed images are highly sensitive and specific in the detection of hemorrhage or fat. Compared with standard T1-weighted fast spin-echo chemical shift fat-suppressed sequences, 3D dual-echo Dixon sequences have superior-quality and requires a shorter time to acquire images. Identifying lipid is important for the diagnosis of fetal masses. In a fetus, a small amount of lipid can be only detected on opposed-phase images.

3.2.5 Echoplanar Imaging

As ecoplanar (EP) sequences demonstrate bone as hypointense structures and delineate the hyperintense cartilaginous epiphyses, they are the only sequences that can depict the fetal skeleton before 27GW. EP sequences are used to obtain an overview of thoracic size and skeletal development. In addition, EP sequences are sensitive to demonstrating hemorrhage, especially when these no longer present as hyperintense lesions on T1WI.

3.2.6 Diffusion-Weighted Imaging

Diffusion-weighted imaging (DWI) has been used to assess ischemic lesions of the white matter of the brain, normal and abnormal developing kidneys, tumors, and ischemic lesions of the placenta.

3.2.7 Three-Dimensional Dataset for Reconstruction

The acquisition of a continuous three-dimensional super-resolution dataset covering the whole fetus allows re-slicing of the stack of images in any desired section plane. These images are useful for the assessment of small intricate structures such as the posterior fossa, bronchial patency, or facial clefts.

3.3 MRI Indications

3.3.1 Approach to the Central Nervous System

T2-weighted sequences are the mainstay of fetal brain evaluation. They are used to obtain orthogonal images through the posterior fossa. T2-weighted sequences allow assessment of global anatomy and development. Sagittal MRI provides excellent images of the brainstem, pons, and cerebellar peduncles in the posterior fossa. T1-weighted sequences provide information about cell density and myelination. Hyperintense on T1WI combined with hypointense on T1WI or EP may characterize methemoglobin or calcification (Figs. 3.3 and 3.4). In Chiari 2 malformation, MRI allows more detailed evaluation of both the brain and spine and is useful for detecting associated central nervous system findings. DWI evaluates brain development and depicts ischemic lesions and hemorrhage. Additional sequences, such as diffusion-tensor imaging and proton MR spectroscopy, are useful assessing the prognosis.

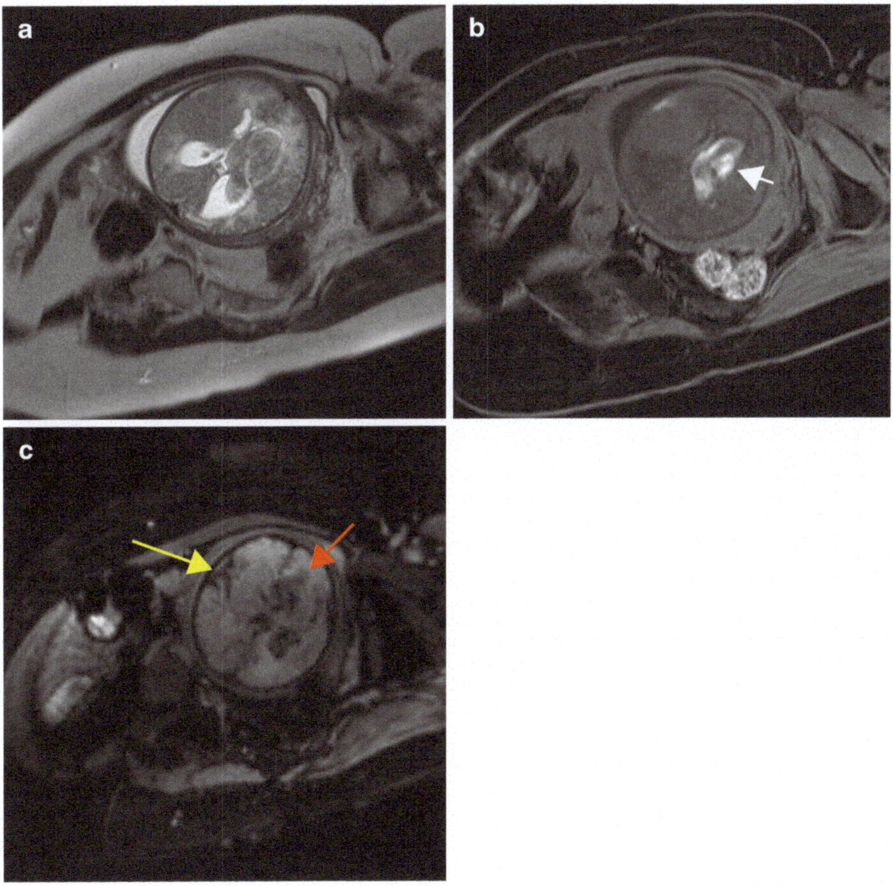

Fig. 3.3 Axial MRI of different sequences of the fetus at 37 weeks with ventriculomegaly and intraventricular hemorrhage. (**a**) T2-weighted image. (**b**) T1-weighted image. (**c**) Echoplanar imaging. Left caudate nucleus shows swelling with ventricular hematoma showing T2-hypointensity/T1-hyperintensity (white arrow). On EP imaging, right Sylvian fissure subarachnoid hemorrhage (yellow arrow) and parenchymal hemorrhage in the left frontal lobe (red arrow) are clear

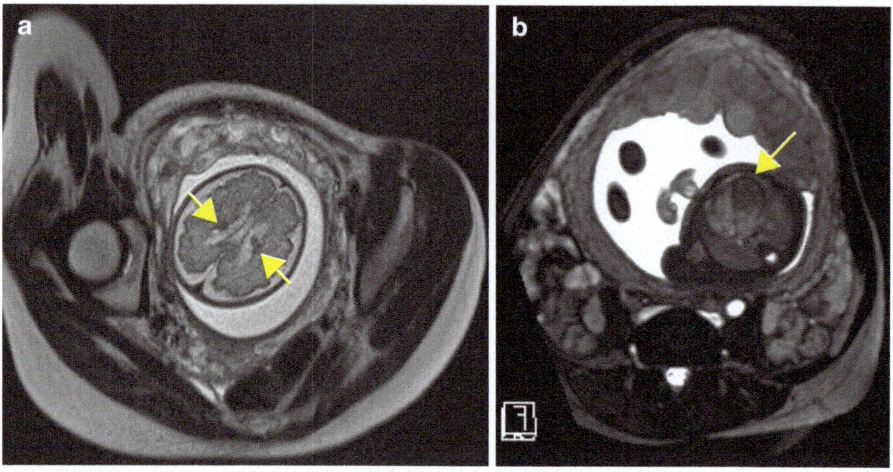

Fig. 3.4 Rhabdomyomas and tuberous sclerosis complex. MRI of the fetus at 29 weeks. (**a**) Axial T2-weighted image shows subependymal nodules (arrows). (**b**) SSFP sequences demonstrate cardiac rhabdomyomas as hypointense area (arrow)

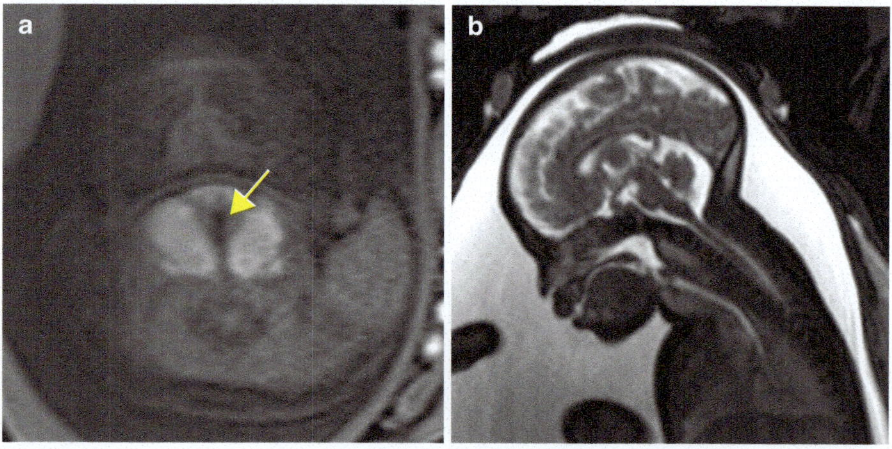

Fig. 3.5 MRI of the fetus at 35 weeks with large goiter. (**a**) On axial T1-weighted image, the large goiter showed hyperintensity and the trachea running in the center was narrowing (arrow). (**b**) Fetal airway patency was assessed with 3D dataset for reconstruction

3.3.2 Approach to the Face and Neck

The superior soft tissue differentiation of MRI and absence of artifact from bone allow for better evaluation of the deep structures of the mouth and neck. In cases of cleft lip, T2-weighted sequences demonstrate the posterior palate consistently, regardless of fetal position. A fetus with giant neck masses, such as teratoma, lymphangioma, or large goiter, may benefit from MRI in order to better assess fetal airway patency (Fig. 3.5). Accurate anatomic evaluation is necessary for planning ex utero intrapartum treatment (EXIT) procedure. This procedure is used when only the baby's head and shoulders are delivered. In the EXIT procedure, the pediatric surgeon establishes access to the airway while the baby continues to receive oxygen through the umbilical cord.

3.3.3 *Approach to the Chest*

MRI is a useful adjunct in the evaluation of fetal chest masses such as cystic adenomatoid malformation, bronchopulmonary sequestration, congenital diaphragmatic hernia (CDH), and other cysts or masses. Space-occupying intrathoracic lesions may adversely affect lung development. MRI provides further information regarding the lesions' structure and prognostic implications. Predicting the outcome in these cases is based on lung volume, lung growth, and development. In left-sided CDH, the presence of liver herniation into the thoracic cavity suggests a poor outcome. MRI can visualize the position of the liver and differentiates meconium-filled bowel loops from cystic lesions within the thoracic cavity. On T2WI, the lungs are more hyperintense than the surrounding musculature. The signal intensity of the lungs increases during gestation reflecting the fluid within the enlarging alveoli. On T1WI, the liver is more hyperintense than the lung. In addition, a fluid-filled small bowel is hypointense but a meconium-filled large bowel will be hyperintensity. So T1-weighted sequence is helpful in confirming the presence of meconium-filled bowel within the thoracic cavity in CDH (Fig. 3.6).

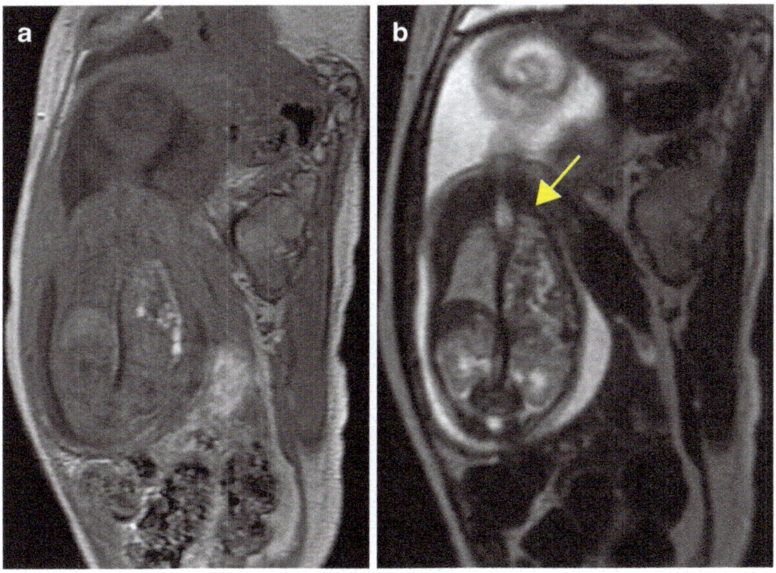

Fig. 3.6 Coronal MRI of the fetus at 28 weeks with congenital diaphragmatic hernia. (**a**) T1-weighted sequence reveal the presence of meconium-filled bowel within the thoracic cavity. (**b**) T2-weighted sequences reveal a tiny left lung at the top of thoracic cavity (arrow)

3.3.4 Approach to the Heart

Fetal echocardiography has clear advantages over MRI for the visualization of cardiac anatomy in real-time, in terms of resolution capability and real-time functional assessment [1]; however, SSFP sequences are superior for demonstrating the cardiovascular system. MRI protocol for studying the fetal heart along body and cardiac planes has been introduced recently [2]. Asplenia is related to cardiovascular anomalies and it is important for evaluation of the spleen. Using US, the spleen is difficult to distinguish from the liver; however, MRI can demonstrate the spleen clearly.

3.3.5 Approach to the Abdominal Wall and Gastrointestinal Tract

Atypical abdominal wall defects, unusual abdominopelvic or abdominal wall masses, and complex laterality disturbances lend themselves well to evaluation by MRI. T2WI provides excellent soft tissue contrast and is the best for anatomic detail.

The meconium is produced after 13WG and slowly migrates from the small bowel to the colon. The meconium contains high levels of protein and minerals, and it appears hypointense on T2WI and hyperintense on T1WI. The course of the colon is easily followed, adding valuable information when an anorectal malformation is suspected. Assessing the caliber and signal changes of the small and large bowels, MRI may better delineate the site of obstruction and bowel atresia with widely dilated bowel loops proximal to the site of stenosis [3]. MRI adds information about the distal bowel. Hyperintense bowel dilatation on T2WI indicates proximal small bowel obstruction, whereas hypointense bowel dilatation on T2WI and hyperintense bowel dilatation on T1WI indicate distal small bowel or colonic obstruction. In cases suggesting esophageal atresia (EA) in the setting of the small stomach or polyhydramnios, MRI is useful to identify the esophageal pouch, a significant positive predictive value for EA when present on fetal MRI; however, half of EA cases have other anomalies. MRI should be considered for searching for other anomalies, specifically target malformations seen in VACTERL association. MRI should be considered to assess the presence of a hyperintense colon on T1WI and further evaluate genitourinary anatomy. A sagittal T2 thin section through the fetal pelvis is useful to evaluate the relationship of the vagina to the perineum. Sagittal T1WI is also useful to visualize a meconium-filled rectum and the relationship of the rectum to the perineum. MRI also allows better evaluation of the organ of origin as well as the extent of an intraabdominal mass and its effect on other organs than US alone.

3.3.6 Approach to Genitourinary Tract

MRI can accurately show many urinary tract anomalies in third-trimester fetuses. It may be a complementary tool in the assessment of bilateral urinary tract anomalies of fetuses, particularly in severe oligohydramnios patients with inconclusive US findings, which are commonly associated with urinary tract malformations (Fig. 3.1). It can also confirm the renal origin of mass. T2WI provides good visualization of the renal pelvis, the bladder, dilated urinary tract, and cystic renal lesions. In cases with genitourinary tract obstruction, MRI is useful for assessing renal dysplasia. Cortical thinning, increased T2-signal intensity, and small cystic change may correlate with renal dysplasia.

DWI can detect the kidneys if renal agenesis is suspected [4].

3.3.7 Approach to the Extremities and Bone

MRI is not as useful in the evaluation of bone abnormalities, but may be performed in cases of suspected visceral abnormalities. EP sequences demonstrate bone as hypointense structures and delineate the hyperintense cartilaginous epiphyses. Thick-slab acquisitions are useful for the assessment of the whole fetus, fetal proportions, and extremities (Fig. 3.2).

3.3.8 Approach to Complex Malformation

Often a fetus will present with malformations of multiple organ systems (Figs. 3.1 and 3.4). While US will usually yield a working diagnosis on which to base further investigations, some malformations may be missed on the initial diagnostic scan.

References

1. Pugasha D, Brugger PC, Bettelheim D, Prayer D. Prenatal ultrasound and fetal MRI: the comparative value of each modality in prenatal diagnosis. Eur J Radiol. 2008;68:214–26.
2. Saleem SN. Feasibility of magnetic resonance imaging (MRI) of the fetal heart using balanced steady-state-free-precession (SSFP) sequence along fetal body and cardiac planes. AJR Am J Roentgenol. 2008;191:1208–15.
3. Shinmoto H, Kashima K, Yuasa Y, Tanimoto A, Morikawa Y, Ishimoto H, et al. MR imaging of non-CNS fetal abnormalities: a pictorial essay. Radiographics. 2000;20:1227–43.
4. Cassart M, Massez A, Metens T, Rypens F, Lambot MA, Hall M, Avni FE. Complementary role of MRI after sonography in assessing bilateral urinary tract anomalies in the fetus. AJR Am J Roentgenol. 2004;182:689–95.

Part II
Genetic Tests

Chapter 4
Prenatal Screening for Fetal Aneuploidy

Akihiko Sekizawa and Ryu Matsuoka

Abstract Traditional prenatal diagnostic tests for fetal chromosomal abnormalities involve the risk of miscarriage. Therefore, to reduce this risk, noninvasive prenatal screening methods have been developed and have improved the detection rates of fetal aneuploidies. Recently, noninvasive prenatal testing (NIPT) was developed, resulting in a fetal aneuploidy detection rate >99% and achieving unparalleled precision as compared with previous prenatal screening methods. Therefore, NIPT has steadily reduced the number of invasive prenatal screens performed.

Keywords Noninvasive prenatal testing · Prenatal screening · Combined test Quadruple screening test · Fetal aneuploidy · Miscarriage

Fetal chromosomal abnormalities account for 25% of congenital diseases, and as the prevalence of congenital chromosomal disease in the fetus increases with maternal age, pregnant women often request prenatal testing to alleviate uncertainty and anxiety. To diagnose fetal chromosomal diseases, it is necessary to obtain a sample of fetal cells and perform chromosomal analysis. However, collecting fetal cells involves the risk of miscarriage. Therefore, to minimize this risk, noninvasive methods to screen pregnant women at high risk of fetal aneuploidies have been developed.

Screening methods for fetal aneuploidies include tests that examine disease incidence rates in individual pregnant women, including maternal serum marker tests and combined tests. By contrast, noninvasive prenatal testing (NIPT) analyzes cell-free DNA (cfDNA) in the maternal plasma and shows higher sensitivity and

A. Sekizawa (✉) · R. Matsuoka
Department of Obstetrics and Gynecology, Showa University School of Medicine, Tokyo, Japan
e-mail: sekizawa@med.showa-u.ac.jp

H. Masuzaki (ed.), *Fetal Morph Functional Diagnosis*, Comprehensive Gynecology and Obstetrics, https://doi.org/10.1007/978-981-15-8171-7_4

specificity. NIPT typically provides clear test results (either positive or negative) for chromosomal diseases, and its use has rapidly increased. Moreover, the kinds of fetal diseases targeted by NIPT are steadily expanding, and NIPT appears to be the ideal screening method for fetal chromosome disease. However, although NIPT is highly accurate, it is not a definitive test of the fetus, as fetal cfDNA represents only ~10% of the total cfDNA in maternal plasma and is derived from villous trophoblasts in the placenta and not directly from the fetus.

4.1 Tests That Estimate the Incidence Rates of Fetal Chromosomal Diseases

Maternal serum marker tests, combined tests, and ultrasound marker tests are used to estimate the incidence rates of fetal aneuploidies. For example, the distributions of ultrasound measurements, such as nuchal translucency (NT), differ between fetuses with normal karyotypes and those with trisomy 21; therefore, NT can be used as a marker to screen for fetal chromosomal abnormalities. Similarly, each maternal serum marker is used, because their concentration distributions differ between a normal fetus and that with a chromosomal disease. Estimation for the incidence rate requires calculation of the likelihood ratio (the disease risk derived from the markers) as the ratio of frequencies of fetuses having a normal karyotype to those having the corresponding chromosomal aneuploidy (Fig. 4.1). In each pregnant woman, the likelihood ratio is calculated based on multiple markers, and the risk of trisomy 21 due to maternal age is multiplied by the likelihoods of each marker in order to provide the incidence risk for each pregnant woman.

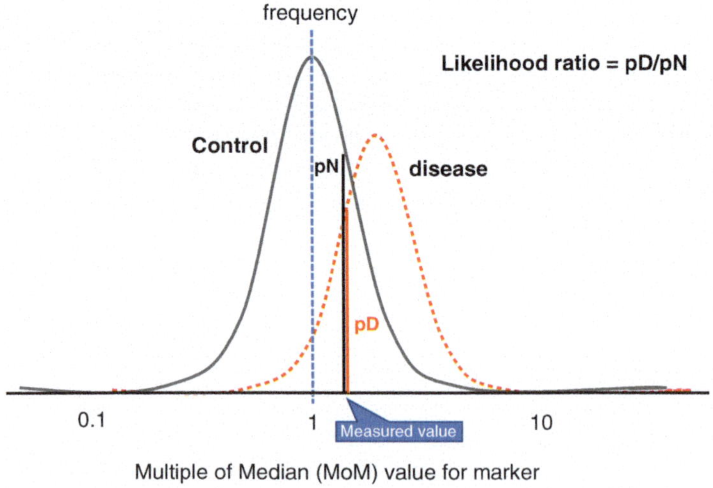

Fig. 4.1 Calculation of likelihood ratios using markers to detect chromosomal abnormalities

The combined test performed during the first trimester (11–13 weeks of gestation) uses three markers: NT, human chorionic gonadotrophin (hCG) concentration, and serum pregnancy-associated plasma protein A (PAPPA) concentration. The quad screen test performed during the second trimester uses four markers: α-fetoprotein (AFP), hCG or free β-hCG, unconjugated estriol, and inhibin A (Table 4.1).

The greater the significance of the difference between healthy and disease distribution curves, the greater the likelihood ratio; therefore, an individual marker with high a likelihood ratio serves as a better marker. However, because the distributions usually overlap, the markers cannot be used for diagnostic purposes. To evaluate the discriminating capacity of a marker, detection rates are often compared at established false-positive rates. At a false-positive rate of 5%, the trisomy 21 detection rate based on maternal age and NT thickness during the first trimester is 68.6%; however, it increases to 78.7% in combined tests that include serum PAPPA and free β-hCG or total hCG concentrations (Table 4.2) [1]. The detection rate using the second-trimester quadruple screen test is 75.0% [2], similar to the combined test, with a report suggesting that combined tests can provide detection rates >90% when used in combination with other early pregnancy ultrasound markers, such as nasal bone development, facial angle, tricuspid flow, and ductus venosus flow [3]. However, although it is relatively easy to manage data accuracy in blood tests, evaluating ultrasound markers is time-consuming, and managing their accuracy and reproducibility is difficult both within and between facilities. Although combined tests are implemented at 11–13 weeks of gestation, quadruple screen tests are

Table 4.1 Markers used to evaluate the possibility of fetal trisomy 21 at different gestational stages

11–13 weeks of gestation (first trimester)	Serum PAPPA concentration Serum free β-hCG or total hCG concentration Thickness of nuchal translucency
≥15 weeks of gestation (second trimester)	Serum AFP concentration Serum hCG or free β-hCG concentration Serum unconjugated estriol concentration Serum inhibin A concentration

hCG human chorionic gonadotrophin, *AFP* α-fetoprotein, *PAPPA* pregnancy-associated plasma protein A

Table 4.2 Screening test performed in the first and second trimester for trisomy 21

	Detection rate with a 5% false-positive rate
Maternal age	32.8%
+AFP + hCG + u-estriol + inhibin A	75.0%
+ NT	68.8%
+ PAPPA + β-hCG	67.2%
+ NT + PAPPA+ β-hCG	78.7%

AFP α-fetoprotein, *hCG* human chorionic gonadotrophin, *u-estradiol* unconjugated estriol, *NT* nuchal translucency, *PAPPA* pregnancy-associated plasma protein A performed at ≥15 weeks of gestation. In places like Japan, where chorionic villus testing is not a widespread practice, there may be little merit in performing combined tests during early pregnancy.

4.2 Fetal Chromosome Tests Using Maternal Plasma cfDNA

(1) History of test development

Based on the discovery that tumor-derived cfDNA circulates in the plasma of patients with malignant tumors [4], Lo et al. [5] hypothesized that fetal cfDNA also circulates in the maternal plasma. They extracted cfDNA from maternal plasma and serum and used it as a template to amplify a Y-chromosome-specific gene using polymerase chain reaction (PCR), subsequently showing that maternal plasma and serum contain fetal DNA. The fetal DNA found in maternal plasma is derived from placental trophoblasts [5], which cover the surface of the villi floating in the intervillous space, where maternal blood circulates. Aged trophoblasts that have finished functioning are shed into the intervillous space, and their DNA enters the maternal circulation, thereby providing the main source of fetal cfDNA in maternal plasma.

Initially, the analysis of maternal plasma cfDNA involved the use of PCR to amplify a specific DNA region. Subsequently, analysis of a Y-chromosome-specific gene revealed that 3–6% of maternal plasma cfDNA is derived from the fetus, and that the fetal cfDNA concentration gradually increases during gestation, decreases sharply after delivery, with a half-life of 16 min, and ultimately becomes undetectable within 2 h of birth [6]. Reported examples of fetal diagnosis include sex determination [7], Rh blood group D antigen (*RHD*) genotyping in RHD-negative women [8], and diagnosis of fetal monogenic diseases [9]. However, despite attempts to detect fetal aneuploids using a variety of approaches, studies using PCR amplification of cfDNA in maternal plasma have not yielded satisfactory results. Nevertheless, this field of study was a major turning point in the advancement of molecular biological analytical techniques, specifically the development of next-generation sequencing (NGS).

A 2008 study reported a novel method for detecting fetal aneuploidy in cfDNA from maternal plasma [10]. Analyzing cfDNA in maternal plasma using NGS allows the detection of DNA fragments as short as several tens of bases, which expands coverage relative to PCR, and demonstrated that the concentration of fetal cfDNA in the maternal plasma is higher than previously reported. The mean concentration of fetal cfDNA in a study of Japanese pregnant women was 13.7%, higher than previously reported in pregnant women in Europe and the United States and thought to be due to the relatively lower body weight of Japanese women [11].

(2) The principle of NIPT

The first report of detection of fetal aneuploidy in maternal plasma cfDNA using NGS technology involved the use of massively parallel sequencing (MPS) [10].

This method evaluates quantitative changes in the proportion of each chromosome-derived component in maternal plasma cfDNA in order to detect numerical alterations of fetal chromosomes.

Specifically, the base sequence of each fragment of maternal plasma cfDNA is read and collated with human genomic information in order to determine its source chromosome; however, this technique does not distinguish whether the sequenced DNA fragment comes from the fetus or the mother. Following analysis of >10 million fragments, the concentration of DNA fragments from each chromosome reflects the length of that chromosome and is constant; therefore, fragments derived from chromosome 21 should account for 1.3% of all fragments. However, when a fetus has trisomy 21, the concentration of cfDNA derived from chromosome 21 in the maternal plasma increases to 1.42% (Fig. 4.2), because when a single trophoblast with trisomy 21 collapses, chromosome 21 releases 1.5-fold more DNA fragments than would be released by a normal karyotype. This allows the detection of chromosomal aneuploidy from changes in DNA-fragment ratios.

Theoretically, the MPS method is able to detect even small differences as the number of DNA fragments analyzed increases. Because NGS allows simultaneous

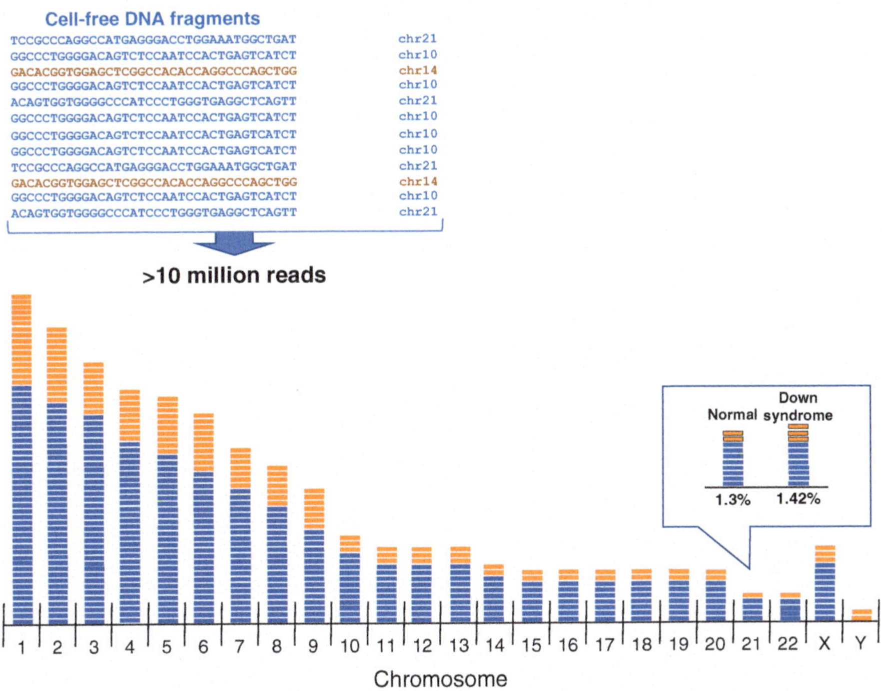

Fig. 4.2 Noninvasive prenatal testing using cell-free DNA in maternal plasma: principle of the massively parallel sequencing method. Cell-free DNA fragments from maternal plasma are sequenced and aligned with the human genome in order to determine the chromosome source. By comparing the number of DNA fragments from each chromosome, relative changes in their levels are evaluated

analysis of a large number of cfDNA fragments, it is possible to detect aneuploidy in fetuses with high accuracy. The test results are often presented as positive, negative, or not reportable and are highly accurate, providing ≥99% sensitivity and specificity [12].

Currently, many studies evaluating methods other than MPS are underway, and methods using single nucleotide polymorphisms (SNPs) have entered practical use. Recently, quantitative PCR, microarrays, and methods to replicate specific DNA regions using polymerases have been developed and applied to screen for aneuploidies involving specific chromosomes. The use of these non-NGS methods is expected to contribute to reducing the cost of NIPT.

(3) Application scope and limitations of NIPT

NIPT detects slight changes in the amounts of each chromosome in the genome by quantitating DNA sequences at high speed using NGS. Therefore, increasing the read count also increases accuracy. Furthermore, counting the number of sequences for each genomic site enables the performance of tests equivalent to microarrays. In practice, it is now possible to test for specific chromosomal microdeletions and duplications, with a test for microdeletions and duplications of ≥7 Mb in clinical use since 2015. Additionally, a reduced-cost test that amplifies DNA in specific regions of certain chromosomes has been clinically applied. Moreover, the diagnosis of genetic diseases and paternity testing is now possible by not just examining changes in genome quantity but also detecting specific gene mutations and SNPs. In one report, integrating the results of haplotype analysis of both parents and NGS analysis of maternal plasma cfDNA allowed sequencing of the entire fetal genome [13].

NIPT analyzes both maternal and trophoblast-derived fetal cfDNA in the maternal circulation. For this reason, changes in the quantity of circulating DNA can influence test accuracy. Specifically, if the mother has chromosomal abnormalities, such as chromosomal mosaicism, microdeletions, and/or microduplications, it is impossible to evaluate the fetus. Additionally, if the mother has a neoplastic disease, abnormal counts might be detected for several chromosomes, making it impossible to evaluate the fetus. Moreover, maternal obesity can decrease fetal cfDNA concentration, leading to an increased failure rate. Furthermore, when a pregnant woman has an autoimmune disease or is being treated with heparin, changes in cfDNA fragmentation and clearance can occur, thereby affecting test accuracy.

Because fetal cfDNA is derived from placental trophoblasts, false positives and false negatives can occur due to confined placental mosaicism or vanishing twin syndrome.

4.3 Accuracy of Prenatal Screening Tests

The conclusive diagnosis of fetal chromosomal diseases requires direct sampling of fetal cells by amniocentesis or chorionic villus sampling; however, these tests involve a risk of miscarriage. Noninvasive prenatal screening tests were developed

Table 4.3 Comparison of the positive and negative predictive values of different screening methods for fetal trisomy 21

		Quadruple test[a]	Combined test[a]	NIPT
Sensitivity		85%	86%	99.7%[b]
Specificity		91.5%	94.4%	99.9%[b]
Prevalence 1/100	PPV	9.2%	13.4%	91.0%
	NPV	99.83%	99.85%	99.997%
Prevalence 1/300	PPV	3.2%	4.9%	76.9%
	NPV	99.95%	99.95%	99.999%
Prevalence 1/1000	PPV	1.0%	1.5%	49.7%
	NPV	99.98%	99.99%	99.999%

PPV positive predictive value, *NPV* negative predictive value
[a]Cut-off value: 1:300, hygroma included
[b]Data from Japan NIPT consortium ($n = 34{,}691$)

as sources of information for pregnant women who are at a crossroads regarding whether to undergo these invasive tests.

Although test accuracy is evaluated based on its sensitivity and specificity, what really matters is the level of accuracy in the positive and negative results (i.e., the positive and negative predictive values). These values depend on the disease prevalence in the population of the patient being tested. Table 4.3 shows the positive and negative predictive values for detecting trisomy 21 using quadruple screening, combined screening, and NIPT. Comparatively, the accuracy of NIPT is overwhelmingly higher [14]; however, in practice, tests are often selected based on cost rather than accuracy alone, thereby limiting the use of NIPT. Reductions in the cost of NIPT and increased reimbursement by insurance companies will significantly influence prenatal screen selection.

4.4 Ethical Aspects of Prenatal Screening Tests

The purpose of prenatal screening is identification of the subset of pregnant women at high risk of having a fetus with chromosomal abnormalities. It is important to consider how much the pregnant woman wants to know about potential fetal illnesses and allow her to make an autonomous and informed decision regarding whether to undergo testing. Additionally, it is important that pregnant women and their partners are able to make informed decisions regarding the pregnancy when the presence of a chromosomal abnormality in the fetus is confirmed.

Because prenatal screening allows noninvasive estimation of the possibility of fetal chromosomal abnormalities, such as trisomy 21, these tests should not be routinely conducted without consideration of their potential impact. There is no social consensus regarding the mass screening of fetal chromosomal diseases in Japan, although some people have expressed concerns about this issue. Appropriate information should be provided to enable the decision to undergo testing to be autonomous and informed, and prenatal counseling is necessary to provide psychological support to anxious pregnant women and support their decision-making processes both before and after screening.

References

1. Wapner R, Thom E, Simpson JL, Pergament E, Silver R, Filkins K, et al. First-trimester screening for trisomies 21 and 18. N Engl J Med. 2003;349(15):1405–13.
2. Wald NJ, Huttly WJ, Hackshaw AK. Antenatal screening for Down's syndrome with the quadruple test. Lancet. 2003;361(9360):835–6.
3. Alldred SK, Takwoingi Y, Guo B, Pennant M, Deeks JJ, Neilson JP, et al. First trimester ultrasound tests alone or in combination with first trimester serum tests for Down's syndrome screening. Cochrane Database Syst Rev (Online). 2017;3:CD012600.
4. Stroun M, Anker P, Lyautey J, Lederrey C, Maurice PA. Isolation and characterization of DNA from the plasma of cancer patients. Eur J Cancer Clin Oncol. 1987;23(6):707–12.
5. Masuzaki H, Miura K, Yoshiura KI, Yoshimura S, Niikawa N, Ishimaru T. Detection of cell free placental DNA in maternal plasma: direct evidence from three cases of confined placental mosaicism. J Med Genet. 2004;41(4):289–92.
6. Lo YM, Zhang J, Leung TN, Lau TK, Chang AM, Hjelm NM. Rapid clearance of fetal DNA from maternal plasma. Am J Human Genet. 1999;64(1):218–24.
7. Sekizawa A, Kondo T, Iwasaki M, Watanabe A, Jimbo M, Saito H, et al. Accuracy of fetal gender determination by analysis of DNA in maternal plasma. Clin Chem. 2001;47(10):1856–8.
8. Lo YM, Hjelm NM, Fidler C, Sargent IL, Murphy MF, Chamberlain PF, et al. Prenatal diagnosis of fetal RhD status by molecular analysis of maternal plasma. N Engl J Med. 1998;339(24):1734–8.
9. Saito H, Sekizawa A, Morimoto T, Suzuki M, Yanaihara T. Prenatal DNA diagnosis of a single-gene disorder from maternal plasma. Lancet. 2000;356(9236):1170.
10. Chiu RW, Chan KC, Gao Y, Lau VY, Zheng W, Leung TY, et al. Noninvasive prenatal diagnosis of fetal chromosomal aneuploidy by massively parallel genomic sequencing of DNA in maternal plasma. Proc Natl Acad Sci U S A. 2008;105(51):20458–63.
11. Suzumori N, Sekizawa A, Ebara T, Samura O, Sasaki A, Akaishi R, et al. Fetal cell-free DNA fraction in maternal plasma for the prediction of hypertensive disorders of pregnancy. Eur J Obstet Gynecol Reprod Biol. 2018;224:165–9.
12. Palomaki GE, Kloza EM, Lambert-Messerlian GM, Haddow JE, Neveux LM, Ehrich M, et al. DNA sequencing of maternal plasma to detect Down syndrome: an international clinical validation study. Genet Med. 2011;13(11):913–20.
13. Kitzman JO, Snyder MW, Ventura M, Lewis AP, Qiu R, Simmons LE, et al. Noninvasive whole-genome sequencing of a human fetus. Sci Transl Med. 2012;4(137):137ra76.
14. Malone FD, Canick JA, Ball RH, Nyberg DA, Comstock CH, Bukowski R, et al. First-trimester or second-trimester screening, or both, for Down's syndrome. N Engl J Med. 2005;353(19):2001–11.

Chapter 5
Diagnostic Tests (Invasive Procedures)

Toshiro Ikeda

Abstract Diagnostic tests, which are performed as screening tests in high-risk cases, refer to invasive techniques such as chorionic villus sampling (CVS), amniocentesis, and cordocentesis (percutaneous umbilical cord blood sampling, PUBS).

Advances in diagnostic techniques that have incorporated molecular genetics now allow the diagnosis of most diseases by means of chromosomal or genetic tests rather than by performing histopathological or enzymatic diagnosis. As a result, highly invasive diagnostic procedures are rarely used.

CVS and amniocentesis are the most frequently used diagnostic tests at present, with amniocentesis more commonly performed. However, as CVS is now more commonly performed via transabdominal rather than transcervical procedure, the fetal loss rate has decreased, so the number of CVS procedures is increasing in various regions.

Cordocentesis is also performed in selected cases due to the ability to diagnose fetal anemia and obtain a rapid chromosomal analysis.

In this chapter, we discuss the specific methods of these tests and their advantages and disadvantages.

Keywords Chorionic villus sampling · Amniocentesis · Cordocentesis · Fetal blood sampling · Invasive prenatal diagnostic procedures

Due to the dissemination of noninvasive prenatal genetic testing (NIPT), various screening tests are slowly being phased out of use as diagnostic tests. Furthermore, advances in diagnostic techniques now allow the diagnosis of most diseases by means of chromosomal or genetic tests rather than by performing histopathological or enzymatic diagnosis. As a result, highly invasive diagnostic techniques are rarely

---

T. Ikeda (✉)
Department of Obstetrics and Gynecology, Kagoshima University, Kagoshima, Japan
e-mail: ikeda@m2.kufm.kagoshima-u.ac.jp

H. Masuzaki (ed.), *Fetal Morph Functional Diagnosis*, Comprehensive Gynecology and Obstetrics, https://doi.org/10.1007/978-981-15-8171-7_5

used. However, retrieval of fetal-derived cells to confirm a diagnosis requires the use of the invasive techniques described in this chapter. The table shows a comparison of frequently used methods.

All of these techniques involve inserting instruments into the pregnant uterus, so aseptic techniques are required. To ensure maximum sterility, the skin and vaginal walls should be adequately disinfected using povidone-iodine or other disinfectants, and the ultrasound probe and ultrasound guide attachment should be covered with a disposable sterile material.

5.1 Chorionic Villus Sampling (Fig. 5.1)

The advantage of Chorionic villus sampling (CVS) is that it can be used to perform confirmatory tests during the earliest stages of pregnancy. This allows couples a great deal of time to make the necessary decisions based on the test outcomes. If couples choose to terminate the pregnancy, it also facilitates the selection of a safer method to do so. The disadvantage is the high miscarriage rate of 1–2%. However, spontaneous miscarriages are common during the period in which CVS is performed, and because the procedure is performed in cases of suspected fetal abnormality, such as increased nuchal translucency, these cases would include fetuses with chromosomal abnormalities or cardiac malformations that would likely have resulted in spontaneous miscarriage. After correcting for these cases, current reports indicate that the increase in the miscarriage rate due to the technique itself is 1 in

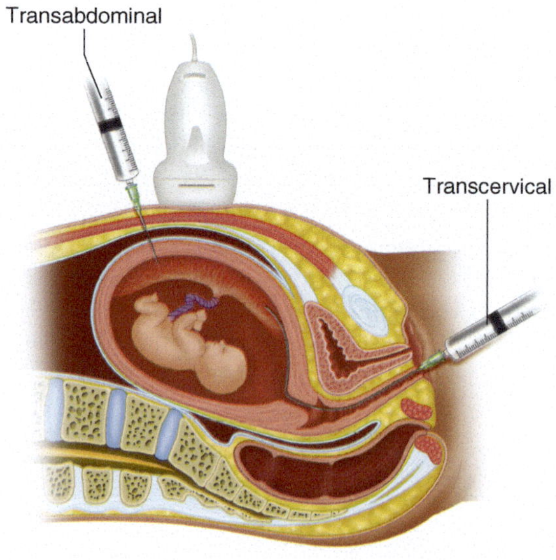

Fig. 5.1 Chollionic villus sampling. (A) Transabdominal, (B) transcervical

370 or lesser, so CVS is as safe as performing amniocentesis. CVS is usually performed via a transcervical or transabdominal approach, with the transabdominal approach becoming popular in recent years due to its increased safety [1, 2].

5.1.1 Approaches for CVS

(a) Transcervical approach

The biggest advantage of the transcervical technique is that it can be performed before gestational week 10, thus allowing collection of the chorionic villi at the earliest stage. Previously, the procedure was performed without ultrasound guidance, but presently, the most popular method involves the insertion of specialized biopsy forceps or catheters via the external cervical os under transabdominal ultrasound guidance, followed by collection of the chorionic tissue. Chorionic villi are abundant during the early weeks of pregnancy, so the tissues can usually be retrieved successfully. Although the procedure has a miscarriage rate of 1–2%, we believe that the miscarriages are primarily caused by bacterial infection. Despite the specification of antibiotics, there has been no obvious decrease in the miscarriage rate.

According to reports, one issue that demands particular caution is the increased rates of fetal limb reduction and oromandibular limb hypogenesis syndrome that are observed when the procedure is performed before 10 weeks [3, 4]. At present, the transabdominal approach discussed below is therefore usually performed from gestational week 10 onward, other than in exceptional cases.

(b) Transabdominal approach

This approach is similar to that used for amniocentesis. However, it is sometimes impossible to perform puncture safely based on the position of the maternal intestines, the placenta, and the umbilical cord attachment site. These issues can sometimes be resolved by either filling or emptying the bladder, although this will only help in ≤10% of patients, so the transabdominal approach must be abandoned in certain cases. When this occurs, it is necessary to determine whether to attempt a transcervical approach or switch to amniocentesis.

The transabdominal approach involves advancing the needle into the chorion and performing aspiration for retrieval. This usually requires the use of an 18 to 21G needle. Various hospitals are devising safer ways to retrieve adequate amounts of chorionic tissue, and recently, the number of hospitals using the double-needle technique to avoid repeated puncture of the uterus has increased. This technique involves puncturing the uterus using a larger 18G needle, then inserting a 20 to 21G needle through the larger needle to perform repeated aspiration to retrieve the required amount of tissue. There are specialized CVS needles that are commercially available, although they may be used in combination with percutaneous transhepatic cholangiography (PTC) needles. A few mL of heparinized saline is drawn up into the syringe that will be used for aspiration, and then the syringe is used to apply continuous suction while gently moving the needle back and forth to retrieve the required amount of chorionic tissue.

The 18G needles are large, so the more that the angle of insertion into the abdominal wall or uterine surface approaches the horizontal (0°), the more likely there will be resistance to the puncture and an inability to advance the needle in the desired direction. This commonly causes needle bevel position errors, and in most cases, the situation can be resolved by rotating the needle by 180°. The use of any needle that is ≥20G usually necessitates the administration of local anesthesia.

The reason the abdominal method has become more mainstream is due to its lower rate of fetal loss, and there has been no obvious increase in risk as compared to amniocentesis when investigating cases other than high-risk groups, such as patients with increased nuchal translucency.

(c) Transvaginal approach

This approach is still not very popular. The transvaginal approach entails puncture of the uterine corpus under ultrasound guidance using a transvaginal probe, similar to the procedure used for transvaginal oocyte retrieval, and retrieving chorionic tissue. This approach may be required to collect chorionic villous tissue from sites that are difficult to reach via the transabdominal and transcervical approaches [5], although it has not become popular due to its perceived high potential for causing intrauterine infection.

5.1.2 Twin Pregnancies

When dealing with monozygotic (monochorionic) twins, a single CVS procedure may be performed. However, when dealing with dichorionic twins that may be dizygotic, a biopsy needs to be taken from each placenta. If the placentas can be clearly differentiated, then it is possible to perform the procedure on each placenta separately. However, if the placentas lie in close proximity to one another, then amniocentesis should be considered.

5.1.3 Chromosomal Mosaicism

When fetal chromosomal analysis is performed by means of CVS, the cell culture must be divided into two or more flasks to facilitate the determination of mosaics (true/false). True mosaicism is detected in 1–2% of cases, although in most cases, this is confined placental mosaicism, and no definitive statements can be made regarding the mosaicism of the fetus. If it is difficult to make a diagnosis, then amniocentesis must be performed for confirmation. An adequate explanation will need to be provided to the patient before the test is performed.

Conversely, mosaicism may not be detected in the small amount of chorionic tissue that is retrieved from a narrow area. To prevent this, some practitioners advocate advancing the needle to ensure collection of chorionic tissue over a wider area, but this leads to the dilemma of inadvertently increasing invasiveness.

5.1.4 *Maternal Cell Contamination*

There is a higher rate of maternal cell contamination during CVS than amniocentesis. It is impossible to completely eliminate maternal cells, such as prolapsed membranes, or maternal skin or uterine muscle layers, but it is important to perform irrigation with culture medium, use equipment such as stereoscopic microscopes, and do the utmost to ensure that only villi are collected. To prevent prolapsed membranes from entering the retrieval site, attention must be paid to ensure that the procedure is performed away from the uterine muscle layers.

5.2 **Amniocentesis** (Fig. 5.2)

Amniocentesis is easier to perform and more widely used than CVS. In most cases, puncture is usually performed via a transabdominal approach using a 21 to 25G needle under ultrasound guidance. To minimize the risk of maternal cell

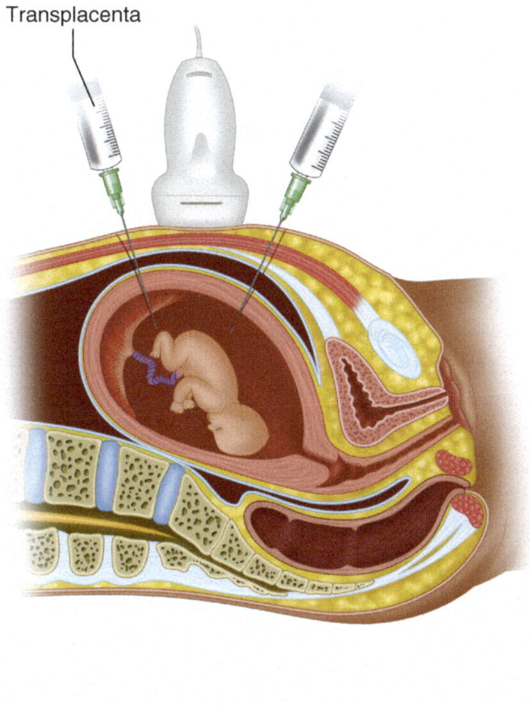

Fig. 5.2 Amniocentesis

contamination, it is preferable to use a specialized amniocentesis needle with a stylet (if one cannot be obtained, then a spinal needle with a stylet or a PTC needle can be used as a substitute). Furthermore, discarding the first 1–2 mL of the aspirate will reduce the number of maternal cells collected.

The procedure can be performed from gestational week 15 onward, although it is increasingly difficult to distinguish between the amnion and chorion from week 16, which significantly reduces the number of puncture attempts. This is why most hospitals perform the procedure from week 16 onward. In addition, in certain cases, despite the ability to see that the needle has entered the amniotic fluid cavity, it may be impossible to perform aspiration. It is not uncommon to be unable to see the needle on ultrasound, but the amnion adopts a tented shape when pressure is applied on the needle. Using a needle that is as sharp as possible and performing the puncture by applying an adequate amount of force at a location where the amnion and chorion have unified reduces this to a significant extent. The needle should be inserted as perpendicularly to the amnion as possible for maximum success.

When performing chromosomal analysis, 10–20 mL of fluid is retrieved, and samples taken for testing mosaicism (true mosaicism, pseudo-mosaicism) should be divided into ≥2 flasks for cell culture.

As discussed in the section on CVS, true mosaicism of the amniotic cells is not necessarily significant for fetal mosaicism, although unlike mosaicism that is detected by means of CVS, confirmatory tests for mosaicism by means of amniocentesis cannot be performed via cordocentesis, which is challenging to perform and a high-risk procedure. Therefore, depending on the case, detailed ultrasound findings and conventional data may be accepted as confirmatory tests.

The rate of fetal loss has been described to be around 0.3%, but the corrected data showed that it was as low as 0.06–0.13% [2, 6, 7].

5.2.1 *Placental Puncture*

It is best to avoid performing placental puncture to reduce the risk of Rh isoimmunization and mother-to-child transmission of infection, although several reports have indicated that the rate of miscarriage does not change when transplacental puncture is performed. There is no need to avoid this procedure until there is no other option. A considerable amount of caution is required when puncturing the lateral uterus or uterine fundus due to the potential for injury to the uterine artery and vein and subsequent hematoma formation, and the risk of inadvertently puncturing the maternal intestines.

In addition, it is necessary to thoroughly confirm the umbilical cord attachment site before puncture. If the placenta is punctured without considering avoidance of the umbilical cord, devastating consequences may occur if the umbilical cord has a velamentous insertion. The umbilical cord attachment site and any large vessels should also be avoided.

5.2.2 *Twin Pregnancies*

A single puncture is sufficient in the case of monozygotic twins (monochorionic). However, when dealing with dichorionic twins that may be dizygotic, a biopsy needs to be taken from the amniotic fluid cavity of each twin. To puncture each individual amniotic fluid cavity with a high degree of certainty, it is possible to inject dye, such as indigo carmine, before puncturing the first cavity to distinguish it from the second cavity. However, the properties of ultrasonic tomography are so advanced that dye injection is not considered to be necessary in most cases (although it may be necessary in cases of multiple pregnancies with ≥3 fetuses). Particular caution is required to ensure that samples are appropriately interpreted for the intended fetus in the case of multiple fetuses of the same sex.

5.2.3 *Early Amniocentesis*

This term refers to amniocentesis performed prior to gestational week 14. This procedure is not usually performed nowadays due to the ability to perform transabdominal CVS safely as it carries the risk of rupture of the membrane (amniotic fluid leakage), fetal deformities, and miscarriages increases.

5.3 Cordocentesis

Cordocentesis (percutaneous umbilical cord blood sampling, PUBS) is performed under ultrasound guidance to collect blood from the umbilical vein. It is commonly performed using a 21 to 23G needle, but a 25G needle is used in some hospitals to perform the procedure. Reports have indicated that the procedure can be performed before week 14, although it is usually difficult to perform before week 18–20.The fetal loss rate was thought to be high, but recently reported 0.6% [8].

(a) Transplacental puncture of the umbilical cord attachment site (Fig. 5.3)

Transplacental puncture of the umbilical vein may be performed near the umbilical cord attachment site if the placenta is attached along the anterior uterine wall. This form of puncture can be performed with the most ease and greatest certainty, so it is preferred. The disadvantage of this technique is that the maternal blood will mix with the fetal blood, which may promote immunosensitization and decrease test accuracy.

(b) Puncture of the umbilical cord attachment site on the posterior uterine wall (Fig. 5.4)

This technique may injure the fetus and is usually difficult to perform, but if the puncture can be performed safely and only the umbilical vein is punctured, then

Fig. 5.3 Cordocentesis (anterior placenta)

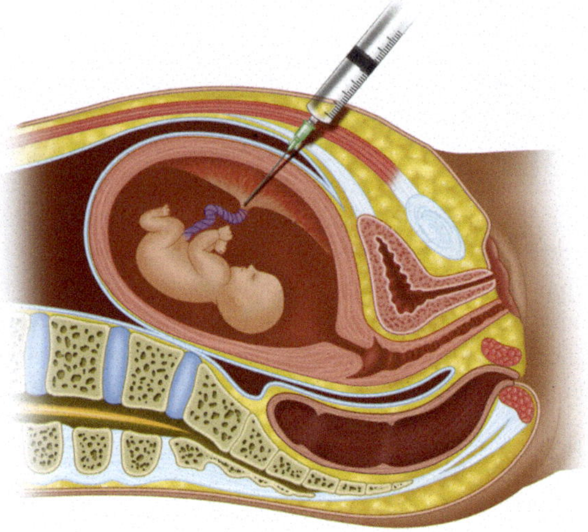

Fig. 5.4 Cordocentesis (posterior placenta)

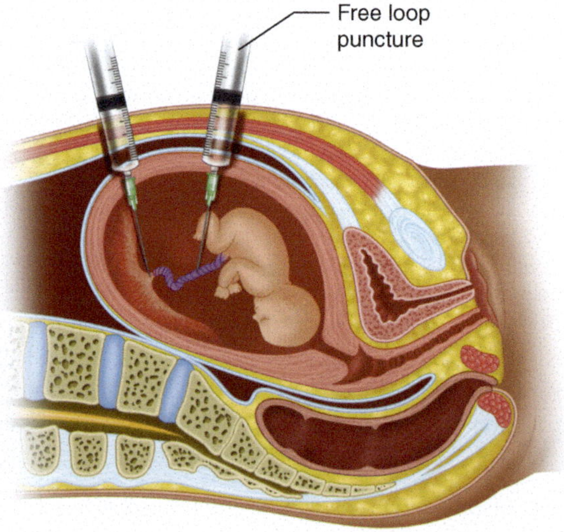

sensitization is unlikely to occur. As with the other methods, it is important to exercise caution regarding contamination with maternal blood located in the intervillous spaces at sites that are close to the placenta.

(c) Free loop puncture (Fig. 5.4)

The issue of sensitization is associated with placental puncture, but it is not uncommon to be able to avoid the placenta. The objective of this technique is to puncture the umbilical cord (the umbilical vein, as a rule) as it is floating in the amniotic fluid. The free loop will move as soon as it is contacted by the tip of the needle, so the trick of this technique is to perform the puncture instantaneously as soon as the needle comes into contact with the cord. Provided that there is an obvious separation between the cord and the placenta, fetal blood will be obtained with absolute certainty. However, it is difficult to perform this technique from the second trimester onward.

5.3.1 *Confirming That Blood Is of Fetal Origin*

It is necessary to rapidly determine whether the blood that has been retrieved is actually of fetal origin. The following methods are useful for detecting erythrocytes of fetal origin.

(a) Blood gas analysis
(b) Erythrocyte morphology (particularly the mean corpuscular volume [MCV] distribution: fetal blood MCV is largely unimodal. If contaminated by maternal blood, there is the simultaneous appearance of an MCV peak that is smaller than that of the fetus.)
(c) Blood type (ABO, RhD)
(d) The Kleihauer-Betke test

So far, the general methods described are summarized in the Table 5.1.

5.4 Other Diagnostic Tests

(a) Coelocentesis

This method involves retrieving coelomic fluid that is present outside the amnion [9]. As its advantages, the procedure can be performed without harming the amnion or chorion, and it can be performed during the early stages of pregnancy. However, this fluid has a high viscosity and cannot be aspirated with needles smaller than 20G. It has not achieved practical application because only a small number of cells are collected, and these cell cultures are difficult. The percentage of contamination by the maternal components is also poorly understood. Preimplantation genetic testing

Table 5.1 Comparisons of common invasive diagnostic tests

		Weeks	Difficulty	Fetal loss[a]
CVS	Transcervical	10~14	Slightly difficult	1~2% (or lesser)
	Transabdominal	10~14	Slightly difficult	–0.11~1.16%
Amniocentesis		15(16~)	Easy	0.06~0.27%
Cordocentesis		18~	Difficult	0.6%~

Although there are various reports on the risks of CVS, it is safer to use the transabdominal approach

[a]Additional risk of fetal loss (exclude spontaneous miscarriage)

(PGT) is usually performed by determining aneuploidy (PGT-A) using next-generation sequencing, and it is expected that this method may be revised in the future.

(b) Fetal muscle biopsy [10]

Reports have indicated that immunohistochemical staining may be used to diagnose suspected cases of Duchenne muscular dystrophy if a biopsy is taken from the fetal gluteal muscle using a needle gun.

(c) Fetal skin biopsy [11]

This is used to diagnose lethal skin diseases. Biopsy forceps are used for this purpose.

(d) Fetal liver biopsy [12]

Reports have indicated that this may be useful in cases of carbamoyl phosphate synthetase deficiency.

(e) Fetal tumor biopsy

5.4.1 Maternal Infections

In the event of antenatal infection with human immunodeficiency virus (HIV) or hepatitis B, or in the case of hepatitis C carriers, it is recommended that noninvasive tests, such as NIPT, perform whenever possible. If invasive tests are required, reports have shown that there is no significant difference in terms of the risk of mother-to-child transmission when amniocentesis is selected over CVS to avoid the placentae in hepatitis B and hepatitis C carriers or patients. Reports have also suggested that the HIV infection rate does not increase as long as patients receive combined antiretroviral therapy, although the evidence for this is insufficient [13]. It is important to explain the risk of inducing fetal infection before performing any test. Ideally, the infection rates for each condition should be explained before the test using the most recent data that is available.

5.4.2 Rh Isoimmunization

After invasive testing is performed on mothers who are Rh(D) negative withs partners who are Rh(D) positive, they will be administered Rh(D) immunoglobulin (RhIG) as prophylaxis against sensitization. If the fetal blood tests and NIPT confirm that the fetus is Rh-negative, then the administration of RhIG is not required, but if the test results are not adequately reliable, then the case must be handled as though the fetus were Rh-positive.

In all cases, the indirect Coombs test and middle cerebral artery peak systolic velocity must be measured periodically after puncture, and the patient should be followed up carefully to ensure that there is no possibility of fetal anemia.

5.4.3 Maternal Risk

Despite being extremely rare, there have been reports of serious maternal complications. These included reports of septicemia that has resulted in maternal death in some cases [14, 15]. These types of complications may be caused by puncture of the maternal intestines when performing transabdominal procedures. Due to the characteristics of ultrasound tomography, it may be challenging to determine whether bowel is lying between the peritoneum and uterus. However, if time is allowed to elapse during the examination, then the peristaltic movements of the bowel will become visible. It is important to perform a thorough examination before puncture to rule out intestinal puncture. There have also been reports of amniotic fluid emboli, but these are even more rare.

Caution is also required during techniques that use the transcervical approach, as this may be associated with the risk of uterine perforation. This is an unavoidable complication, so obtaining appropriate informed consent before the procedure is important.

References

1. Caughey AB, Hopkins LM, Norton ME. Chorionic villus sampling compared with amniocentesis and the difference in the rate of pregnancy loss. Obstet Gynecol. 2006 Sep;108(3 Pt 1):612–6.
2. Salomon LJ, Sotiriadis A, Wulff CB, Odibo A, Akolekar R. Risk of miscarriage following amniocentesis or chorionic villus sampling: systematic review of literature and updated meta-analysis. Ultrasound Obstet Gynecol. 2019 Oct;54(4):442–51.
3. Firth HV, Boyd PA, Chamberlain P, MacKenzie IZ, Lindenbaum RH, Huson SM. Severe limb abnormalities after chorion villus sampling at 56-66 days' gestation. Lancet. 1991 Mar 30;337(8744):762–3.
4. Firth H. Chorion villus sampling and limb deficiency–cause or coincidence? Prenat Diagn. 1997 Dec;17(13):1313–30.
5. Sidransky E, Black SH, Soenksen DM, Jones SL, Dorfmann AD, Schulman JD. Transvaginal chorionic villus sampling. Prenat Diagn. 1990 Sep;10(9):583–6.
6. Eddleman KA, Malone FD, Sullivan L, Dukes K, Berkowitz RL, Kharbutli Y, Porter TF, Luthy DA, Comstock CH, Saade GR, Klugman S, Dugoff L, Craigo SD, Timor-Tritsch IE, Carr SR, Wolfe HM, D'Alton ME. Pregnancy loss rates after midtrimester amniocentesis. Obstet Gynecol. 2006 Nov;108(5):1067–72.
7. Odibo AO, Gray DL, Dicke JM, Stamilio DM, Macones GA, Crane JP. Revisiting the fetal loss rate after second-trimester genetic amniocentesis: a single center's 16-year experience. Obstet Gynecol. 2008 Mar;111(3):589–95.

8. Tanvisut R, Wanapirak C, Piyamongkol W, Sirichotiyakul S, Tongprasert F, Srisupundit K, Luewan S, Traisrisilp K, Jatavan P, Tongsong T. Cordocentesis-associated fetal loss and risk factors: experience of 6650 cases from a single center. Ultrasound Obstet Gynecol. 2020.
9. Jurkovic D, Jauniaux E, Campbell S, Pandya P, Cardy DL, Nicolaides KH. Coelocentesis: a new technique for early prenatal diagnosis. Lancet. 1993 Jun 26;341(8861):1623–4.
10. Evans MI, Greb A, Kunkel LM, Sacks AJ, Johnson MP, Boehm C, Kazazian HH Jr, Hoffman EP. In utero fetal muscle biopsy for the diagnosis of Duchenne muscular dystrophy. Am J Obstet Gynecol. 1991 Sep;165(3):728–32.
11. Holbrook KA, Smith LT, Elias S. Prenatal diagnosis of genetic skin disease using fetal skin biopsy samples. Arch Dermatol. 1993 Nov;129(11):1437–54.
12. Murotsuki J, Uehara S, Okamura K, Yajima A, Oura T, Miyabayashi S. Fetal liver biopsy for prenatal diagnosis of carbamoyl phosphate synthetase deficiency. Am J Perinatol. 1994 Mar;11(2):160–2.
13. Gagnon A, Davies G, Wilson RD, GENETICS COMMITTEE. Prenatal invasive procedures in women with hepatitis B, hepatitis C, and/or human immunodeficiency virus infections. J Obstet Gynaecol Can. 2014 Jul;36(7):648–53.
14. Erez Y, Ben-Shushan A, Elchalal U, Ben-Meir A, Rojansky N. Maternal morbidity following routine second trimester genetic amniocentesis. Fetal Diagn Ther. 2007;22(3):226–8. Epub 2007 Jan 17
15. Thorp JA, Helfgott AW, King EA, King AA, Minyard AN. Maternal death after second-trimester genetic amniocentesis. Obstet Gynecol. 2005 May;105(5 Pt 2):1213–5.

Part III
Genetic Disorders

Chapter 6
Mendelian Disease

Yoshiki Kudo

Keywords Mendelian law · Autosomal dominant disease · Autosomal recessive disease · X-linked dominant disease · X-linked recessive disease · Y-linked disease

Among human genetic diseases, those caused by abnormality of a single gene and which obeys mendelian law in principle are called mendelian disease or monogenic disease. When diseases are classified according to the mode of inheritance based on mendelian law of inheritance, they are autosomal dominant disease, autosomal recessive disease, X-linked dominant disease, X-linked recessive disease and Y-linked disease.

6.1 Mendelian Law

Mendelian law is the law of genetics, published by Mendel, consisting of the rules of dominance, the rules of segregation and the rules of independence. This is derived from the results obtained from the pea mating experiments. Mendel conducted experiments using multiple varieties of peas to cross pure pea expressing different traits and found seven traits (seed shape, seed colour, pod shape, pod colour, flower colour, flowering position, stem length). Mendel first focused on the fact that there are tall and low peas. He then collected only the tall seeds from there and raised them separately. Looking at the height of the grown ones, he collected only the seeds of the raised ones and sowed the following year. By continuing this for several years, it has become possible to harvest tall pea seeds. Shorter ones were similarly selected over the years, successfully harvesting the shorter ones.

Y. Kudo (✉)
Department of Obstetrics and Gynecology, Hiroshima University, Hiroshima, Japan
e-mail: yoshkudo@hiroshima-u.ac.jp

H. Masuzaki (ed.), *Fetal Morph Functional Diagnosis*, Comprehensive Gynecology and Obstetrics, https://doi.org/10.1007/978-981-15-8171-7_6

6.1.1 Discovering the Law of Dominance

Mendel then discovered the law dominance by means of the following experiments. He raised the tall pea seeds and pollinated the stamens of the blooming flowers with pollen of the short pea seeds. Conversely, the pistils of short flowers were pollinated with high pollens. And when they sowed the harvested seeds, they were all tall.

6.1.2 Discovering the Law of Segregation

Mendel then self-pollinated the peas and sown the following year. As a result, the proportion of tall was three and the proportion of short was one. Mendel performed the same experiment on several traits, besides the height, including those with and without wrinkled pea seeds. In the same way, if we crossed the wrinkled and the unwrinkled, the next year only the unwrinkled was harvested. When the seeds were raised the following year, the percentage of wrinkles was three and one was unwrinkled. Similarly, the same conclusion was obtained when the seed colour was crossed between yellow and green.

6.1.3 Discovering the Law of Independence

Mendel crossed together things with multiple traits, such as the height of peas and the presence or absence of wrinkles. As a result, there was no correlation between the manner of inheritance of each trait, and the rule of dominance and the law of separation were established for each trait. This is called the law of independence, but it turned out that it only holds under certain conditions.

As a result, (1) Inheritance-determining substances are inherited after mating. (2) Each plant has two genetic components. This is what we now call a gene. We think that there is basically one pair of genes, each inherited from the father and mother one by one. (3) There are separate genes for the features. Mendel argued that when gametes were formed, the two genes behaved like elementary particles and split into germ cells to contain only one member of each pair. During this process, the two genes do not undergo any changes and do not mix. Now we call it an allele. In pure plants, the alleles are the same. If at least one of the two genes is present, the one that exhibits its characteristics is called dominant inheritance, and that gene is called the dominant gene. In addition, recessive inheritance appears only when both have the same allele, and the related genes are called recessive genes. (4) At the time of mating, one of the parental alleles is inherited by offspring. The probability of which one is inherited is half. Those with the same allele are called homozygous, and those with different alleles are called heterozygous.

Mendelian laws of inheritance were unknown to anyone at the time of its publication. Mendel's law was independently rediscovered by De Vries, Chelmak and Korens afterwards, and put together by Korens into three laws. Later, with the progress of chromosome research, it was recognized that the gene was an entity on the chromosome, and the idea of the current gene was developed.

6.2 Mendelian Disease

It became clear that the law of inheritance holds for not only plants but also all living things. Although few can be applied simply to mendelian rules of inheritance, humans also have traits that obey the rules described above. Mendelian disease is thought to be caused by an abnormality in one of the genes. Mendelian diseases are classified according to the mode of inheritance based on mendelian law and are mainly autosomal dominant disease, autosomal recessive disease, X-linked recessive disease and X-linked dominant disease.

6.2.1 Autosomal Dominant Disease

In an autosomal dominant trait, only one abnormal allele is abnormal and the trait is expressed; that is, heterozygotes and homozygotes for the abnormal gene are affected.

In general, the following rules apply: (1) One of the affected parents is affected. (2) Affected heterozygous parents and unaffected parents have an average of the same number of affected and unaffected children; that is, the risk of developing an affected child is 50%. (3) Unaffected children born to affected parents do not transmit the trait to their offspring. (4) Males and females have the same probability of contracting.

In the family tree (Fig. 6.1), there may be several people in each generation who have the same illness. The affected individuals are considered to be the same heterozygous and may transmit the mutated allele to the next generation. However, even within the same family, even with the same genotype, there are individual differences in the degree of symptoms and tend to vary from severe to mild.

To date, more than 2000 autosomal dominant diseases have been found. Representative diseases include Huntington disease, Marfan syndrome, achondroplasia, neurofibromatosis type II and familial colon polyposis (Table 6.1).

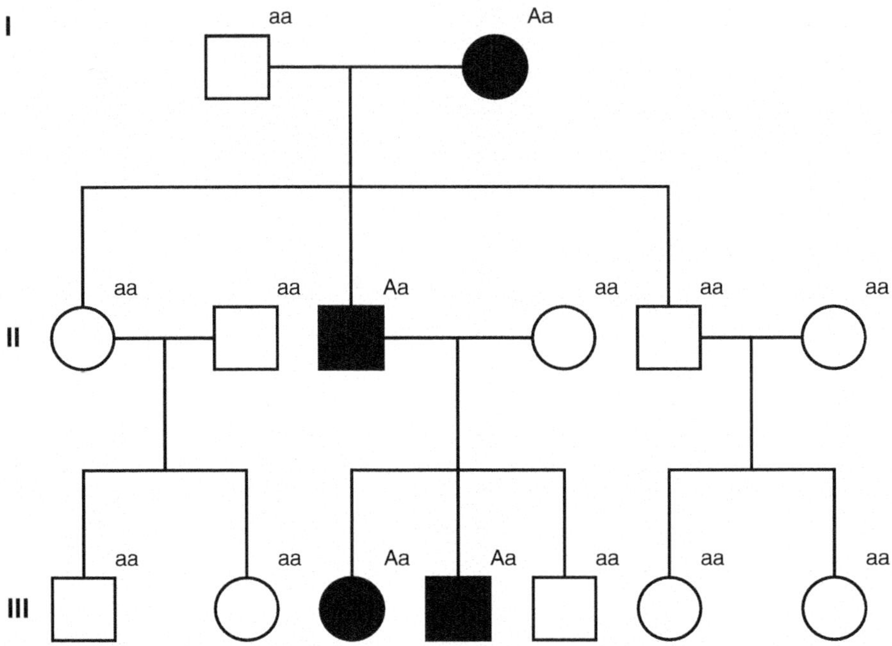

Fig. 6.1 Inheritance pattern of autosomal dominant mendelian disorder

Table 6.1 Examples of autosomal dominant disorder

Disorder	Phenotype	OMIM number
Achondroplasia	Dwarfism due to incomplete development of long bones	100800
Brachydactyly	Malformed hand with short fingers	112500
Camptodactyly	Little finger bow	114200
Crouzon syndrome	Malformation of the central part of the face	123500
Ehlers-Danlos syndrome	Abnormal connective tissue, joint laxity	130000
Familial hypercholesterolaemia	Elevated blood cholesterol level, heart disease	144010
Polycystic kidney disease	Renal failure	173900
Huntington disease	Neurodegeneration	143100
Hypercalcaemia	Increased blood calcium level	143880
Marfan syndrome	Abnormal connective tissue, arterial rupture	154700
Nail-patella syndrome	Nail and patella defects	154700
Porphyria	Abnormal porphyrin metabolic process, neuropsychiatric symptoms	176200

6.2.2 Autosomal Recessive Disease

The disease occurs only when the mutated allele is homozygous (Fig. 6.2). Heterozygous states do not cause disease and become carriers. This is quite different from an autosomal dominant disease that develops at heterozygosity. The difference between patients in the same family and the degree of symptoms is similar and less variable, unlike the autosomal dominant genetic disease. The same incidence rate in men and women is common for the autosomal disease.

In general, the following genetic rules apply: (1) If an affected child is born to a normal parent, both parents are heterozygous. On average, one-quarter of offspring are affected, half are heterozygotes, and one-quarter are normal. Thus, the likelihood of a child not being disturbed (i.e. being normal or a carrier) is three-quarters, and the likelihood of an unaffected child being a carrier is two-thirds. (2) The offspring of the affected parent and the normal genotype parent are all phenotypically normal heterozygotes. (3) On average, half of affected parents and heterozygous offspring are affected, and the other half are heterozygotes. (4) If both parents are affected, all children are affected. (5) Males and females are equally likely to be affected. (6) Heterozygotes have a normal phenotype but carry an abnormal gene.

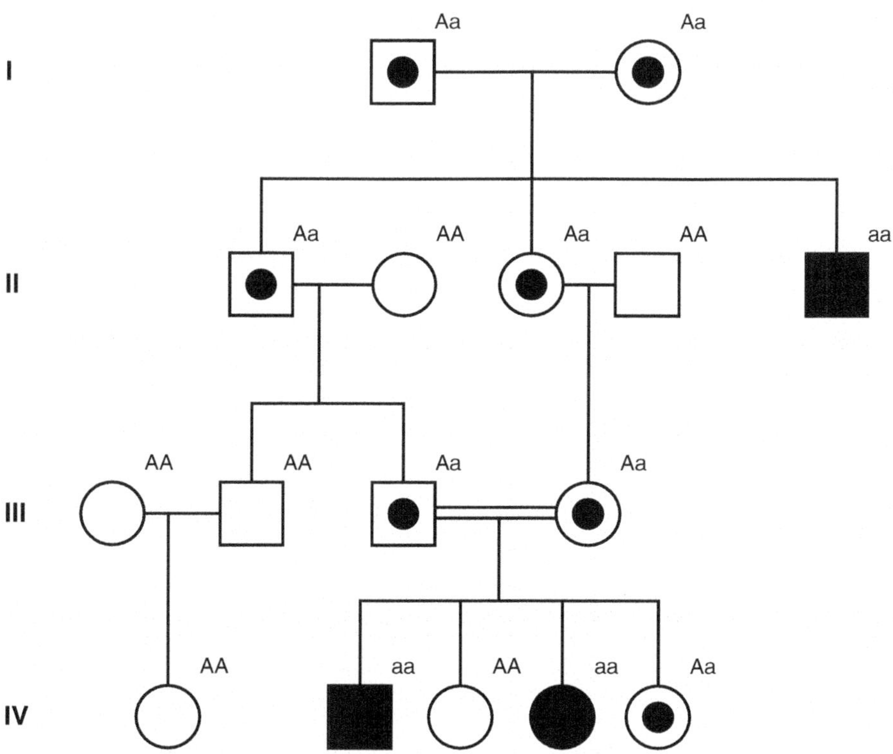

Fig. 6.2 Inheritance pattern of autosomal recessive mendelian disorder

(7) Relatives are more likely to carry the same variant allele, so when relatives get married, they are more likely to have an affected child.

So far, more than 600 types of autosomal recessive inheritance have been found, and typical diseases include major congenital metabolic disorders such as phenylketonuria and albinism (Table 6.2).

6.2.3 X-Linked Recessive Disease

Because it is related to the gene present on the X chromosome, males and females have different rates of incidence (Fig. 6.3). In addition, the gene on the father's X chromosome is transmitted to the daughter, but not to the son. On the other hand, mothers have two X chromosomes, but whether the child is a boy or a girl, it will transmit an allele on either X chromosome. The wild-type allele on the X chromosome is X^A, and the mutant gene is X^a. When male inherits the mutant gene X^a, the disease will be reflected even X^a itself is a recessive gene because of one hemizygote. Therefore, most patients with X-linked recessive genetic disease are male. X^AX^A is normal for female genotypes, and X^AX^a is a carrier and usually does not cause disease. X^aX^a causes disease like male; however, it is very few because father's genotype is limited to X^aY. However, one of the two X chromosomes in a woman has stopped functioning and is in an inactivated state, so even a woman with X^AX^a rarely develops a mild illness.

Table 6.2 Examples of autosomal recessive disorder

Disorder	Phenotype	OMIM number
Albinism	Absence of skin, eye, and hair pigments	203100
Ataxia telangiectasia	Neurodegeneration	208900
Bloom syndrome	Dwarfism, skin redness, high cancer rate	210900
Cystic fibrosis	Decreased organ function due to regression of secretory glands	219700
Fanconi Anaemia	Developmental delay, heart failure, transition to leukaemia	227650
Galactosaemia	Galactose accumulation in the liver, mental retardation	230400
Phenylketonuria	Excessive accumulation of phenylalanine in blood, mental retardation	261600
Sickle cell anaemia	Haemoglobin abnormalities, vascular damage	141900
Thalassaemia syndrome	Abnormal production of haemoglobin	141800
Xeroderma Pigmentosum	Lack of DNA repair enzymes, UV damage, skin cancer	278700
Tay-Sachs Disease	Ganglioside metabolism abnormality in neurons, early death	272800

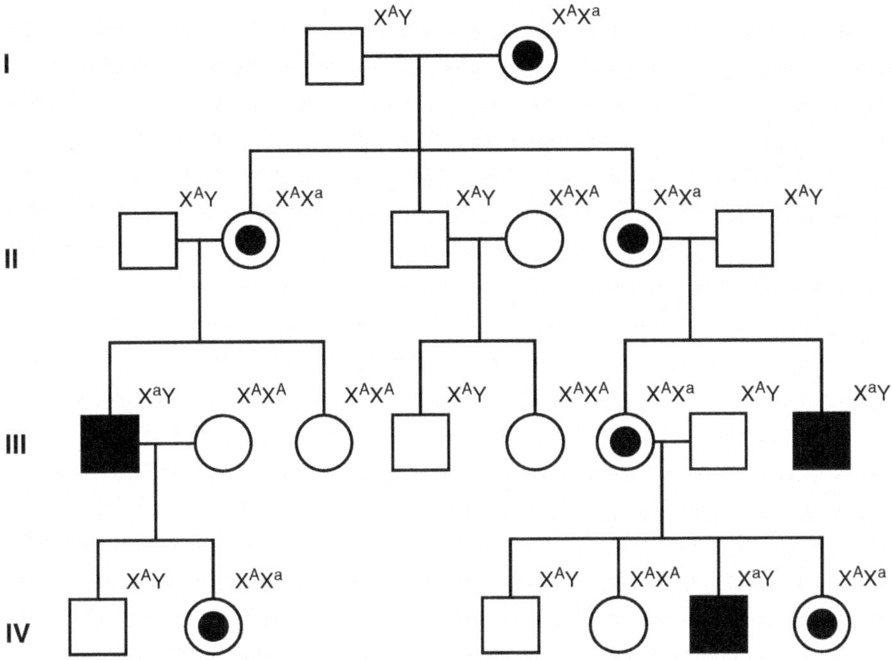

Fig. 6.3 Inheritance pattern of X-linked recessive mendelian disorder

In general, the following genetic rules apply: (1) Almost all affected individuals are male. (2) Heterozygous women usually have a normal phenotype, but because they are carriers, half of the offspring inherit the abnormal gene. (3) Half of the sons of female carriers are affected, and half of the daughters are carriers. (4) The trait is not passed on to the son from the affected man. (5) All daughters of affected men are carriers. (6) The female carrier and the daughter of a normal male are not affected, but half are carriers.

Occasionally, women with heterozygotes for an X-linked mutation may develop some trait, but rarely become more severe in affected men. There are about 600 types of X-linked recessive inheritance, and typical diseases include haemophilia, Duchenne muscular dystrophy and colour blindness (Table 6.3).

6.2.4 X-Linked Dominant Diseases

The X-linked dominant trait is carried on the X chromosome and is very rare. Males are usually more severe, and some X-linked dominant disorders are often fatal in men. Women with only one abnormal allele are affected, but less severe.

In general, the following genetic rules apply: (1) From an affected man, all daughters carry the trait, but not their sons. (2) Half of the offspring of a

Table 6.3 Examples of X-linked recessive disorder

Disorder	Phenotype	OMIM number
Adrenoleukodystrophy	Adrenal insufficiency and mental decline	300100
Green colour blindness	Insensitivity to green light	303800
Red colour blindness	Insensitivity to red light	303900
Fabry disease	Metabolic disorders due to enzyme deficiency	301500
Glucose-6-phosphate dehydrogenase deficiency	Severe anaemia	305900
Haemophilia A	Deficiency of blood coagulation factor VIII	306700
Haemophilia B	Deficiency of blood coagulation factor IX	306900
Ichthyosis	Skin disease	308100
Muscular dystrophy	Duchenne type, extreme muscle fatigue	310200

heterozygous affected woman inherit the trait, regardless of gender. (3) From a homozygous affected woman, the trait is inherited in all offspring.

Because women can be heterozygous or homozygous, more females have the trait than men. If the disorder is fatal in men, the gender difference is even greater. Typical diseases are Rett syndrome and Alport syndrome. In Rett syndrome, all affected individuals are women, and boys die in utero.

6.3 Cases Not Applicable to Mendelian Law of Segregation

Inherited disorders are usually isolated according to the principles of Mendelian Law, but this rule may not apply in some cases. The probable causes are as follows.

6.3.1 Decrease in Penetration

In the case of an autosomal dominant genetic disease, it is a principle that each generation has a diseased individual and that there is no jump between generations. However, when actually conducting a family survey, a certain percentage of jumping phenomena are observed. The penetrance can be expressed by using the genotype Aa as the denominator and the actual sick person as the numerator. Gene expression is suppressed by methylation of DNA. Genotype is predicted to be sick if Aa, but inactivation of the mutant gene by DNA methylation may be unaffected for some reason. This phenomenon is called “imperfect penetration”.

6.3.2 Difference in Expression

In autosomal dominant diseases, it is known that even if the disease is caused by the same causative gene, there is a large difference in the severity and the content of the symptoms, and even in the same family, the expression is different. If the symptoms are very mild compared to severe cases, they may not be noticed as a disease or may not be recognized as the same disease.

6.3.3 Gonad Mosaic

In autosomal dominant genetic diseases, the principle is that the causative gene is transmitted from the first generation to the next generation. However, there may be multiple siblings with disease in one generation, even though none have been sick before the parent generation. It is unlikely that the same mutation would occur coincidentally during meiosis (the sperm or egg production process), so it would be one that occurred during the gonad development stage of the parent (when the parent was in the womb of the grandmother). It is considered that the mutation occurred in the part. However, after this generation, the traits of the disease will be transmitted according to the laws of Mendelian inheritance.

6.3.4 Difference in Age of Onset

There are quite a few hereditary diseases that occur after adulthood. Even with the same illness, there are individual differences between those who become ill in adolescence and those who become ill in old age. Therefore, even if a genotype predicts that they will have a genetic disease, they may be late in onset and end their life without waiting for the disease to develop. On the other hand, it is known that the newer generations become more severe from generation to generation, and the newer generations become sick at younger generations, such as neurodegenerative diseases. This is called "expression promotion phenomenon".

6.3.5 Genetic Heterogeneity

Examination of the causative gene has revealed that a disease that was previously thought to be the same genetic disease is actually caused by a different gene. In genetics, there are diseases that are consistent with an autosomal dominant inheritance pattern, and diseases that have a mixture of autosomal recessive inheritance and X-linked recessive inheritance.

Further Reading

Connor M, Ferguson-Smith M. Essential medical genetics. 5th ed. Oxford: Blackwell Science; 1997.
Gelehrter TD, Collins FS, Ginsburg D. Principles of medical genetics. 2nd ed. Baltimore: Williams and Wilkins; 1998.

Chapter 7
Neuroimaging and Genetics in Brain Maldevelopment

Ritsuko K. Pooh

Abstract Fetal brain malformations diagnosed in early pregnancy are limited to cranial bifidum, spinal bifidum, and holoprosencephaly. Other brain dysmorphic disorders occur after the first trimester because neuronal growth, including proliferation, migration, and post-migrational development, starting from 3 months of gestation. Recent advanced technology with three-dimensional (3D) ultrasound has accelerated prenatal neuroimaging. Trans-fontanelle brain imaging by transabdominal or transvaginal ultrasound has been introduced in routine clinical practice. A combination of 3D ultrasound and the trans-fontanelle procedure has guided us to the systematic neuroimaging. However, congenital brain abnormalities cannot be classified only by morphological imaging diagnosis, but are now being categorized based on causal genetic factors. In this chapter, the author describes the imaging diagnoses and genetic causes and of fetal cerebral disorders.

Keywords Fetus · Brain · Abnormality · Neurulation · Prosencephalic Malformations of cortical development · Proliferation · Migration · Brain damage

7.1 Introduction

The embryonic premature central nervous system (CNS) structure develops rapidly into the mature structure during the fetal period. Various developmental disorders and unexpected events in this rapid change of development result in multiple phenotypes of fetal CNS abnormalities. For understanding fetal CNS diseases, basic knowledge of relevant genes and the development of the central nervous system is essential. In each stage of CNS growth (Fig. 7.1), significant disorders occur

R. K. Pooh (✉)
Fetal Brain Center, CRIFM Clinical Research Institute of Fetal Medicine PMC, Osaka, Japan

H. Masuzaki (ed.), *Fetal Morph Functional Diagnosis*, Comprehensive Gynecology and Obstetrics, https://doi.org/10.1007/978-981-15-8171-7_7

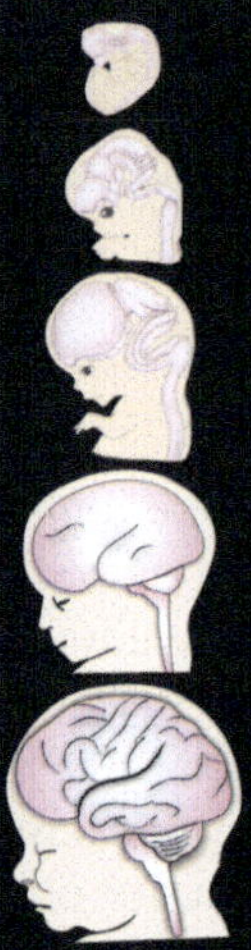

Developmental stage	Representative Cerebral Disorders
Neurulation (3-4 weeks' gestation)	Cranial and spinal dysraphism (Craniorachischisis totalis, Anencephaly, Myelomeningocele, Myeloschisis)
Procencephalic development (2-3 months' gestation)	Holoprosencephaly, Agenesis of the corpus callosum, Agenesis of the septum pellucidum,
Neuronal proliferation (3-4 months' gestation)	Micrencephaly, Macrencephaly
Neuronal migration (3-5 months' gestation)	Lissencephaly, Pachygyria, Focal cortical dysplasia, Heterotopias (periventricular nodular heterotopia and band heterotopias), Polymicrogyria, Schizencephaly,
Organization (5 months' gestation – years postnatal)	Idiopathic mental retardation, Learning disability, Link to epilepsy and autism
Myelination (Birth – years postnatal)	Range of disorders including adrenoleukodystrophy

Fig. 7.1 The developmental stage and representative cerebral disorders during the fetal period

according to development. The first stage is neurulation, followed by prosencephalic development. In neuronal proliferation stage, more than twice the surviving neurons of 100 billions of neurons in the adult brain were produced in the first and early second trimesters. The peak time of neuronal proliferation is 3–4 months of gestation, and the site producing neurons is mainly ventricular and subventricular zones. After that, neurons are differentiated and migrating to their final position. After neuronal migration, organization and myelination occur. Meanwhile, programmed cell death (apoptosis) arises from the middle of gestation for adjusting the number of neural cells to the target size. Cortical maldevelopment, so-called malformations of cortical development (MCDs), is a representative of developmental delay, mental retardation, severe epilepsy, and one of the hot topics in the field of pediatric neurology. Many gene mutations have been identified as being responsible for cortical maldevelopment during the developing processes of neuronal proliferation, migration, and post-migration. Therefore the classification of neuronal disorders has been modified according to etiology and focal gene mutation. Unexpected events such as hemodynamic disorder can be the causal factors for intrauterine brain disorders. They make brain structural phenotypes disorders more complicated.

Most of the congenital abnormalities have been diagnosed in the first trimester by recent advanced prenatal ultrasound [1–3]. However, brain malformations diagnosed in early pregnancy are limited to cranial bifidum, spinal bifidum, and holoprosencephaly. Other brain dysmorphic disorders occur after the first trimester because neuronal growth, including proliferation, migration, and post-migrational development, starting from 3 months of gestation. Recent advanced technology with three-dimensional (3D) ultrasound has accelerated prenatal neuroimaging.

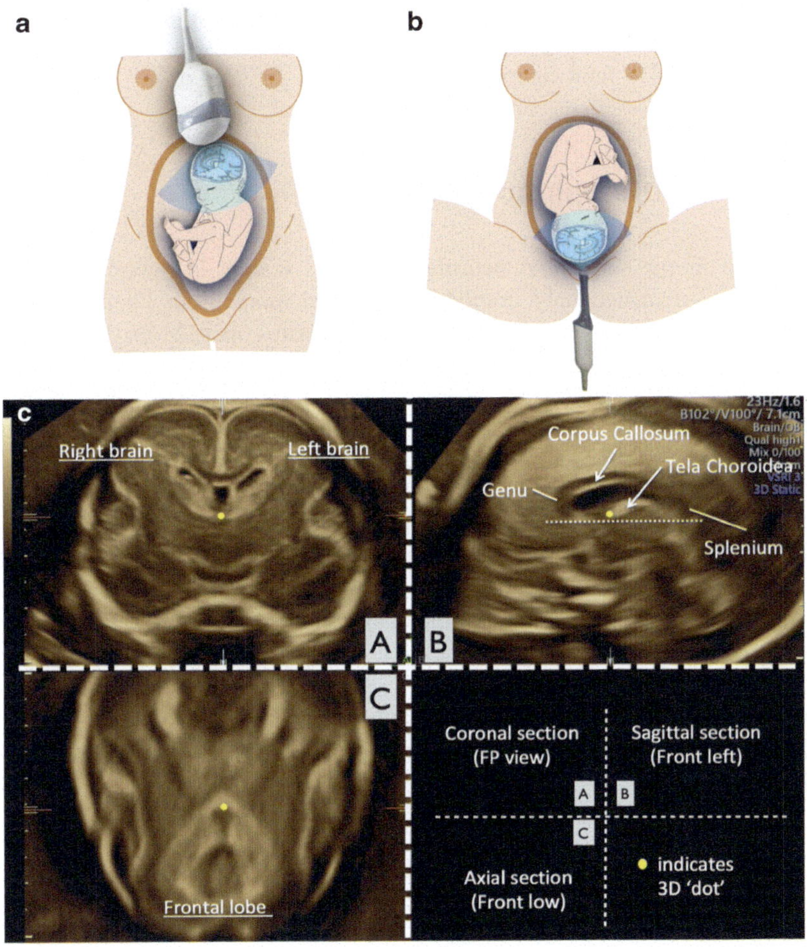

Fig. 7.2 Transabdominal and transvaginal neurosonography and 3D orthogonal brain image. (**a**) Transabdominal neurosonography for breech presented fetus, utilizing the anterior fontanelle as an ultrasound window. (**b**) Transvaginal neurosonography. (**c**) 3D orthogonal brain image for obtaining cerebral orientation. After auto-scanning while observing the coronal section of the fetal brain with 3D ultrasound, three orthogonal sections are displayed immediately after acquisition. On the vertical three-sectional image, the upper left is shown as Plane A, the top right is Plane B, and the lower left is Plane C. The coronal, sagittal, and axial cutting sections of the brain are depicted in these A, B, and C cross-sections respectively. Manual rotation in the x, y, and z directions on the image is performed. In the sagittal section in Plane B, always turn the frontal lobe of the brain toward the left of the image. Secondly, in the axial section of Plane C, the frontal lobe is directed toward the lower side of the image. After these manipulations, in plane A's coronal section, the right side of the screen is the left fetal brain, and the left side of the screen is the right fetal brain

Trans-fontanelle brain imaging by transabdominal or transvaginal ultrasound (Fig. 7.2) has been introduced in routine clinical practice. A combination of 3D ultrasound and the trans-fontanelle procedure has guided us to the systematic neuroimaging. However, congenital brain abnormalities cannot be classified only by morphological imaging diagnosis, but are now being categorized based on causal genetic factors. In this chapter, the author describes the imaging diagnoses and genetic causes and of fetal cerebral disorders.

7.2 Cranial Dysraphism (Neurulation Disorder)

Disturbance in the sequential neurulation events results in neural tube defects (NTDs), such as anencephaly, cranial bifidum, and spina bifida. Phenotypes varies depending on the region of the neural tube that remains open. More than 200 genes are known to cause NTDs in mice. The occurrence pattern in humans has a multifactorial polygenic or oligogenic etiology [4, 5]. In anencephaly, the complete or incomplete absence of the brain and calvaria is seen. Craniorachischisis is characterized by anencephaly accompanied by a contiguous bony defect of the spine and exposure of neural tissue. Early pathogenesis of encephalocele is not well understood. Encephalocele has been often classified as one of "neural tube defects." However, it is controversial whether encephalocele is NTD or a post-neurulation defect. From the mice model experiment, Rolo et al. showed that the encephalocele does not result from failure of neural tube closure, but rather from a later disruption of the surface ectoderm covering the already closed neural tube, allowing the brain to herniate [6]. Although the exact pathogenesis of encephalocele remains unknown, multifactorial inheritance, single gene mutation, specific teratogens (valproic acid), maternal diabetes, and environmental factors can be considerable etiology. Due to normal maternal serum alpha-fetoprotein levels in cases with skin-covered encephalocele, neurosonography is a powerful tool for detection during pregnancy.

7.3 Holoprosencephaly (Prosencephalic Disorder)

Holoprosencephaly is the representative of prosencephalic disorders. The incidence of holoprosencephaly is 1 out of 15,000–20,000 live births. However, the initial incidence may be more than 60-fold higher in aborted human embryos [7, 8]. Holoprosencephalies are mainly classified into three varieties; alobar, semilobar, and lobar types. Seventy-five percent of holoprosencephaly has normal karyotype, but trisomy 13, 18, and some other chromosomal aberrations have been associated with holoprosencephaly. Mainly, trisomy 13 is the most common. *Sonic Hedgehog (SHH)* on 7q36, *ZIC2* on 13q32, *SIX3* on 2p21, and *TGIF* on 18p11.3 were identified as responsible genes for holoprosencephaly [9–12], and other relevant genes were reported. For patients with normal karyotype results, approximately 22% have identified point mutations of the above four genes or pathogenic copy number variation (microdeletion), including those four genes [10]. Failure of the prosencephalon and diencephalon during the early first trimester (5–6 weeks) results in holoprosencephaly. Facial abnormalities such as cyclopia, ethmocephaly, cebocephaly, flat nose, cleft lip, and palate are invariably associated with holoprosencephaly [13].

7.4 Agenesis of the Corpus Callosum

The corpus callosum (CC) is the most extensive fiber-tract in the brain, connecting the bilateral cerebral hemispheres, and facilitating the integration of motor and sensory information as well as influencing higher cognition [14]. *FGF8* is an essential gene for early forebrain patterning, development of commissural plate, and forebrain commissures. *EMX1, NFIA, ZIC2,* and *SIX3* genes are responsible for subsequent development of the corpus callosum, the hippocampal and anterior commissure. By 20 post-conception weeks (18 gestational weeks), the final shape of the CC is complete, although axonal growth continues even after birth. Early cerebral development is associated with cortical development by a combination of morphogenetic gradients that together with developing thalamocortical circuits [15, 16].

Agenesis of the corpus callosum (ACC) is a common brain malformation that occurs either isolated or associated with congenital syndromes. ACC includes complete ACC (total absence of CC, Fig. 7.3), partial ACC, and hypoplastic CC (thin CC but has a normal anterior to a posterior extent) [14]. The causes of ACC are associated with an abnormality in each step of neuronal and glial proliferation, midline patterning, callosal neuron migration and specification, axon guidance, and post-guidance [14]. Various copy number variations (CNV) are related to ACC, 1q42-q44 deletion [17, 18], 4p16.3 deletion (Wolf-Hirschhorn syndrome) [19], 8p rearrangements [20–22], 17p13,3 deletion (Miller-Dieker lissencephaly syndrome) [23, 24], and others.

Mutations in the *ARX* gene [25–28] are responsible for X-linked lissencephaly with an absent corpus callosum and ambiguous genitalia (XLAG). *L1CAM* mutations cause L1 syndrome [29], CRASH (Corpus Callosum Hypoplasia, Retardation, Adducted Thumbs, Spastic Paraparesis, and Hydrocephalus) syndrome [30], and MASA (Mental retardation, aphasia, shuffling gait, adducted thumbs) syndrome [29]. As an *L1CAM* (L1 cell adhesion molecule) gene is located on Xq28, the mostly male baby is affected. L1 gene is essential for the development of CNS, in adhesion among neurons. Individuals with L1 syndrome have various disorders of severe mental retardation, lower limb spasticity, and paraplegia.

Causative genes have not been identified in some of the syndromes with ACC. Aicardi syndrome [31], characterized by agenesis of the corpus callosum, infantile spasms, and chorioretinal lacunae (including microphthalmia, coloboma), is X-linked dominant and requires a pair of the X chromosome. Therefore, the affected fetuses are mostly females, but males with Kleinfelter syndrome (XXY) can be affected. An age-adjusted prevalence is 0.63 per 100,000 females [32]. Occasionally, intrahemispheric cysts (Fig. 7.3) or pericallosal lipoma is associated with ACC.

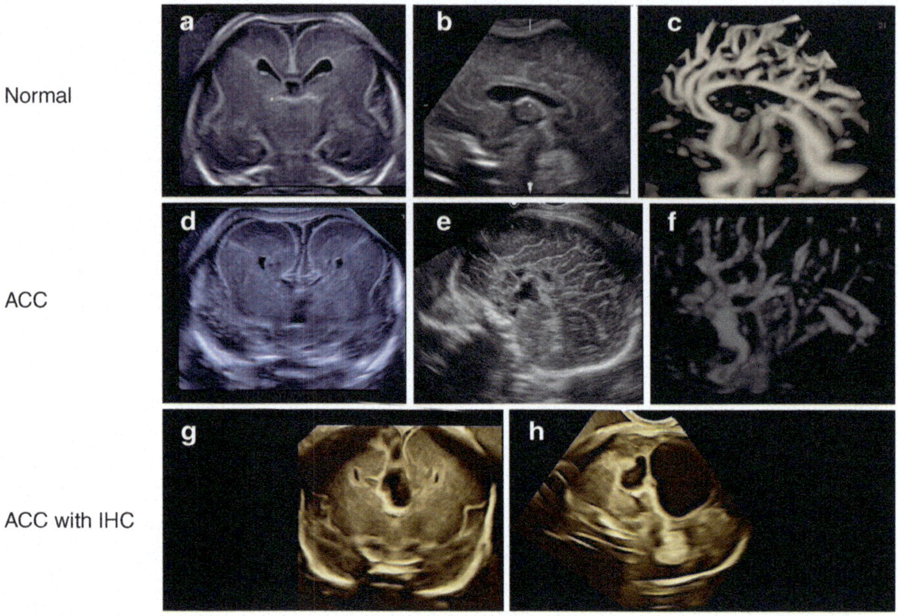

Fig. 7.3 Agenesis of the corpus callosum. (**a**), (**b**), and (**c**) are 20-week-coronal brain, 28-week-sagittal brain, and 29-week-3D angiography (sagittal view). The pericallosal artery is running along with the corpus callosum. (**d**) shows a 20-week-coronal image of ACC. (**e**) shows a 28-week-sagittal image of ACC. Absent of CC is apparent, and sulci form radially. (**f**) demonstrates 3D angiography in the ACC case. The pericallosal artery is not demonstrated, and the branches are running radially. (**g**) and (**h**) demonstrate intracranial cysts (IHC), in the coronal and sagittal section, in the case of ACC

7.5 Malformations of Cortical Development (Disorders of Proliferation, Migration, and Post-migration)

The cerebral cortical development is a complex dynamic process in the three stages [33]. In the first stage, stem cells proliferate in number and differentiate into neurons or glial cells in the ventricular and subventricular zones. The second stage is the migration phase. The neurons are tangentially migrating toward the brain surface with inside-out mode. This third stage is the organization in the six layers of the cortex [34].

After birth, abnormal cortical development is gradually noticed with signs of developmental disabilities and epilepsy and malformations of cortical development (MCD) has been investigated with molecular genetics and MR imaging [35]. MCD is classified into three groups by the three developmental steps of proliferation, migration, and post-migration. More than 100 genes were clarified, being responsible for one or more types of MCD.

a) *Proliferation disorders (MCD group I)*

Microcephaly is one of the neuronal proliferation disorders. Microcephaly is a developmental disorder secondary to abnormal development or degeneration of normal growth and subsequent loss of neuronal cells [36]. Microcephaly vera (true microcephaly or primary microcephaly) results in postnatal intellectual disability. Infants with microcephaly vera had been thought to have no significant brain malformations despite small cerebri, but at present, it is considered that the phenotypes are not always uniform. There is a continuum between patients that have microcephaly with regular gyral/sulcal pattern, and microcephaly complicated with other malformation [37–39]. Other types of microcephalies are consistently associated with abnormal brain structures, such as microlissencephaly.

The causes of microcephaly include infections by rubella virus, cytomegalovirus (CMV), ZIKA virus and toxoplasmosis, and genetic mutations. The responsible gene mutations for microcephalies were reported, such as Microcephalin (*MCPH1* [38, 40, 41]), *ASPM* [42], *CDK5RAP2* [43], *CENPJ* [35, 43, 44], *STIL* [39, 44], *WDR62* [37, 39, 45, 46], and *CEP152* [47] and others. It is often quite hard to observe intracranial structure in cases with microcephaly because cranial fontanelles and sutures are very narrow due to microcephaly. Therefore ultrasound neuroimaging via sutures and fontanelles as ultrasound windows is quite tricky. Microcephaly is one of the indications for MR imaging.

b) *Neuronal Migration Disorders (MCD group II)*

As a consequence of migration, the brain is matured with gyration/sulcation from the late 7 months' gestation. The fastest increase in the number of major gyri occurs between 26 and 28 weeks of gestation. This further gyral elaboration continues during the third trimester and shortly after birth. Neuronal migration is controlled by a complex series of chemical guidance and signals. When these signals are absent or incorrect, neurons cannot end up where they should belong to. This can result in structurally abnormal or missing areas in any site of intracranial structure, such as the cerebral hemispheres, cerebellum, brainstem, or hippocampus and types of neuronal migration disorders includes lissencephaly, agyria, pachygyria, microgyria, micropolygyria, neuronal heterotopias (including band heterotopia and periventricular nodular heterotopia), and schizencephaly. Neuronal migration disorders, the aberration of gyral development, usually cause seizures and neurological function disturbances from early days after birth. Migration disorder appears conspicuously on the surface of cerebral hemispheres in the late pregnancy. Therefore it does not seem to be possible to detect migration disorder before gyration. Toi and his colleagues [48] reported regular gyri/sulci pattern during fetal life, depicted by transabdominal ultrasound imaging. During the latter half of the second trimester, the cortical structure macroscopically develops, and the most distinct morphological difference appears to be the different structure of Sylvian fissure [49–51]. Thus, the Sylvian fissure is one of the landmarks indicating cortical development by regular migration. Changing the appearance of Sylvian fissure according to cerebral development is remarkable, and Poon et al. [52] proposed the Sylvian fissure angle and described the significant decrease of the angle with advancing gestational age. Furthermore, Pooh et al. [53] demonstrated 22 cases with MCDs between 18 and 30 weeks of gestation and show the delayed development of the Sylvian fissure angle in 22 cases with migration disorder.

Lissencephaly is characterized as a malformation of cortical development associated with abnormal neuronal cell migration and abnormal cerebral gyral/sulcal formation. Lissencephaly spectrum includes agyria (smooth brain), pachygyria, and subcortical band heterotopia. Lissencephaly was conventionally divided into two types; type I with a smooth surface of the brain and type II with cobblestone appearance. After that, many responsible genes were clarified, and classification has been changed by etiology, as below.

Classic lissencephaly

- *LIS1* (17p13.3): lissencephaly due to *PAFAH1B1* gene mutation, which subdivides into Miller-Dieker syndrome
- *DCX*: lissencephaly due to doublecortin mutation
- Isolated lissencephaly, without other known genetic defects

Cobblestone lissencephaly

- *POMGnT1* [54, 55]: Muscle-eye-brain disease (MEB), Walker-Warburg syndrome
- *Fukutin* [56–59]: Fukuyama syndrome

X-linked lissencephaly

- *ARX* gene (Xq22.13) [60–63] mutation

Lissencephaly with cerebellar hypoplasia

- *Reelin* gene (7q22.1) [64–66]: Norman-Roberts syndrome

Microlissencephaly [35, 67–72]

- Lissencephaly + microcephaly

However, owing to recent rapid progress in molecular genetics, a conventional classification system has been insufficient to distinguish various patterns of lissencephaly, and a new imaging-based classification system was proposed in 2017 for prediction of most likely causative gene mutation [73].

Several reports on the prenatal diagnosis of lissencephaly have been published [48, 51, 74–78]. Without a previous history of an affected child, it is quite hard to diagnose reliably as lissencephaly until 26–28 weeks of gestation. However, Fig. 7.4b shows the microlissencephaly in midgestation. In this case, migration disorder was strongly suspected from 19 weeks of gestation.

c) *Post-migrational disorders (MCD group III)*

Polymicrogyria is the representative MCD relevant to the post-migrational disorder. 1p36.3 mutation, 22q11.2 mutation, and *mTOR* genes are associated with polymicrogyria. Etiology may be from prenatal ischemic, teratogenic or infectious brain

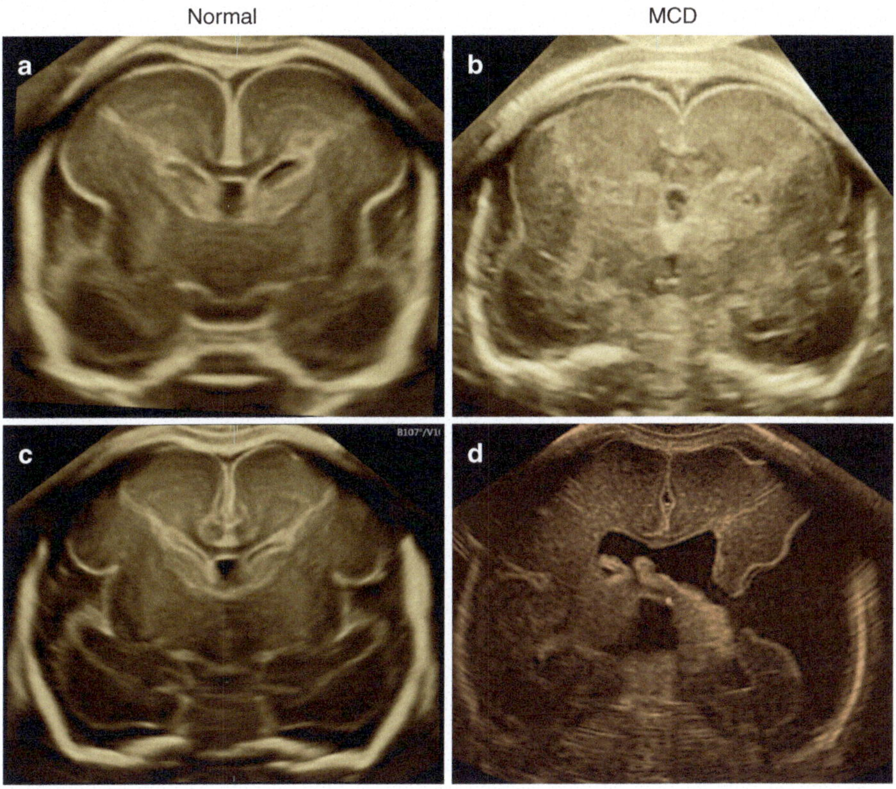

Fig. 7.4 MCD in midgestation. (**a**) and (**c**) are standard coronal brain images at 23 and 27 weeks of gestation, respectively. (**b**) shows microlissencephaly at 23 weeks of gestation. Note premature Sylvian fissures. (**d**) shows Schizencephaly at 27 weeks of gestation. Split-brain is seen, lined by pia-ependyma, with communication between the subarachnoid space laterally and the lateral ventricle

injury. Perisylvian bilateral polymicrogyria [79, 80] is commonly associated with schizencephaly.

Schizencephaly is a disorder characterized by congenital cerebral clefts, which is lined by pial-ependyma, with communication between the subarachnoid space laterally and the ventricular system medially. Unilateral schizencephaly occurs in 63% and bilateral in 37%. Possible cause is a disruption of vascular development during cerebral development, genetic origins including *WDR62* gene mutation [45, 81], which causes microcephaly as well as schizencephaly in some cases [45, 46], indicating relations between processes underlying proliferation and the genesis of schizencephaly, and *COL4A1* gene mutation associated with schizencephaly as well as other CNS abnormalities [82–84]. Figure 7.4d shows prenatal neuroimaging in the case of schizencephaly at midgestation.

7.6 Ventriculomegaly

Fetal ventriculomegaly is defined when an atrial width diameter is 10 mm or higher by prenatal neurosonography. Fetal ventriculomegaly is categorized in mild (10–12 mm), moderate (13–15 mm), or severe (>15 mm) ventriculomegaly. The incidence of mild to moderate ventriculomegaly is approximately 1%. Mild ventriculomegaly is likely a normal variant when other intracranial morphologies, extra-CNS structures, and genetic testing are all normal [85].

"Ventriculomegaly" and "hydrocephalus" are the terms that indicate the pathological condition with lateral ventricular dilation, not the pathology per se. Hydrocephalus is mostly associated with increased intracranial pressure by cerebrospinal fluid (CSF) flow pathway occlusion or stenosis, and neurosonography reveals the enlarged ventricles with dangling choroid plexus. In contrast, normal-pressure hydrocephalus (NPH) is associated with enlarged ventricles with no increase of intracranial pressure, with the normal appearance of choroid plexus. Hydrocephalus due to congenital cerebral aqueduct stenosis is common but secondary ventriculomegaly can arise, in association with vascular disease, cortical maldevelopment, intracranial tumor, or cysts, intracerebral/intraventricular hemorrhage, encephalopathy, meningitis, Chiari malformation due to myelomeningocele, and other CNS deformities.

By recent advances in sequencing technologies to date, four genes have been known to cause Mendelian diseases in which congenital hydrocephalus is the primary clinical feature [86]; *L1CAM, AP1S2* (X-linked) and *CCDC88C* [87], *MPDZ* [88] (autosomal recessive). Furthermore, more than 100 genes have been identified as the causal factors of genetic disorders with hydrocephalus or ventriculomegaly [89].

L1CAM [30, 90–92] located at Xq28 mediates cell to cell adhesion, the guidance of neurite outgrowth, myelination, bundling and pathfinding, long-term potentiation, neuronal cell survival and migration, and synaptogenesis [93]. *L1CAM* mutations result in invariable neurological phenotypes, such as hydrocephalus, and agenesis or hypoplasia of the corpus callosum, and adducted thumbs (Fig. 7.5). Due to X-linked recessive inheritance, the male fetus from carrier mother has a 50% chance to be affected.

CSF flow pathway is also affected by abnormal beating or asynchronism of the ependymal cilia lining the ventricular system. Therefore, ciliopathies such as Bardet-Biedl syndrome (*CEP290* [94]), Meckel syndromes (*MKS1, TMEM67* [95–97]), and Joubert syndromes (*TMEM216* [98], *CC2D2A* [99]) are associated with ventriculomegaly.

A group of muscular dystrophies are associated with the aberrant glycosylation of α-dystroglycan and collectively termed dystroglycanopathies [89, 100]. Dystroglycanopathies are often associated with CNS and eye pathology. In cases of dystroglycanopathy, neuronal cell migration disorder results in cortical maldevelopment and subsequent ventriculomegaly. Representative dystroglycanopathies are muscle–eye–brain disease (*POMGnT1*), Walker-Warburg syndrome (*POMT1, PONT2*, and *B3GALNT2*), and Fukuyama congenital muscular dystrophy (*FKTN*).

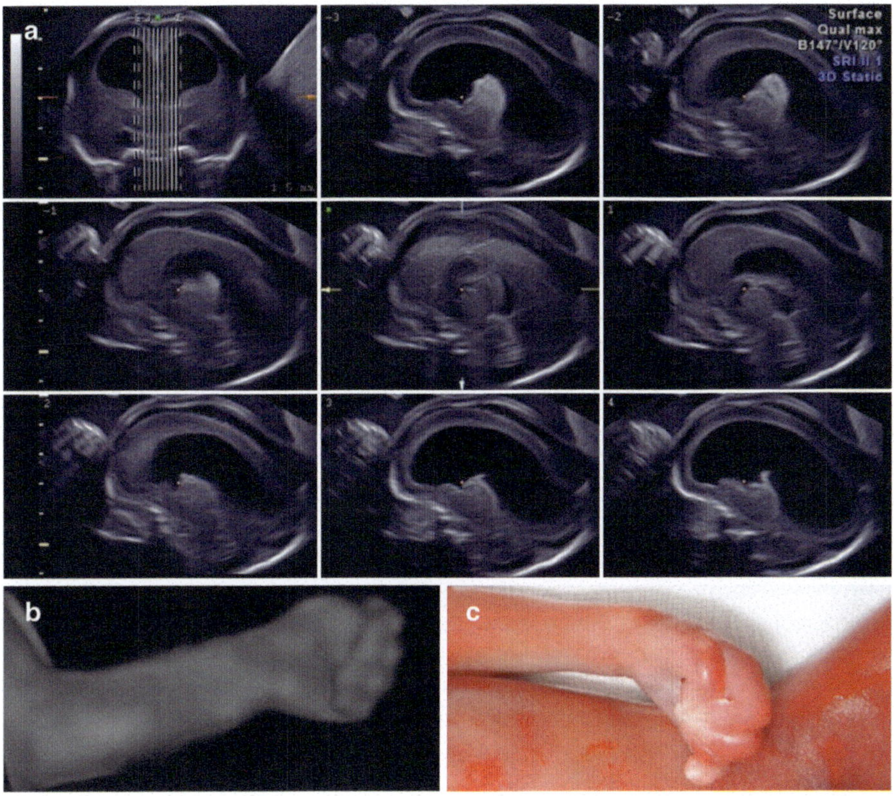

Fig. 7.5 X-linked hydrocephalus by *L1CAM* gene mutation at 20 weeks of gestation. (**a**) 3D tomographic images in the sagittal section. (**b**) Adducted thumb by three ultrasound. (**c**) The adducted thumb after the termination of pregnancy at 21 weeks

PI3K-AKT-mTOR pathway genes have also been identified in several other overgrowth syndromes. The megalencephaly-polymicrogyria-polydactyly-hydrocephalus (MPPH) syndrome and megalencephaly-capillary malformation-polymicrogyria (MCAP) syndromes are a spectrum of megalencephaly-associated syndromes [89, 101] characterized by megalencephaly, progressive ventriculomegaly, Chiari malformation, and polymicrogyria. The morphological mechanism for ventriculomegaly in megalencephaly-associated syndromes has been explained that megalencephaly induces polymicrogyria and cerebellar overgrowth, leading to oppression of the posterior fossa and cerebellar tonsillar herniation, which obstructs CSF flow.

Mutations of growth factors such as *FGFR3* (Thanatophoric dysplasia) can lead to ventriculomegaly with enlarged and hyperconvoluted temporal lobe [102].

There are various shapes of the enlarged ventricle, according to etiology. "Isolated" ventriculomegaly is often described when there are no other structural abnormalities. However, many cases that are antenatally diagnosed as "isolated"

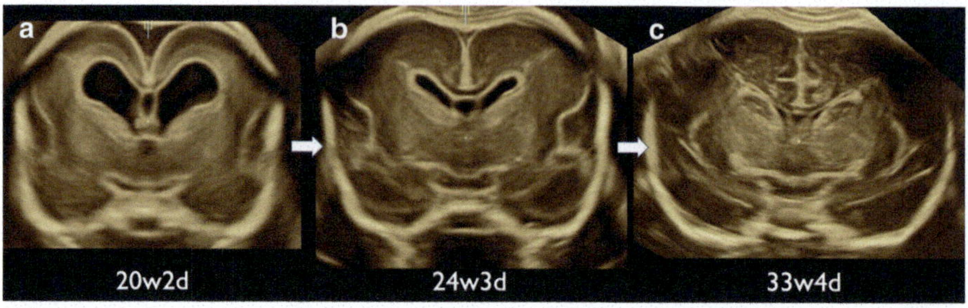

Fig. 7.6 Spontaneous resolution of ventriculomegaly. At 20 weeks of gestation (**a**), conspicuous ventriculomegaly was found, and atrial width was 15 mm at that time. However, longitudinal observation throughout gestation shows spontaneous resolution of ventriculomegaly week by week, as shown in (**b**) and (**c**). The baby was born at term with an Apgar score of 10, and no neurological deficit was recorded up to 1 year after birth

have been ultimately found to have other CNS abnormalities or responsible gene mutations after birth. Detailed observation of intracerebral and extra-CNS morphology may lead to the identification of causes and prognostic evaluation far more than AW measurement. For investigating causal factors, chromosomal microarray, exome sequencing, or genome sequencing, as well as viral infection analysis, may be recommendable. Furthermore, longitudinal study during the fetal period by neurosonography is quite important because some of the isolated cases have spontaneous resolution during pregnancy, as shown in Fig. 7.6.

7.7 In Utero Brain Injury and Damage

In the case with neonatal cerebral palsy and encephalopathy, "When did the causal event occur, antepartum, intrapartum or postpartum?" is the controversial question because it includes the medico-socio-legal-ethical problems. Brain insults may be related to prenatal events such as cerebral hemorrhage, encephalopathy, and migration disorder, as shown in Fig. 7.7. The timing of insult cannot always be determined. Occasionally the causative event for encephalopathy may be measured, for example, co-twin demise or intervention for twin-to-twin transfusion syndrome in cases of monochorionic twins. It is a hard task, however, to grasp prenatal evidence of brain injury, which predict cerebral palsy after birth. Neuroimaging by ultrasound or MRI is the most reliable modality for detecting silent encephalopathy. In many cases with cerebral palsy with acquired brain insults, especially, term-delivered infants with re-assuring fetal heart rate monitoring and good Apgar score at delivery are not suspected of having a brain injury and often overlooked for months or years.

Intracranial hemorrhage is a rare condition during pregnancy and has also been called a fetal stroke after 2004 [103–106]. The exact incidence is hard to confirm because it may be underdiagnosed, and various descriptions have been used in

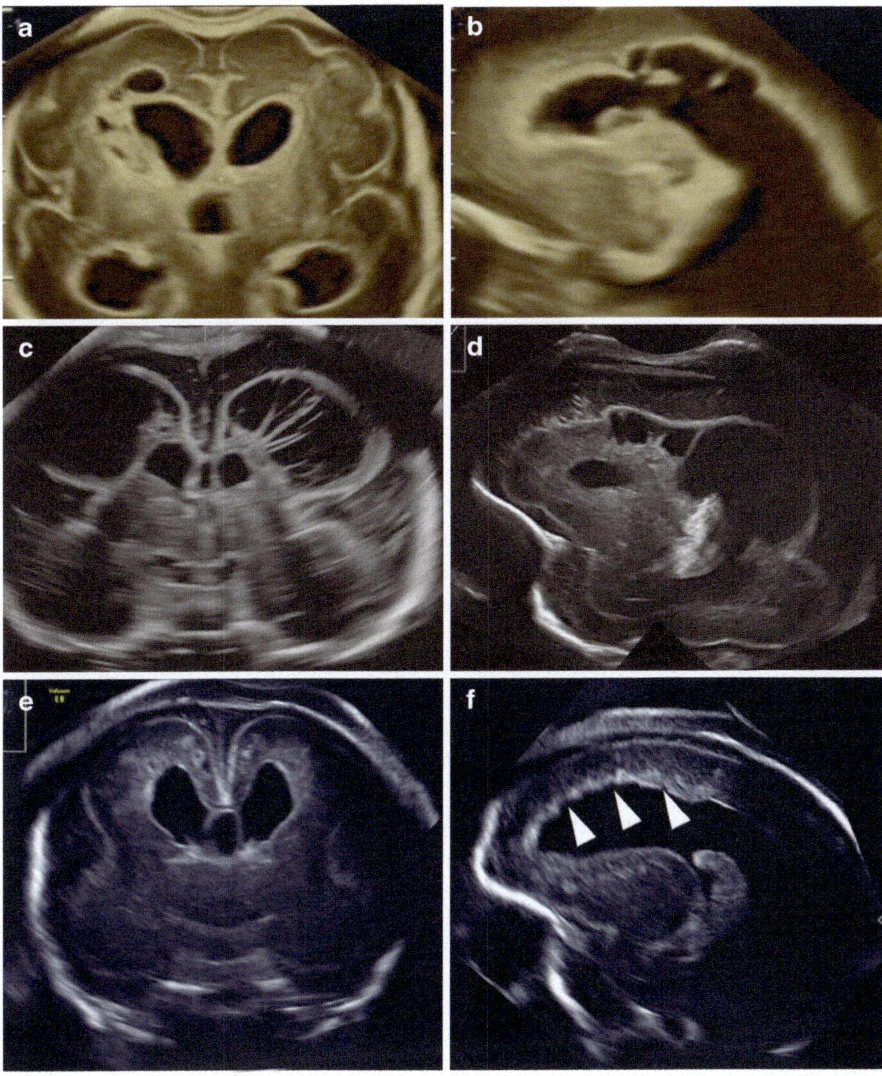

Fig. 7.7 Brain damage with various causes, in coronal (left) and parasagittal (right) images. (**a**), (**b**) Porencephalic change with intraventricular hemorrhage (secondary IVH) after cerebral hemorrhage at 32 weeks of gestation. Porencephalic cystic change associated with ventriculomegaly is seen in the right cerebrum. Hyperechogenesity of the inside ventricular wall indicates intraventricular hemorrhage. (**c**), (**d**) Destructive encephalopathy after intervention for twin-to-twin transfusion syndrome at 28 weeks of gestation. Note the thin cerebral parenchyma due to destructive encephalopathy. Note most of the cerebral parenchyma disappear, and remnant cerebral tissue is demonstrated as thin membranes. (**e**), (**f**) Multiple cerebral hemorrhages are seen in (**e**). In the parasagittal section (**f**), periventricular heterotopia is seen (arrowheads). (**g**), (**h**) Massive intracranial hemorrhage with porencephalic change due to *COL4A1* gene mutation. (**g**) shows the anterior coronal image at 20 weeks of gestation. Bilateral massive intracranial hemorrhage is seen with unilateral conspicuous porencephalic change. (**h**) shows the sagittal section

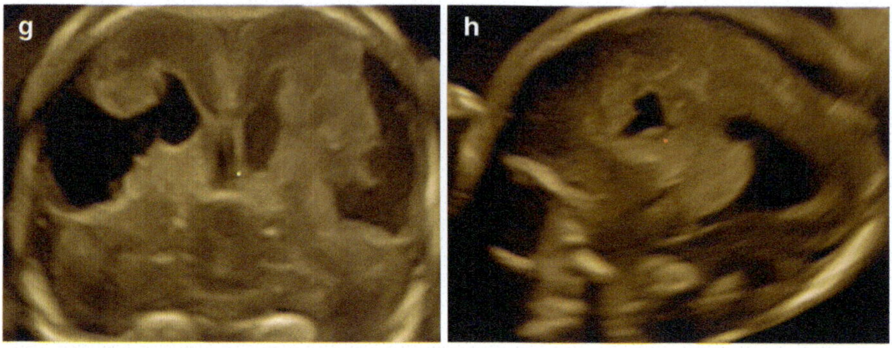

Fig. 7.7 (continued)

published reports, such as fetal stroke, fetal cerebrovascular disorder, or perinatal brain injury [107]. One report defined fetal stroke as an event between the 14th week of gestation and labor onset and cited an incidence of about 17–35 of 100,000 live births [103]. Another report described an incidence of 0.5–1.0/1000 pregnancies [108]. It was reported in 1985 that autopsy in a series of stillborn babies revealed 6% had fetal intracranial hemorrhage [109].

Various etiologies of fetal intracranial hemorrhage are considered, including idiopathic, alterations of maternal and fetal blood pressure, fetomaternal hemorrhage, placental abnormalities, umbilical abnormalities, in utero infection, gene mutations, trauma, alloimmune and idiopathic thrombocytopenia, von Willebrand's disease, specific medications (warfarin) or illicit drug (cocaine) abuse, seizure, fetal conditions including congenital factor X and factor-V deficiencies, intracranial tumor, twin to twin transfusion, the demise of a monochorionic co-twin, and vascular diseases. Recent reports have described *COL4A1* and *COL42A* gene mutations strongly related to perinatal cerebral hemorrhage and porencephaly [110–116]. Prenatal sonogram demonstrated variable echogenicity of the ventricular wall, echogenicity of the parenchyma, avascular intracranial mass, porencephalic cysts, hyperechoic acute clot adherent to bulky/nodular choroid plexus, hyperechoic clot outlining cerebral cortex, hyperechoic nodular ependyma, and increased periventricular white matter echogenicity in cases with intracranial hemorrhage. Ventriculomegaly is often associated with intracranial hemorrhage.

Intraventricular hemorrhage (IVH), arising from intraventricular events such as vascular malformation or tumor involving the choroid plexus, is defined as primary IVH. Primary IVH is approximately 30%, and the rest of 70% is secondary IVH. The cause of secondary IVH is mostly intraparenchymal bleeding, which is expanding into the ventricular system. The grading for fetal IVH is the same as that used for preterm infants. The grading system most commonly used for IVH in the infant was first reported by Papile et al. [117]. Grade I is isolated to the periventricular (subependymal) germinal matrix, Grade II implies IVH (10–50%) without ventricular dilatation, Grade III is IVH (>50% or with ventriculomegaly), and Grade IV is with parenchymal hemorrhage or periventricular hemorrhagic infarction [118]. Grading is helpful for discussions regarding prognosis.

7.8 Future Perspective

Owing to recent advances in ultrasound technology, a systematic approach to the fetal brain has been possible, as shown in this article. The rapid development of molecular genetics has revealed that more than a hundred genetic mutations are associated with congenital brain abnormalities. Many congenital brain disorders are deeply and complicatedly associated with developmental steps, genetic factors, and environmental factors, and many kinds of insults and events during fetal life. Previously, prenatal counseling was performed by a morphology-based diagnosis. However, at present, it is not possible to diagnose by morphology alone, and finding the cause by chromosomal microarray, exome/genome sequencing, is becoming essential for prenatal genetic counseling in cases with fetal brain abnormalities, and multidisciplinary team approach should be required [119]. A combination of molecular genetics and detailed neurosonography has established "neurosonogenetics," a new field in multidisciplinary perinatal neurology, for prompt prenatal/postnatal management and care and prevention and treatment in the future [120, 121].

References

1. Pooh RK, Kurjak A. 3D/4D sonography moved prenatal diagnosis of fetal anomalies from the second to the first trimester of pregnancy. J Matern Fetal Neonatal Med. 2012;25(5):433–55. https://doi.org/10.15386/cjmed-437.
2. Pooh RK, Shiota K, Kurjak A. Imaging of the human embryo with magnetic resonance imaging microscopy and high-resolution transvaginal 3-dimensional sonography: human embryology in the 21st century. Am J Obstet Gynecol. 2011;204(1) https://doi.org/10.1016/j.ajog.2010.07.028.
3. Pooh RK. Sonoembryology by 3D HDlive silhouette ultrasound – What is added by the "see-through fashion"? J Perinat Med. 2016;44(2) https://doi.org/10.1515/jpm-2016-0008.
4. Copp AJ, Greene NDE. Genetics and development of neural tube defects. J Pathol. 2010; https://doi.org/10.1002/path.2643.
5. Greene NDE, Copp AJ. Development of the vertebrate central nervous system: formation of the neural tube. Prenat Diagn. 2009; https://doi.org/10.1002/pd.2206.
6. Rolo A, Galea GL, Savery D, Greene NDE, Andrew J. Novel mouse model of encephalocele: post-neurulation origin and relationship to open neural tube defects. DMM Dis Model Mech. :2019. https://doi.org/10.1242/dmm.040683.
7. Cohen MM. Perspectives on holoprosencephaly: Part I. Epidemiology, genetics, and syndromology. Teratology. 1989; https://doi.org/10.1002/tera.1420400304.
8. Matsunaga E, Shiota K. Holoprosencephaly in human embryos: epidemiologic studies of 150 cases. Teratology. 1977; https://doi.org/10.1002/tera.1420160304.

9. Cohen MM. Holoprosencephaly: clinical, anatomic, and molecular dimensions. Birth Defects Res Part A – Clin Mol Teratol. 2006; https://doi.org/10.1002/bdra.20295.
10. Roessler E, Muenke M. The molecular genetics of holoprosencephaly. Am J Med Genet Part C Semin Med Genet. 2010; https://doi.org/10.1002/ajmg.c.30236.
11. Robbins DJ, Nybakken KE, Kobayashi R, Sisson JC, Bishop JM, Thérond PP. Hedgehog elicits signal transduction by means of a large complex containing the kinesin-related protein costal2. Cell. 1997; https://doi.org/10.1016/S0092-8674(00)80331-1.
12. Robbins DJ, Fei DL, Riobo NA. The hedgehog signal transduction network. Sci Signal. 2012; https://doi.org/10.1126/scisignal.2002906.
13. Blaas HGK. Holoprosencephaly. In: Obstetric imaging: fetal diagnosis and care. 2nd ed; 2017. https://doi.org/10.1016/B978-0-323-44548-1.00039-5.
14. Edwards TJ, Sherr EH, Barkovich AJ, Richards LJ. Clinical, genetic and imaging findings identify new causes for corpus callosum development syndromes. Brain. 2014; https://doi.org/10.1093/brain/awt358.
15. O'Leary DDM, Chou SJ, Sahara S. Area patterning of the mammalian cortex. Neuron. 2007; https://doi.org/10.1016/j.neuron.2007.10.010.
16. Hoerder-Suabedissen A, Hayashi S, Upton L, et al. Subset of cortical layer 6b neurons selectively innervates higher order thalamic nuclei in mice. Cereb Cortex. 2018; https://doi.org/10.1093/cercor/bhy036.
17. Puthuran MJ, Rowland-Hill CA, Simpson J, et al. Chromosome 1q42 deletion and agenesis of the corpus callosum [3]. Am J Med Genet. 2005; https://doi.org/10.1002/ajmg.a.30888.
18. Filges I, Röthlisberger B, Boesch N, et al. Interstitial deletion 1q42 in a patient with agenesis of corpus callosum: phenotype-genotype comparison to the 1q41q42 microdeletion suggests a contiguous 1q4 syndrome. Am J Med Genet Part A. 2010; https://doi.org/10.1002/ajmg.a.33330.
19. Righini A, Ciosci R, Selicorni A, et al. Brain magnetic resonance imaging in Wolf-Hirschhorn syndrome. Neuropediatrics. 2007; https://doi.org/10.1055/s-2007-981685.
20. O'Driscoll MC, Black GCM, Clayton-Smith J, Sherr EH, Dobyns WB. Identification of genomic loci contributing to agenesis of the corpus callosum. Am J Med Genet Part A. :2010. https://doi.org/10.1002/ajmg.a.33558.
21. Heide S, Keren B, Billette de Villemeur T, et al. Copy number variations found in patients with a corpus callosum abnormality and intellectual disability. J Pediatr. 2017; https://doi.org/10.1016/j.jpeds.2017.02.023.
22. Schell-Apacik CC, Wagner K, Bihler M, et al. Agenesis and dysgenesis of the corpus callosum: clinical, genetic and neuroimaging findings in a series of 41 patients. Am J Med Genet Part A. 2008; https://doi.org/10.1002/ajmg.a.32476.
23. Chen CP, Chang TY, Guo WY, et al. Chromosome 17p13.3 deletion syndrome: ACGH characterization, prenatal findings and diagnosis, and literature review. Gene. 2013; https://doi.org/10.1016/j.gene.2013.09.044.
24. Chen CP, Chien SC. Prenatal sonographic features of Miller-Dieker syndrome. J Med Ultrasound. 2010; https://doi.org/10.1016/j.jmu.2010.11.002.
25. Kitamura K, Yanazawa M, Sugiyama N, et al. Mutation of ARX causes abnormal development of forebrain and testes in mice and X-linked lissencephaly with abnormal genitalia in humans. Nat Genet. 2002; https://doi.org/10.1038/ng1009.
26. Kato M, Das S, Petras K, et al. Mutations of ARX are associated with striking pleiotropy and consistent genotype-phenotype correlation. Hum Mutat. 2004; https://doi.org/10.1002/humu.10310.
27. Dobyns WB, Berry-Kravis E, Havernick NJ, Holden KR, Viskochil D. X-linked lissencephaly with absent corpus callosum and ambiguous genitalia. Am J Med Genet. 1999; https://doi.org/10.1002/(SICI)1096-8628(19991008)86:4<331::AID-AJMG7>3.0.CO;2-P.
28. Bonneau D, Toutain A, Laquerrière A, et al. X-linked lissencephaly with absent corpus callosum and ambiguous genitalia (XLAG): clinical, magnetic resonance imaging, and neuropathological findings. Ann Neurol. 2002; https://doi.org/10.1002/ana.10119.

29. Fransen E, Vits L, Van Camp G, Willems PJ. The clinical spectrum of mutations in L1, a neuronal cell adhesion molecule. Am J Med Genet. 1996; https://doi.org/10.1002/(SICI)1096-8628(19960712)64:1<73::AID-AJMG11>3.0.CO;2-P.
30. Yamasaki M, Thompson P, Lemmon V. CRASH syndrome: mutations in L1CAM correlate with severity of the disease. Neuropediatrics. 1997; https://doi.org/10.1055/s-2007-973696.
31. Aicardi J. Aicardi syndrome. In: Brain and development; 2005. https://doi.org/10.1016/j.braindev.2003.11.011.
32. Lund C, Bjørnvold M, Tuft M, Kostov H, Røsby O, Selmer KK. Aicardi syndrome: an epidemiologic and clinical study in Norway. Pediatr Neurol. 2015; https://doi.org/10.1016/j.pediatrneurol.2014.10.022.
33. Parrini E, Conti V, Dobyns WB, Guerrini R. Genetic basis of brain malformations. Mol Syndromol. 2016; https://doi.org/10.1159/000448639.
34. Guerrini R, Dobyns WB. Malformations of cortical development: clinical features and genetic causes. Lancet Neurol. 2014; https://doi.org/10.1016/S1474-4422(14)70040-7.
35. Desikan RS, Barkovich AJ. Malformations of cortical development. Ann Neurol. 2016;80(6):797–810. https://doi.org/10.1002/ana.24793.
36. Gilmore EC, Walsh CA. Genetic causes of microcephaly and lessons for neuronal development. Wiley Interdiscip Rev Dev Biol. 2013; https://doi.org/10.1002/wdev.89.
37. Yu TW, Mochida GH, Tischfield DJ, et al. Mutations in WDR62, encoding a centrosome-associated protein, cause microcephaly with simplified gyri and abnormal cortical architecture. Nat Genet. 2010; https://doi.org/10.1038/ng.683.
38. Jackson AP, Eastwood H, Bell SM, et al. identification of microcephalin, a protein implicated in determining the size of the human brain. Am J Hum Genet. 2002; https://doi.org/10.1086/341283.
39. Nicholas AK, Khurshid M, Désir J, et al. WDR62 is associated with the spindle pole and is mutated in human microcephaly. Nat Genet. 2010; https://doi.org/10.1038/ng.682.
40. Trimborn M, Bell SM, Felix C, et al. Mutations in microcephalin cause aberrant regulation of chromosome condensation. Am J Hum Genet. 2004; https://doi.org/10.1086/422855.
41. Brunk K, Vernay B, Griffith E, et al. Microcephalin coordinates mitosis in the syncytial Drosophila embryo. J Cell Sci. 2007; https://doi.org/10.1242/jcs.014290.
42. Bond J, Roberts E, Mochida GH, et al. ASPM is a major determinant of cerebral cortical size. Nat Genet. 2002; https://doi.org/10.1038/ng995.
43. Bond J, Roberts E, Springell K, et al. A centrosomal mechanism involving CDK5RAP2 and CENPJ controls brain size. Nat Genet. 2005; https://doi.org/10.1038/ng1539.
44. Kumar A, Girimaji SC, Duvvari MR, Blanton SH. Mutations in STIL, encoding a pericentriolar and centrosomal protein, cause primary microcephaly. Am J Hum Genet. 2008; https://doi.org/10.1016/j.ajhg.2009.01.017.
45. Bilgüvar K, Öztürk AK, Louvi A, et al. Whole-exome sequencing identifies recessive WDR62 mutations in severe brain malformations. Nature. :2010. https://doi.org/10.1038/nature09327.
46. Kaya B, Ali Kemal O, Angeliki L, et al. Whole-exome sequencing identifies recessive WDR62 mutations in severe brain malformations. Nature. 2011;
47. Guernsey DL, Jiang H, Hussin J, et al. Mutations in centrosomal protein CEP152 in primary microcephaly families linked to MCPH4. Am J Hum Genet. 2010; https://doi.org/10.1016/j.ajhg.2010.06.003.
48. Toi A, Lister WS, Fong KW. How early are fetal cerebral sulci visible at prenatal ultrasound and what is the normal pattern of early fetal sulcal development? Ultrasound Obstet Gynecol. 2004; https://doi.org/10.1002/uog.1802.
49. Pooh RK. The role of imaging detection of congenital defects in the era of PGT-A and NIPT. J Perinat Med. 2019; https://doi.org/10.1515/jpm-2019-2501.
50. Pooh RK. Fetal brain imaging. Ultrasound Med Biol. 2017; https://doi.org/10.1016/j.ultrasmedbio.2017.08.1416.
51. Pooh RK. Fetal neuroimaging of neural migration disorder. Ultrasound Clin. 2008; https://doi.org/10.1016/j.cult.2008.09.007.

52. Poon LC, Sahota DS, Chaemsaithong P, et al. Transvaginal three-dimensional ultrasound assessment of Sylvian fissures at 18–30 weeks' gestation. Ultrasound Obstet Gynecol. 2019;54(2) https://doi.org/10.1002/uog.20172.
53. Pooh RK, Machida M, Nakamura T, et al. Increased Sylvian fissure angle as early sonographic sign of malformation of cortical development. Ultrasound Obstet Gynecol. 2019;54(2) https://doi.org/10.1002/uog.20171.
54. Yoshida A, Kobayashi K, Manya H, et al. Muscular dystrophy and neuronal migration disorder caused by mutations in a glycosyltransferase, POMGnT1. Dev Cell. 2001; https://doi.org/10.1016/S1534-5807(01)00070-3.
55. Hehr U, Uyanik G, Gross C, et al. Novel POMGnT1 mutations define broader phenotypic spectrum of muscle-eye-brain disease. Neurogenetics. 2007; https://doi.org/10.1007/s10048-007-0096-y.
56. Godfrey C, Clement E, Mein R, et al. Refining genotype-phenotype correlations in muscular dystrophies with defective glycosylation of dystroglycan. Brain. 2007; https://doi.org/10.1093/brain/awm212.
57. Kobayashi K, Nakahori Y, Miyake M, et al. An ancient retrotransposal insertion causes Fukuyama-type congenital muscular dystrophy. Nature. 1998; https://doi.org/10.1038/28653.
58. Toda T, Kobayashi K, Kondo-Iida E, Sasaki J, Nakamura Y. The Fukuyama congenital muscular dystrophy story. Neuromuscul Disord. 2000; https://doi.org/10.1016/S0960-8966(99)00109-1.
59. Takeda S. Fukutin is required for maintenance of muscle integrity, cortical histiogenesis and normal eye development. Hum Mol Genet. 2003; https://doi.org/10.1093/hmg/ddg153.
60. Friocourt G, Kanatani S, Tabata H, et al. Cell-autonomous roles of ARX in cell proliferation and neuronal migration during corticogenesis. J Neurosci. 2008; https://doi.org/10.1523/JNEUROSCI.1067-08.2008.
61. Friocourt G, Poirier K, Rakić S, Parnavelas JG, Chelly J. The role of ARX in cortical development. Eur J Neurosci. 2006; https://doi.org/10.1111/j.1460-9568.2006.04629.x.
62. Sherr EH. The ARX story (epilepsy, mental retardation, autism, and cerebral malformations): one gene leads to many phenotypes. Curr Opin Pediatr. 2003; https://doi.org/10.1097/00008480-200312000-00004.
63. Colasante G, Simonet JC, Calogero R, et al. ARX regulates cortical intermediate progenitor cell expansion and upper layer neuron formation through repression of Cdkn1c. Cereb Cortex. 2015; https://doi.org/10.1093/cercor/bht222.
64. Folsom TD, Fatemi SH. The involvement of Reelin in neurodevelopmental disorders. Neuropharmacology. 2013; https://doi.org/10.1016/j.neuropharm.2012.08.015.
65. Tissir F, Goffinet AM. Reelin and brain development. Nat Rev Neurosci. 2003; https://doi.org/10.1038/nrn1113.
66. Chen Y, Beffert U, Ertunc M, et al. Reelin modulates NMDA receptor activity in cortical neurons. J Neurosci. 2005; https://doi.org/10.1523/JNEUROSCI.1951-05.2005.
67. Kato M. Genotype-phenotype correlation in neuronal migration disorders and cortical dysplasias. Front Neurosci. 2015; https://doi.org/10.3389/fnins.2015.00181.
68. Fallet-Bianco C, Laquerrière A, Poirier K, et al. Mutations in tubulin genes are frequent causes of various foetal malformations of cortical development including microlissencephaly. Acta Neuropathol Commun. 2014; https://doi.org/10.1186/2051-5960-2-69.
69. Laquerriere A, Gonzales M, Saillour Y, et al. De novo TUBB2B mutation causes fetal akinesia deformation sequence with microlissencephaly: an unusual presentation of tubulinopathy. Eur J Med Genet. 2016; https://doi.org/10.1016/j.ejmg.2015.12.007.
70. Harding BN, Moccia A, Drunat S, et al. Mutations in citron kinase cause recessive microlissencephaly with multinucleated neurons. Am J Hum Genet. 2016; https://doi.org/10.1016/j.ajhg.2016.07.003.
71. Barkovich AJ, Ferriero DM, Barr RM, et al. Microlissencephaly: a heterogeneous malformation of cortical development. Neuropediatrics. 1998; https://doi.org/10.1055/s-2007-973545.
72. Poirier K, Martinovic J, Laquerrière A, et al. Rare ACTG1 variants in fetal microlissencephaly. Eur J Med Genet. 2015; https://doi.org/10.1016/j.ejmg.2015.06.006.

73. Di Donato N, Chiari S, Mirzaa GM, et al. Lissencephaly: expanded imaging and clinical classification. Am J Med Genet Part A. 2017; https://doi.org/10.1002/ajmg.a.38245.
74. McGahan JP, Grix A, Gerscovich EO. Prenatal diagnosis of lissencephaly: Miller-Dieker syndrome. J Clin Ultrasound. 1994; https://doi.org/10.1002/jcu.1870220908.
75. Greco P, Resta M, Vimercati A, et al. Antenatal diagnosis of isolated lissencephaly by ultrasound and magnetic resonance imaging. Ultrasound Obstet Gynecol. 1998; https://doi.org/10.1046/j.1469-0705.1998.12040276.x.
76. Kojima K, Suzuki Y, Seki K, et al. Prenatal diagnosis of lissencephaly (type II) by ultrasound and fast magnetic resonance imaging. Fetal Diagn Ther. 2002; https://doi.org/10.1159/000048003.
77. Fong KW, Ghai S, Toi A, Blaser S, Winsor EJT, Chitayat D. Prenatal ultrasound findings of lissencephaly associated with Miller-Dieker syndrome and comparison with pre- and postnatal magnetic resonance imaging. Ultrasound Obstet Gynecol. 2004; https://doi.org/10.1002/uog.1777.
78. Gha S, Fong KW, Toi A, Chitayat D, Pantazi S, Blaser S. Prenatal US and MR imaging findings of lissencephaly: review of fetal cerebral sulcal development. Radiographics. 2006; https://doi.org/10.1148/rg.262055059.
79. Leventer RJ, Jansen A, Pilz DT, et al. Clinical and imaging heterogeneity of polymicrogyria: a study of 328 patients. Brain. 2010; https://doi.org/10.1093/brain/awq078.
80. Stutterd CA, Leventer RJ. Polymicrogyria: a common and heterogeneous malformation of cortical development. Am J Med Genet Part C Semin Med Genet. 2014; https://doi.org/10.1002/ajmg.c.31399.
81. Manzini MC, Walsh CA. The genetics of brain malformations. In: The genetics of neurodevelopmental disorders; 2015. https://doi.org/10.1002/9781118524947.ch7.
82. Smigiel R, Cabala M, Jakubiak A, et al. Novel COL4A1 mutation in an infant with severe dysmorphic syndrome with schizencephaly, periventricular calcifications, and cataract resembling congenital infection. Birth Defects Res A Clin Mol Teratol. 2016; https://doi.org/10.1002/bdra.23488.
83. Watanabe J, Okamoto K, Ohashi T, et al. Malignant hyperthermia and cerebral venous sinus thrombosis after ventriculoperitoneal shunt in infant with schizencephaly and COL4A1 Mutation. World Neurosurg. 2019; https://doi.org/10.1016/j.wneu.2019.04.156.
84. Errata to Intracranial hemorrhage and tortuosity of veins detected on susceptibility-weighted imaging of a child with a type IV collagen α1 mutation and schizencephaly (Singapore Med J 14,3 223-226, 2014 10.2463/mrms.2014-0060). Magn Reson Med Sci. :2015. https://doi.org/10.2463/mrms.2014-0060er.
85. Fox NS, Monteagudo A, Kuller JA, Craigo S, Norton ME. Mild fetal ventriculomegaly: diagnosis, evaluation, and management. Am J Obstet Gynecol. 2018; https://doi.org/10.1016/j.ajog.2018.04.039.
86. Shaheen R, Sebai MA, Patel N, et al. The genetic landscape of familial congenital hydrocephalus. Ann Neurol. 2017; https://doi.org/10.1002/ana.24964.
87. Ekici AB, Hilfinger D, Jatzwauk M, et al. Disturbed Wnt signalling due to a mutation in CCDC88C causes an autosomal recessive non-syndromic hydrocephalus with medial diverticulum. Mol Syndromol. 2010; https://doi.org/10.1159/000319859.
88. Al-Dosari MS, Al-Owain M, Tulbah M, et al. Mutation in MPDZ causes severe congenital hydrocephalus. J Med Genet. 2013; https://doi.org/10.1136/jmedgenet-2012-101294.
89. Kousi M, Katsanis N. The genetic basis of hydrocephalus. Annu Rev Neurosci. 2016; https://doi.org/10.1146/annurev-neuro-070815-014023.
90. Itoh K, Fushiki S. The role of L1cam in murine corticogenesis, and the pathogenesis of hydrocephalus. Pathol Int. 2015; https://doi.org/10.1111/pin.12245.
91. Takahashi S, Makita Y, Okamoto N, Miyamoto A, Oki J. L1CAM mutation in a Japanese family with X-linked hydrocephalus: a study for genetic counseling. Brain Dev. 1997; https://doi.org/10.1016/S0387-7604(97)00079-X.
92. Jouet M, Rosenthal A, Armstrong G, et al. X–linked spastic paraplegia (SPG1), MASA syndrome and X–linked hydrocephalus result from mutations in the L1 gene. Nat Genet. 1994; https://doi.org/10.1038/ng0794-402.

93. Adle-Biassette H, Saugier-Veber P, Fallet-Bianco C, et al. Neuropathological review of 138 cases genetically tested for X-linked hydrocephalus: evidence for closely related clinical entities of unknown molecular bases. Acta Neuropathol. 2013; https://doi.org/10.1007/s00401-013-1146-1.
94. Rachel RA, Yamamoto EA, Dewanjee MK, et al. CEP290 alleles in mice disrupt tissue-specific cilia biogenesis and recapitulate features of syndromic ciliopathies. Hum Mol Genet. 2015; https://doi.org/10.1093/hmg/ddv123.
95. Iannicelli M, Brancati F, Mougou-Zerelli S, et al. Novel TMEM67 mutations and genotype-phenotype correlates in meckelin-related ciliopathies. Hum Mutat. 2010; https://doi.org/10.1002/humu.21239.
96. Abdelhamed ZA, Natarajan S, Wheway G, et al. The Meckel-Gruber syndrome protein TMEM67 controls basal body positioning and epithelial branching morphogenesis in mice via the non-canonical Wnt pathway. DMM Dis Model Mech. 2015; https://doi.org/10.1242/dmm.019083.
97. Leightner AC, Hommerding CJ, Peng Y, et al. The meckel syndrome protein meckelin (TMEM67) is a key regulator of cilia function but is not required for tissue planar polarity. Hum Mol Genet. 2013; https://doi.org/10.1093/hmg/ddt054.
98. Valente EM, Logan CV, Mougou-Zerelli S, et al. Mutations in TMEM216 perturb ciliogenesis and cause Joubert, Meckel and related syndromes. Nat Genet. 2010; https://doi.org/10.1038/ng.594.
99. Xiao D, Lv C, Zhang Z, et al. Novel CC2D2A compound heterozygous mutations cause Joubert syndrome. Mol Med Rep. 2017; https://doi.org/10.3892/mmr.2016.6007.
100. Johnson K, Bertoli M, Phillips L, et al. Detection of variants in dystroglycanopathy-associated genes through the application of targeted whole-exome sequencing analysis to a large cohort of patients with unexplained limb-girdle muscle weakness. Skelet Muscle. 2018;8(1):1–12. https://doi.org/10.1186/s13395-018-0170-1.
101. Mirzaa GM, Rivière JB, Dobyns WB. Megalencephaly syndromes and activating mutations in the PI3K-AKT pathway: MPPH and MCAP. Am J Med Genet Part C Semin Med Genet. 2013; https://doi.org/10.1002/ajmg.c.31361.
102. Itoh K, Pooh R, Kanemura Y, Yamasaki M, Fushiki S. Brain malformation with loss of normal FGFR3 expression in thanatophoric dysplasia type I. Neuropathology. 2013; https://doi.org/10.1111/neup.12036.
103. Dicuonzo F, Palma M, Fiume M, et al. Cerebrovascular disorders in the prenatal period. J Child Neurol. 2008; https://doi.org/10.1177/0883073808318054.
104. Özduman K, Pober BR, Barnes P, et al. Fetal stroke. Pediatr Neurol. 2004; https://doi.org/10.1016/j.pediatrneurol.2003.08.004.
105. Elchalal U, Yagel S, Gomori JM, et al. Fetal intracranial hemorrhage (fetal stroke): does grade matter? Ultrasound Obstet Gynecol. 2005; https://doi.org/10.1002/uog.1969.
106. Huang YF, Chen WC, Tseng JJ, Ho ESC, Chou MM. Fetal intracranial hemorrhage (fetal stroke): report of four antenatally diagnosed cases and review of the literature. Taiwan J Obstet Gynecol. 2006; https://doi.org/10.1016/S1028-4559(09)60211-4.
107. Putbrese B, Kennedy A. Findings and differential diagnosis of fetal intracranial haemorrhage and fetal ischaemic brain injury: what is the role of fetal MRI? Br J Radiol. 2017; https://doi.org/10.1259/bjr.20160253.
108. Kutuk MS, Yikilmaz A, Ozgun MT, et al. Prenatal diagnosis and postnatal outcome of fetal intracranial hemorrhage. Child's Nerv Syst. 2014; https://doi.org/10.1007/s00381-013-2243-0.
109. Sims ME, Turkel SB, Halterman G, Paul RH. Brain injury and intrauterine death. Am J Obstet Gynecol. 1985; https://doi.org/10.1016/0002-9378(85)90503-4.
110. Lichtenbelt KD, Pistorius LR, De Tollenaer SM, Mancini GM, De Vries LS. Prenatal genetic confirmation of a COL4A1 mutation presenting with sonographic fetal intracranial hemorrhage. Ultrasound Obstet Gynecol. 2012; https://doi.org/10.1002/uog.11070.

111. Garel C, Rosenblatt J, Moutard ML, et al. Fetal intracerebral hemorrhage and COL4A1 mutation: promise and uncertainty. Ultrasound Obstet Gynecol. 2013; https://doi.org/10.1002/uog.12268.
112. Vermeulen RJ, Peeters-Scholte C, Van Vugt J, et al. Fetal origin of brain damage in 2 infants with a COL4A1 mutation: fetal and neonatal MRI. Neuropediatrics. 2011; https://doi.org/10.1055/s-0031-1284388.
113. de Vries LS, Pistorius L, Lichtenbelt KD, Koopman C, Meuwissen MEC, Mancini GMS. COL4A1 mutation: expansion of the phenotype. Pediatr Res. 2011; https://doi.org/10.1038/pr.2011.406.
114. Meuwissen MEC, Halley DJJ, Smit LS, et al. The expanding phenotype of COL4A1 and COL4A2 mutations: clinical data on 13 newly identified families and a review of the literature. Genet Med. 2015; https://doi.org/10.1038/gim.2014.210.
115. De Vries LS, Koopman C, Groenendaal F, et al. COL4A1 mutation in two preterm siblings with antenatal onset of parenchymal hemorrhage. Ann Neurol. 2009; https://doi.org/10.1002/ana.21525.
116. Colin E, Sentilhes L, Sarfati A, et al. Fetal intracerebral hemorrhage and cataract: think COL4A1. J Perinatol. 2014; https://doi.org/10.1038/jp.2013.135.
117. Papile LA, Burstein J, Burstein R, Koffler H. Incidence and evolution of subependymal and intraventricular hemorrhage: a study of infants with birth weights less than 1,500 gm. J Pediatr. 1978; https://doi.org/10.1016/S0022-3476(78)80282-0.
118. Vergani P, Strobelt N, Locatelli A, et al. Clinical significance of fetal intracranial hemorrhage. Am J Obstet Gynecol. 1996; https://doi.org/10.1053/ob.1996.v175.a73598.
119. Van den Veyver IB. Prenatally diagnosed developmental abnormalities of the central nervous system and genetic syndromes: a practical review. Prenat Diagn. 2019;39(9):666–78. https://doi.org/10.1002/pd.5520.
120. Pooh RK. The study of early pregnancy with genetic and high-resolution ultrasound. J Perinat Med. 2013;
121. Pooh RK. Sonogenetics in fetal neurology. Semin Fetal Neonatal Med. 2012; https://doi.org/10.1016/j.siny.2012.07.005.

Chapter 8
Muscular Dystrophy

Miwako Nagasaka and Mariko Taniguchi-Ikeda

Abstract Muscular dystrophy is one of the main intractable, inherited neuromuscular diseases. Owing to respiratory failure and cardiac complications, the life expectancy of patients is shortened in certain types of muscular dystrophies. More than 50 genes are known to cause muscular dystrophy, and the prognosis of patients varies according to the type and the age of onset of the disease. One parent or both parents are usually carriers of the genetic mutation that causes the disease. Despite the extensive research and clinical trials being performed worldwide, few radical treatments are available at present. On the other hand, with the advancements in genetic diagnostic tests and promising treatments for some types of muscular dystrophies, there is an increasing need for the prenatal diagnosis of muscular dystrophies in couples who already have a child with muscular dystrophy, or have a family member with muscular dystrophy. In this chapter, we discuss prenatal genetic tests for the three most well-known muscular dystrophies, namely, myotonic dystrophy, Duchenne muscular dystrophy, and Fukuyama congenital muscular dystrophy.

Keywords Muscular dystrophy · Gene therapy · Prenatal diagnosis · Genetic counseling · Preimplantation genetics · Ethical issues · Intractable diseases
Universal screening for the newborn

M. Nagasaka
Department of Clinical Genetics, Fujita Health University Hospital, Toyoake, Aichi, Japan
e-mail: nagasaka@fujita-hu.ac.jp

M. Taniguchi-Ikeda (✉)
Department of Pediatrics, Takatsuki General Hospital, Osaka, Japan
e-mail: mtani@fujita-hu.ac.jp

H. Masuzaki (ed.), *Fetal Morph Functional Diagnosis*, Comprehensive Gynecology and Obstetrics, https://doi.org/10.1007/978-981-15-8171-7_8

8.1 Introduction

Muscular dystrophy is a group of hereditary neuromuscular diseases that mainly affect the skeletal muscle, which are caused by progressive necrosis and/or the lack of muscle fiber regeneration. Patients show progressive muscle weakness, leading to muscle atrophy, resulting in decreased activities of daily living and quality of life. In some muscular dystrophies, cardiac function and pulmonary function are gradually affected, which can cause serious complications in patients and may be life-threatening. Usually, respiratory support and feeding tubes are required for patients in the end-stage of disease for severe types of muscular dystrophy. Other complications include scoliosis, joint contractures, and dysphagia. In some muscular dystrophies, neurological symptoms, such as intellectual disability and epilepsy are also observed. Therefore, the main symptoms are motor dysfunction associated with skeletal muscle defects, but it is a systemic disease that often involves systemic physical functions, including the central nervous system (CNS), and hence requires multidisciplinary management. The patient and the patient's family members all require continuous medical and social support. Therefore, parents or couples should be provided information regarding any options available to have an unaffected child in their subsequent pregnancies. Moreover, with the recent progress in therapies for some of the muscular dystrophies, it may be very important to identify the causative genetic alterations, as this may enable early and appropriate medical intervention for the patients. However, it is sometimes very difficult to make sufficient time to provide detailed information to clients in a regular clinic. Therefore, for such cases, genetic counseling can provide the necessary information to clients (see Part 5, Chap. 22 for detailed information).

8.2 Genetic Causes of Muscular Dystrophy

More than 50 causative genes of muscular dystrophy have been elucidated to date, and approximately 25 genes are known to cause congenital muscular dystrophy (Table 8.1) [1, 2]. From the functional view of these causative genes, muscular dystrophies are caused not only by sarcolemmal proteins, such as dystrophin and sarcoglycan, but by extracellular matrix proteins, basement membrane proteins, and some glycosylation enzymes that post-translationally modify these proteins [1]. The severity and disease onset vary according to the disease type or mutations. Muscular dystrophy is mainly classified into congenital muscular dystrophy (CMD), limb-girdle muscular dystrophy (LGMD), dystroglycanopathies, myotonic dystrophies, and others, including the Emery-Dreifuss type, fascioscapulohumeral type, and unclassified types. CMDs are mainly caused by extracellular matrix proteins and basement membrane proteins. LGMDs are mainly caused by sarcolemmal proteins, and usually have a later onset. The inheritance pattern of muscular dystrophies is mainly classified into four categories, i.e., autosomal dominant (AD) inheritance, autosomal recessive (AR) inheritance, X-linked recessive (XLR) inheritance, and

Table 8.1 Genetic classification for muscular dystropies

Disease	Inheritance pattern	Causative gene	Protein
Congenital muscular dystrophy (CMD)			
Dystroglycanopathies			
Fukuyama CMD	AR	*FKTN*	Fukutin
Muscle-eye-brain disease	AR	*FKRP*	Fukutin-related protein
Walker Warburg syndrome		*LARGE*	LARGE
	AR	*POMT1*	Protein O-mannosyl-transferase 1
	AR	*POMT2*	Protein O-mannosyl-transferase 2
	AR	*B4GAT1*	Beta-1,4-glucuronyl-transferase 1
	AR	*TMEM5*	Ribitol β1,4-Xylosyl-transferase
	AR	*B3GALNT2*	β-1,3-N-acetylgalactosaminyltransferase 2
	AR	*POMGnT1*	Protein O-linked-mannose
	AR	*POMGnT2*	β-1,2-N-acetylglucosaminyltransferase 1/2
	AR	*SGK196*	Protein O-mannose kinase
	AR	*ISPD*	Isoprenoid synthase domain
CMD due to glycosylation disorder	AR	*DPM2*	Dolichyl-phosphate mannosyl-transferase
		DPM3	Polypeptide 2/3
Primary alpha dystroglycanopathy	AR	*DAG*	Alpha dystroglycan
Merosinopathy	AR	*LAMA2*	Merosin
Collagenopathies			
Ullrich CMD	AD/AR	*COL6A1/A2/A3*	Alpha 1/2/3 type VI collagen
Bethlem myopathy	AD/AR	*COL6A1/A2/A3*	Alpha 1/2/3 type VI collagen
Multiminicore disease	AR	*SEPN1/RYR1*	Selenon, Ryanodine receptor 1
LMNA-associated CMD	AR	*LMNA*	Lamin A/C
CMD due to mitochondrial structural anomaly	AR	*CHKB*	Choline kinase beta
CMD with generalized lipodystrophy	AR	*PTRF*	Polymerase I and transcript release factor
Integrin α7 CMD	AR	*ITGA7*	Integrin alpha 7
Ingegrin α9 CMD	AR	*ITGA9*	Ingegrin alpha 9
Rigid spine CMD	AR	*SEPN1*	Selenoprotein 1
Facioscapulohumeral MD 1	AD	*DUX4*	Double homeobox 4
Facioscapulohumeral MD 2	AD	*SMCHD1*	Facioscapulohumeral alpha 2

(continued)

Table 8.1 (continued)

Disease	Inheritance pattern	Causative gene	Protein
Scapuloperoneal MD	AD	*PABP2*	Palenoprotein 2
Oculopharyngeal MD	AD/AR	*PABN1*	Palenoprotein 1
Limb girdle muscular dystrophy (LGMD)			
LGMD 1A	AD	*MYOT*	Myotilin
LGMD 1B	AD	*LMNA*	Lamin A/C
LGMD 1C	AD	*CAV3*	Caveolin-3
LGMD 1D	AD	*DNAJB6*	Co-choaperone DNAJB6
LGMD 1E	AD	*DES*	Desmin
LGMD 1F	AD	*TNPO3*	Transportin-3
LGMD 1G	AD	*HNRDL*	Heterogenious nuclear ribonucleoprotein D-like protein
LGMD 1H	AD	*Unknown*	Unknown
LGMD 2A	AR	*CAPN3*	Calpain-3
LGMD 2B	AR	*DYSF*	Dysferlin
LGMD 2C	AR	*SGCG*	γ-sarcoglycan
LGMD 2D	AR	*SGCA*	α-sarcoglycan
LGMD 2E	AR	*SGCB*	β-sarcoglycan
LGMD 2F	AR	*SGCD*	δ-sarcoglycan
LGMD 2G	AR	*TCAP*	Titin-cap (telethonin)
LGMD 2H	AR	*TRIM32*	Tripartite motif-containing 32
LGMD 2I	AR	*FKRP*	Fukutin-related protein
LGMD 2J	AR	*TTN*	Titin
LGMD 2K	AR	*POMT1*	Protein O-mannosyl-transferase 1
LGMD 2L	AR	*ANO5*	Anoctamin 5
LGMD 2M	AR	*FKTN*	Fukutin
LGMD 2N	AR	*POMT2*	Protein O-mannosyl-transferase 2
LGMD 2O	AR	*POMGNT1*	Protein O-linked-mannose
LGMD 2P	AR	*DAG1*	Alpha dystroglycan
LGMD 2Q	AR	*PLEC1*	Plectin-1
Emery-Dreifuss	XLR	*EMD*	Emerin
	AD	*LMNA, SYNE1,2*	Lamin A/C, Spectrin repeat containing, nuclear envelope 1/2 (nesprin 1/2)
	AR	*LMNA/C*	Lamin A/C
Myotonic dystrophy type 1	AD	*DM1*	DPMK1
Myotonic dystrophy type 2	AD	*DM2*	DPMK2
Dystrophinopathy			
Duchenne muscular dystrophy	*XLR*	DMD	Dystrophin
Becker muscular dystrophy	*XLR*	DMD	

See GeneTable for the updated information from Neuromuscular Disorders mitochondrial disease (we will not discuss mitochondrial diseases in this chapter). For a detailed explanation of the inheritance patterns, please see Chap. 6. There are still some types of muscular dystrophies for which the causative genes have not yet been identified. For such cases, a genetic diagnosis can sometimes be performed by a research-based test, in which genetic tests are performed on the whole family to identify the causative gene.

In the AD inheritance pattern, the father or mother is usually affected, i.e., one copy of the altered gene in each cell is sufficient to cause the disease. Although there are de novo cases, we will not discuss such cases in this chapter. The recurrence rate of AD diseases in offspring is 50%. Children of either sex can inherit the condition. Myotonic dystrophy (DM), facioscapulohumeral muscular dystrophy, and LGMD type 1 (LGMD1) are mainly known to have an AD inheritance pattern. Particularly, in DM, which is the most common AD muscular dystrophy, the possibility of congenital DM is the biggest concern in couples who desire a prenatal diagnosis. In the case of an AD disease, besides a high risk of recurrence, the expansion of triplet repeats inside the responsible gene, particularly from the mother's allele, can sometimes cause a severer form of muscular dystrophy in the next generation.

In AR forms of disease, basically the father and mother are both carriers. The recurrence risk in the offspring 25%. Children of either sex can inherit the condition. In AR disease, both copies of the causative gene have to be pathogenic to cause symptoms. A person who has one copy of the gene with a pathogenic variant is termed as a carrier, and basically the person is asymptomatic. Spinal muscular atrophy, congenital muscular dystrophies, such as Fukuyama congenital muscular dystrophy (FCMD; also known as an alpha-dystroglycanopathy), merosin-negative muscular dystrophy (classified as a merosinopathy), Ullrich-type muscular dystrophy, and LGMD type 2 (LGMD2) are the main known types of muscular dystrophy with AR inheritance patterns. The incidence is the highest (1 in 35,000 birth) for FCMD in Japan [3].

For X-linked recessive diseases, basically the mother is a carrier, and the male offspring are affected. These conditions are caused by a pathogenic variant in a gene on the X chromosome. As females have two X chromosomes, even if one copy of the gene is affected, females generally do not show symptoms. On the other hand, males have one copy of the X chromosome, and hence only boys manifest symptoms. Female carriers sometimes show symptoms later in life, which is generally considered to be caused by skewed X-chromosome inactivation or aging [4]. Some female carriers who manifest severe forms of disease sometimes have translocation of the X chromosome. The recurrence risk is 50% of born male offspring. Fifty percent of female offspring will inherit the mutated gene, which means that 50% of born female offspring are carriers. Duchenne muscular dystrophy (DMD), Becker muscular dystrophy (BMD), Emery-Dreifuss muscular dystrophy, and X-linked myotubular myopathy are the main muscular dystrophies known to have an XLR inheritance pattern. For carrier genetic tests, the results of the proband are essential, because only 60% of variants can be diagnosed as DMD by commercially available genetic tests, and even if a variant was detected, it is unclear whether the genetic changes in the asymptomatic carriers are truly disease-associated in the absence of information about the proband.

8.3 Diagnosis and Clinical Management of Muscular Dystrophies

Although treatments for muscular dystrophies are gradually being developed, there are still many types of muscular dystrophies for which only palliative treatments are available. Muscular dystrophy may present symptoms from early infancy or later in adulthood depending on the type, and symptoms vary according to the disease or the types of genetic variants. For a clinical diagnosis, clinical signs such as reduced muscle tone and delayed motor development milestones are initially important. The onset of symptoms and complications, such as cardiac involvement or CNS symptoms, will assist in making a correct diagnosis. Blood tests, such as checking possible increases in the levels of serum creatine kinase, aldolase, aspartate aminotransferase, and alanine aminotransferase, are also important. Muscle biopsy and imaging analyses, such as computed tomography, magnetic resonance imaging (MRI), and electromyography, are able to specify some types of muscular dystrophies, as the distribution of affected muscle varies according to the types of muscular dystrophy. Brain MRI also helps to detect certain types of muscular dystrophies, such as FCMD. However, advancements in molecular genetic techniques in recent years have led to the identification of new responsible genes, as well as the development of detailed variant databases for the muscular dystrophies. Therefore, genetic diagnosis has replaced muscle biopsy and imaging techniques as the key diagnosis method for these diseases. Muscle biopsies are still very useful for detailed pathological analyses, but such invasive diagnostic procedures are restricted to patients in whom a diagnosis cannot be easily made. Some genetic tests are commercially available. At present, genetic diagnostic testing for some muscular dystrophy genes are covered by national health insurance in Japan.

For some types of muscular dystrophies that result in symptoms from the neonatal period to early childhood, a definitive clinical diagnosis can sometimes be very difficult. Preborn fetal echography findings can sometimes be nonspecific, so genetic testing during the fetal period is usually performed for a definitive diagnosis in suspected patients with a previous family history.

8.4 Recent Progress in Treatments for Muscular Dystrophy

In recent years, the development of radical therapies for certain types of neuromuscular disorders has progressed dramatically. The most striking advancement is gene therapy for spinal muscular atrophy (SMA). Although SMA is not a muscular dystrophy, the dramatic advancement in the clinical use of gene therapies and chemical compounds for SMA is expected to accelerate the development of therapies for other intractable diseases, including the muscular dystrophies [5]. Particularly for DMD, many researchers all over the world are aiming to develop radical therapies, including gene therapies and small chemical compounds. Antisense oligonucleotide therapy has already been partially approved in the United States and Europe. Japanese pharmaceutical companies are also conducting clinical trials for antisense therapy for DMD (see current trials in DMD [6] below). Antisense oligonucleotide therapy aims to delete exons of dystrophin, leading to the correction of codons and the restoration of an in-frame dystrophin protein, although it is not the full-length protein. This exon-skipping therapy strategy was invented by Matsuo et al., and is now applied for many genetic diseases [7, 8]. Theoretically, patients with particular types of deletions in DMD exons (it is at present suitable for skipping exons 51, 45, and 53) may benefit from this therapy, and their symptoms become milder, as in BMD. Antisense therapy targeting abnormal splicing is called splice-modulation therapy. For FCMD, the use of antisense oligonucleotides for the correction of abnormal splicing is a promising therapy [9]. This therapy restores the normal expression of *fukutin*, which is the causative gene of FCMD, and is applicable for all FCMD patients [10]. Adeno-associated virus (AAV) gene therapy is also approaching clinical use. Regarding gene delivery therapies, although there are various issues, such as immune responses, cost, the large size of dystrophin, and the duration of efficacy, clinical trials for patients are now ongoing, and a recent study reported that preclinical trials using AAV8 and AAV9 were overall successful in terms of clinical and histological outcomes [11]. Other treatment strategies include anti-inflammatory methods against muscle cell necrosis or fibrosis. Oral corticosteroids are an approved treatment and are now one of the standard therapies for DMD, but the long-term administration of steroids may be harmful to many organs. Therefore, many other anti-inflammatory chemicals have been investigated to replace corticosteroid therapy [12]. There is a nationwide muscular dystrophy registry called registration of muscular dystrophy (REMUDY) in Japan, which registers various types of muscular dystrophy patients so that they will be efficiently introduced to clinical trials when they become available [13].

8.5 Ethical Standards for the Prenatal Diagnosis of Muscular Dystrophy

In Japan, the ethics committee of each facility discusses whether a prenatal diagnosis for muscular dystrophy is applicable for each case, based on the Genetic Diagnosis Guidelines for Genetic Counseling and Prenatal Diagnosis established by the Japan Society of Human Genetics [14]. Preimplantation diagnosis is not yet a common genetic test in Japan, but has been conducted in clinical studies by some facilities that have been certified by the Japan Society of Obstetrics and Gynecology. The approach to preimplantation diagnosis varies among countries because of historical, religious, and social backgrounds. In this chapter, we describe prenatal genetic tests that are presently performed in Japan for three well-known muscular dystrophies, i.e., DMD, DM1, and FCMD.

8.6 Prenatal Genetic Testing

8.6.1 Duchenne Muscular Dystrophy

Form of inheritance: XLR; responsible gene: dystrophin (*DMD*) gene on Xp21.2

Both DMD and BMD are caused by abnormalities in dystrophin, which is a giant protein located under the cell membrane of muscle cells. DMD is the most common muscular dystrophy in the world (incidence: 1 in 5000 boys). The phenotypes of DMD are severer because dystrophin is not synthesized, whereas those of BMD are milder owing to the existence of partial dystrophin proteins. Patients (usually boys) with DMD first manifest symptoms, such as frequent falls and delayed motor milestones, at 1–2 years of age, and gradually develop Gower's sign, which is a characteristic maneuver of requiring the help of the hands to push on the knees to provide sufficient momentum to become upright, because of the weakness of their pelvic and proximal lower limb muscles, and is a typical sign of DMD [15]. Patients gradually lose independent ambulation by the age of 12 years. A third of DMD patients are known to have intellectual disabilities, such as autistic spectrum disorders. Cardiac complications owing to dilated cardiomyopathy are observed in every patient in the end-stages of DMD. Depending on the X-chromosome inactivation pattern, women may have mosaicism of dystrophin expression in the skeletal muscle and may present symptoms, so carriers also require appropriate medical care. In particular, dilated cardiomyopathy is reported to occur in 8–18% of female manifesting carriers [16]. Cardiomyopathies and skeletal muscle symptoms can also be exacerbated or manifested during pregnancy or delivery, and hence careful management during the perinatal period is also important.

8.6.1.1 Molecular Genetic Testing

Approximately 60% of DMD cases are caused by exonic deletions, and 10% are caused by duplications in the *DMD* gene. The remaining 30% are caused by microdeletions, insertions, and point mutations in the *DMD* gene. By detecting these deletions/duplications by multiplex ligation-dependent probe amplification (MLPA), about 70% of DMD patients can be confirmed by a simple blood test. However, MLPA cannot detect mutations of microdeletions/duplications insertions, single nucleotide substitutions, or splicing abnormalities, so analysis using next-generation sequencing, direct sequencing, or muscle biopsy is required. For the genetic diagnosis chart, see Fig. 8.1 [17, 18].

Regarding recurrence, if the mother is a carrier, 50% of the male sibs will be affected, and 50% of the female sibs will be carriers.

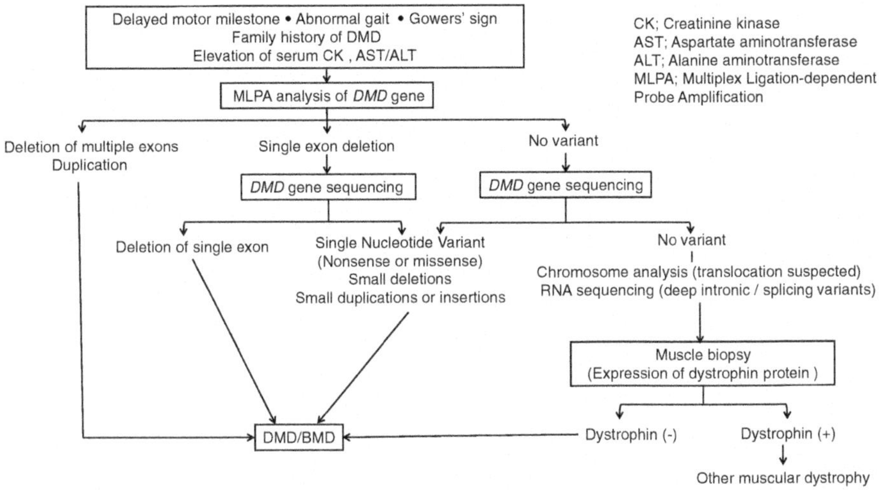

Fig. 8.1 Molecular testing strategy for DMD. MLPA analysis identifies deletions and duplications encompassing one or more exons, which account for 70% of all DMD cases. Direct sequencing will identify mutations in 25% of cases. Together with chromosome analysis, mutations can be identified in almost all DMD patients. *CK* creatine kinase, *AST* aspartate aminotransferase, *ALT* alanine aminotransferase, *MLPA* multiplex ligation-dependent probe amplification

8.6.1.2 Prenatal Diagnosis

The sex of the fetus is determined by a chorionic villus sample test or amniotic fluid test. If the karyotype is 46, XY, DNA is extracted and target gene variants are analyzed. On the other hand, gonadal mosaicism cannot be denied even when the mother is not a carrier. Although there are various opinions regarding gonadal mosaicism of the *DMD* gene, there is a report that the mother's gonadal mosaicism rate for new mutations is 14% [19], and the fact that the mother's peripheral blood is not informative is the limitation of this test. Basically, a prenatal diagnosis should be performed when the proband is genetically confirmed as having DMD, so that the mother's carrier diagnosis is also genetically confirmed. Therefore, when the mother is not a carrier, a prenatal genetic test is not commonly offered. However, it should be considered if there is a need for a prenatal genetic test, and the mother is thought to be a noncarrier but may have germline mosaicism. An institution's ethics committee and genetic counseling unit will discuss the need for genetic testing and the appropriate support for families who will undergo genetic testing. Japanese Consortium of Neurology announced the guidelines for prenatal genetic testing for neuromuscular disorders [20], which stated that BMD is not applicable for prenatal genetic testing in Japan, considering the high life expectancy of milder patients with BMD. However, there are patients who are genetically diagnosed as having BMD who have clinically intermediate types of BMD, and manifest severer phenotypes.

For patients with such intermediate types, whether prenatal genetic testing is applicable should be carefully discussed. Appropriate genetic counseling and support for the family during and after the test are essential.

8.6.1.3 Preimplantation Diagnosis

The first case of diagnosis by preimplantation genetic testing (PGT) in Japan was for DMD. It is performed only within facilities approved to perform preimplantation diagnosis and unbiased genetic counseling, and it requires ethical review by the Japan Society of Obstetrics and Gynecology. The facilities that can perform preimplantation diagnosis are limited, and there are regional discrepancies. Japan PGT Consortium [21] was established in 2017, and this consortium has announced reduction of the regional discrepancies, and promotion and standardization PGT in Japan. There are ethical opinions and conflicts regarding PGT, such as the living rights of the fetus, and furthermore, there are opinions regarding whether it is reasonable to offer expensive tests and make profits from patients' families who have no other alternatives (please see chapter on PGT). PGTs are accompanied by in vitro fertilization, and hence compared to prenatal testing, the mother is able to avoid termination of a pregnancy.

8.6.2 DM1

Form of inheritance: AD; responsible gene: myotonin protein kinase-1 (*DMPK*) gene on 19q13

DM1 It is a systemic disease mainly affecting skeletal muscle, smooth muscle, eyes, heart, and the endocrine and central nervous systems [22]. The prevalence of DM1 is the quite high among the muscular dystrophies (1 in 10,000 births). There are three types, namely, mild DM1, classic DM1, and congenital DM1. Mild DM1 shows mild symptoms, such as only cataracts, or very mild myotonia, so patients sometimes remain undiagnosed. For classic DM1 and congenital DM1, patients require both social support and medical support throughout their lives. Cardiac abnormalities as well as skeletal muscle wasting and myotonia are progressive and sometimes life-threatening. For congenital DM1, early death owing to respiratory deficiency can occur. Cognitive impairment is observed in all patients, but is severer in congenital DM1. There are many cases in which mothers with classic DM1 raise their children who have congenital DM1. Therefore, supporting healthy family members is also important.

DM1 is caused by expansion of the CTG triplet repeat within the 3′ untranslated region (UTR) of the *DMPK* gene. In recent years, it has been demonstrated that mRNA transcribed from an abnormally expanded repeat sequence affects the splicing of other mRNAs and causes various clinical symptoms. The number of CTG repeats within the *DMPK* gene in normal individuals is 5–34, and symptoms manifest when the repeats exceed 50. Individuals with 35–49 CTG repeats are asymptomatic (termed as a premutation), but if an expansion of repeat number occurs in their offspring, the offspring will manifest symptoms. This repeat expansion (also termed as anticipation) is more likely to occur when the mother is the premutation carrier, although there are a small number of cases in which the father was the premutation carrier. A larger number of repeats correlate with severer and earlier onset of disease. The age of onset and symptoms vary among individuals, but roughly 50–150 CTG repeats result in milder symptoms. Usually, up to 1000 CTG repeats are termed as the classic, or adult type, and more than 1000 repeats are termed as congenital DM1.

In mild cases, the mother may be diagnosed after her infant is diagnosed with congenital DM1. Pregnancy with a DM1 fetus often causes polyhydramnios, which is likely to result in premature birth. The use of ritodrine hydrochloride as a preventive treatment for possible premature birth can cause rhabdomyolysis, and therefore it is usually contraindicated for pregnant mothers with DM1. Magnesium sulfate is also usually contraindicated for pregnant mothers with DM1, because of the high risk of causing respiratory depression. In addition, at the time of caesarean section, care must be taken regarding the use of anesthetics and muscle relaxants, as the risk for atonic bleeding is higher in pregnant mothers with DM1.

During pregnancy, the mother's symptoms, such as muscle weakness, myotonia, and muscle pain may temporarily worsen, and other complications, such as placenta previa, urinary tract infections, and diabetes have also been reported. It is strongly recommended for pregnant women with DM1 to be transferred to a medical center that has well-equipped departments of neurology, and obstetrics and gynecology, as well as a neonatal intensive care unit.

8.6.2.1 Molecular Genetic Testing

Analysis of CTG repeat number in the *DMPK* gene by polymerase chain reaction (PCR), followed by visualization by Southern blotting (see Fig. 8.2a, b).

Regarding the recurrence rate, if the mother is affected, about 50% of her children will be normal, about 30% will have classic DM1, and about 20% will have congenital DM1. It has been suggested that if the first child has congenital DM1, subsequent affected children will also have congenital DM1 [23].

8.6.2.2 Prenatal Diagnosis

Owing to the limitation in the amount of genomic DNA that can be extracted from fetal tissue, triplet repeat-primed PCR (TP-PCR) is the preferred method for checking the presence or absence of an expanded allele. Expanded alleles cannot be detected by conventional PCR methods because the repeat length is too long to be amplified by conventional PCR (Fig. 8.2c). Therefore, repeat length analysis (fragment analysis) of the PCR products (Fig. 8.2d) only detects the normal alleles. On

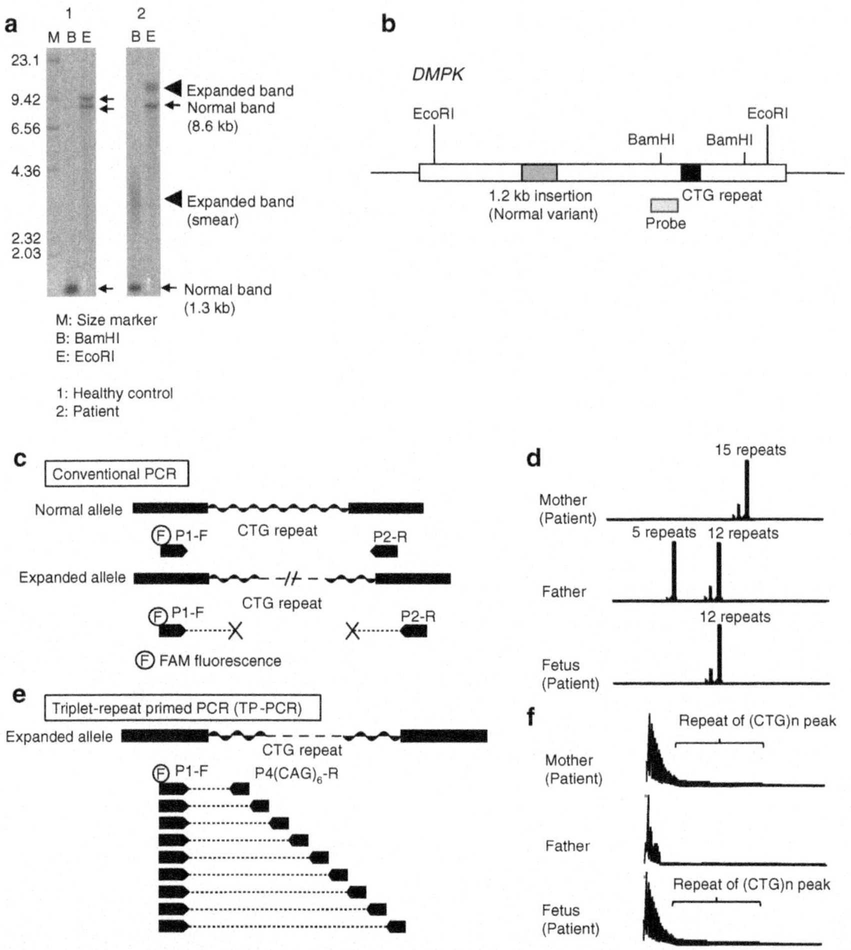

Fig. 8.2 Molecular diagnosis strategy for DM1. (**a**) Results of Southern blot analysis of a DM1 patient. Autoradiography images were kindly provided by Bio Medical Laboratory, Saitama, Japan. (**b**) Schema of restriction enzyme cleavage sites in the *DMPK* gene for Southern blot analysis of a DM1 patient. As there are polymorphisms in the EcoRI sites, there may be one or two bands. If there is an expanded repeat, smear bands are observed in the BamHI lane. As the size of the restriction enzyme fragment of BamHI in the normal allele is short, the distribution range of the expanded number of repeats will spread as a smear in the higher molecular weight region. (**c**) Diagram of genotyping by conventional PCR. The primers P1-F and P2-R bind to specific gene regions that closely flank the CTG repeat, and amplify only the normal alleles as only alleles with short repeat lengths can be amplified. For large alleles exceeding 100 CTG repeats, PCR using the primers P1-F and P2-R cannot amplify the product. (**d**) Fragment analysis of the patient and the parents by conventional PCR. The mother and the fetus were diagnosed as having DM1, so their expanded allele cannot be detected by conventional PCR. (**e**) Diagram of TP-PCR. Primer P4-(CTG)6-R can anneal to random complementary regions of the CTG tract within the *DMPK* gene. Specificity is dictated by the fluorescent locus-specific primer (P1). (**f**) In TP-PCR, the presence of an expanded allele can be identified by PCR amplification using CTG recognition primers of various sizes depending on the CAG sequences. The presence of the expanded allele is determined by detection of this (CTG)n repeat peaks. FAM, 6-carboxyfluorescein

the other hand, TP-PCR is able to detect a specific wave pattern in the expanded allele (Fig. 8.2e). However, this test has a limitation in that the exact CTG repeat length cannot be clarified [24]. Although conventional PCR can be utilized as a supportive diagnosis only when the repeat length of the two alleles differs between couples, combining TP-PCR and conventional PCR increases the accuracy of diagnosis (Fig. 8.2d).

The majority of congenital DM1 is of maternal origin, and it is generally suggested that the larger the number of repeats of the affected mother, the higher the chance of having congenital DM1. However, precise prediction of the age of onset is not possible [25], and it is difficult to accurately determine postnatal symptoms from the results of TP-PCR. Therefore, whether prenatal diagnosis is applicable or not should be determined for each case.

8.6.2.3 Preimplantation Diagnosis

Many cases of preimplantation diagnosis of DM1 have been reported by the Japan Society of Obstetrics and Gynecology. The number of CTG repeats considered to be appropriate to perform PGT is controversial, with 200–300 repeats generally being considered as borderline at present. For the reasons described in the prenatal diagnosis section, preimplantation diagnosis, which mainly determines the presence or absence of a disease, is a more favorable method for DM1 than prenatal diagnosis. Considering the risk of maternal symptom exacerbations owing to pregnancy, it may be helpful to provide information on preimplantation diagnosis by genetic counseling, according to the wishes of the family. However, PGT has the risk of allele drop-out (ADO) [26], which is a loss of one allele during PCR amplification of DNA, as the test has to be performed using genomic DNA with few copy numbers. ADO can hence lead to a misdiagnosis, and therefore great caution must be taken to ensure that the test results were obtained as a result of the biallelic amplification of both alleles.

It is important to increase the accuracy rate of genetic diagnosis of DM1 using the whole genome amplification method that has high amplification efficiency and high stability, by combining the direct method for the analysis of pathogenic variants and the indirect method by haplotype analysis using short tandem repeat.

8.6.3 FCMD

Form of inheritance: AR; responsible gene: *FKTN* on 9q31

FCMD is the second most common childhood muscular dystrophy in Japan. Symptoms include muscular dystrophy, and brain and eye anomalies. Disease onset is usually in early infancy or from the fetal stage, and brain MRI displays typical signs, such as a cobblestone appearance of the cerebral cortex, and cerebellar cysts. Ninety percent of FCMD patients do not gain ambulation, and the life expectancy is shorter than that of DMD patients. Complications include joint contractures, scoliosis, cardiomyopathy, and epilepsy. Intellectual disability is mild to severe. Patients hence require a large amount of support from their family. FCMD is caused by a 3-kb SINE-VNTR-*Alu* (SVA)-type retrotransposon insertion in the 3′-untranslated region of *FKTN*. This variant is thought to be a founder variant that was inherited from one Japanese ancestor approximately 100 generations ago. Therefore, FCMD is found almost exclusively in Japan, although there have been some reports that these founder mutations are also observed in China and Korea [27]. This is a splicing disease caused by the loss of function of the protein product, because the SVA insertion causes aberrant splicing, which accounts for almost all FCMD patients in Japan. Some patients have complex heterozygous mutations of retrotransposon insertion mutations and point mutations. The most frequent point mutation is one that causes abnormal splicing in intron 5 [28], and the second most frequent is a nonsense mutation caused by a point mutation in exon 3. Patients with compound heterozygous mutations have severer symptoms than the typical homozygous mutation. The *FKTN* gene product is a glycosyltransferase for ribitol 5-phosphoric acid, which is involved in the modification of α-dystroglycan, and FCMD belongs to a group of congenital α-dystroglycanopathies [29].

8.6.3.1 Molecular Genetic Diagnosis

Diagnosis is possible in approximately 87% of patients by checking the 3-kb retrotransposal insertion(s) by PCR. A definitive diagnosis is confirmed when an insertion mutation is found in one allele and muscle symptoms are observed. Other mutant alleles can be detected by commercial tests, or research base. Carrier genetic tests can also be performed by PCR, but health insurance does not cover the test. The carrier frequency is of 1 in 90 Japanese, and the recurrence rate of FCMD is 25% in siblings.

8.6.3.2 Prenatal Diagnosis

Prenatal genetic testing is indicated for families who wish to do so. Besides the identification of the founder 3-kb SVA insertion mutation by PCR, diagnosis is also confirmed by microsatellite DNA polymorphism analysis surrounding the *FKTN* gene region in affected children and fetuses (Fig. 8.3). Therefore, it is important to perform genetic counseling before pregnancy, analyze the variants in the parents and patients, and prepare for the prenatal diagnosis.

8.6.3.3 PGT

According to a report by the Japan Society of Obstetrics and Gynecology, PGT for FCMD has been approved and performed in a few cases. In addition to the above-mentioned diseases, prenatal diagnosis of merosin deficiency, muscle-eye-brain

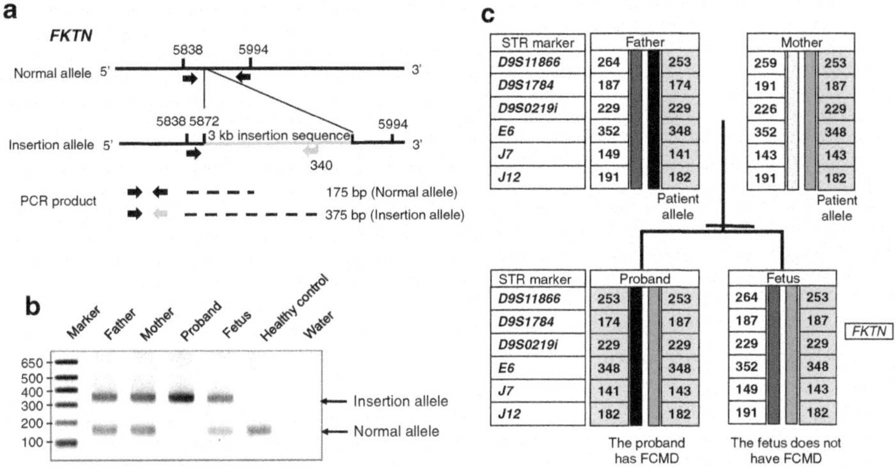

Fig. 8.3 Example of the prenatal diagnosis of FCMD. (**a**) Schema of insertion PCR for FCMD. Three primers are used in one reaction mixture to simultaneously detect both the normal and insertion alleles. One primer pair bridges the normal and insertion sequence, resulting in the amplification of a 375-bp product. The second pair generates a 157-bp product from the normal FKTN gene sequence [27]. (**b**) Results of electrophoresis of the insertion PCR products. Blood samples from the father and mother, and the fetus show two bands, suggesting that the parents were heterozygous carriers. The proband shows a single band, suggesting homozygosity of the insertion allele. (**c**) Haplotype analysis using short tandem repeats close to the FKTN gene. STR polymorphisms located close to the *FKTN* gene are used to determine the haplotype of the patient allele. The *FKTN* gene is located between *D9S1784* and the *D9S0219i*

disease, Walker-Warburg syndrome, and congenital muscular dystrophy types 1C and 1D, etc., has been performed in Europe and the United States. It is expected that the number of diseases for which prenatal diagnoses can be performed will increase in the future with the development of clinical tests [29].

8.7 Summary

In this chapter, we introduced the presently known genetic information regarding muscular dystrophies together with information regarding PGT for three representative muscular dystrophies. In recent years, gene therapy has become the first choice for some intractable diseases. Antisense oligonucleotide therapy and gene replacement therapy using AAV are also being tested in clinical trials. These treatments are mostly effective when introduced early in patients' lives [30, 31]. To provide efficient and timely treatments to patients, universal screening or newborn screening for the muscular dystrophies might help such patients to receive treatment earlier and more efficiently in the future. In some areas of the United States, as well as in Taiwan and China, prepregnancy carrier testing is provided to healthy couples upon request. Together with the advancements in preborn testing and preimplantation testing, radical treatments have become increasingly available for patients with muscular dystrophies. Therapies for more types of muscular dystrophies are expected to be developed in the near future. Therefore, newborn screening might help to identify patients before they manifest symptoms, so that they can receive treatment faster, leading to less complications and a higher quality of life [32–34]. However, it is also important to consider the other side of the meaning of genetic testing, as these tests might lead to the discrimination of carriers, or this information might affect family planning, or relationships, or the future lives of these patients. Therefore, it is very important to provide accurate information as well as appropriate knowledge, including ethical issues, and set up an adequate system for genetic counseling to provide such information.

Acknowledgments We would like to thank Dr. Yasuhiro Takeshima for advice on the diagnosis and genetic testing of DMD. We would like to thank Mr. Tatsuro Ikeda for drawing the figures and Helena Akiko Popiel for proofreading of the manuscript. Images of autoradiography in Fig. 8.2 were kindly provided by Bio Medical Laboratories, Inc. Our research introduced in this study was partially supported by AMED (to MTI, 18ek0109318h0001) and a Grant-in-aid for Scientific research (Kaken-hi 18K07790).

References

1. Mercuri E, et al. Muscular dystrophies. Lancet. 2019;394:2025–38.
2. Kang PB, et al. Evidence-based guideline summary: evaluation, diagnosis, and management of congenital muscular dystrophy: Report of the guideline development subcommittee of the American Academy of Neurology and the Practice Issues Review Panel of the American Association. Neurology. 2015;85:1432–3.
3. Fukuyama Y, et al. Congenital progressive muscular dystrophy of the Fukuyama type – clinical, genetic and pathological considerations. Brain and Development. 1981;3(1):1–29.
4. Minks J, et al. A skewed view of X chromosome inactivation. J Clin Invest. 2008;118:20–3.
5. Treatment for Spinal Muscular Atrophy (Cure SMA). https://www.curesma.org/treatment/
6. TREAT-NMD. Neuromuscular Network. https://treat-nmd.org/
7. Matsuo M, et al. Exon skipping during splicing of dystrophin mRNA precursor due to an intraexon deletion in the dystrophin gene of Duchenne muscular dystrophy Kobe. J Clin Invest. 1991;87:2127–31.
8. Van Deutekom JCT, Van Ommen GJB. Advances in Duchenne muscular dystrophy gene therapy. Nat Rev Genet. 2003;4:774–83.
9. Taniguchi-Ikeda M, et al. Pathogenic exon-trapping by SVA retrotransposon and rescue in Fukuyama muscular dystrophy. Nature. 2011;478:127–31.
10. Kobayashi K. An ancient retrotransposal insertion causes Fukuyama-type congenital muscular dystrophy. Nature. 1998;394:388–92.
11. Chamberlain, J. R. & Chamberlain, J. S. Progress toward gene therapy for Duchenne muscular dystrophy. Mol Ther 25, 1125–1131 (2017).
12. Miyatake S, et al. Anti-inflammatory drugs for Duchenne muscular dystrophy: focus on skeletal muscle-releasing factors. Drug Des Dev Ther. 2016;10:2745–58.
13. Registry of Muscular Dystrophy (REMUDY). http://www.remudy.jp/english/
14. The Japan Society of Human Genetics. Guidelines for genetic counseling and prenatal diagnosis. J Hum Genet. 1995;40(1)

15. Darras BT, et al. Dystrophinopathies summary genetic counseling GeneReview Scope. GeneReviews® 1–35 (2018).
16. Bushby K, et al. 107th ENMC International Workshop: the management of cardiac involvement in muscular dystrophy and myotonic dystrophy. 7th–9th June 2002, Naarden, the Netherlands. Neuromuscul Disord. 2003;13:166–72.
17. Takeshima Y, et al. Mutation spectrum of the dystrophin gene in 442 Duchenne/Becker muscular dystrophy cases from one Japanese referral center. J Hum Genet. 2010;55:379–88.
18. Birnkrant DJ, et al. Diagnosis and management of Duchenne muscular dystrophy, part 1: diagnosis, and neuromuscular, rehabilitation, endocrine, and gastrointestinal and nutritional management. Lancet Neurol. 2018;17:251–67.
19. Bakker E, et al. Germinal mosaicism increases the recurrence risk for 'new' Duchenne muscular dystrophy mutations. J Med Genet. 1989;26:553–9.
20. Guideline for the prenatal genetic tests for Neuromuscular Diseases from Japanese society of Neurology. https://www.neurology-jp.org/guidelinem/sinkei_gl.html
21. Japan PGT Consortium. http://www.fujita-hu.ac.jp/~japco/patient/pgd/index.html
22. Bird TD. Myotonic dystrophy type 1 summary genetic counseling suggestive findings. GeneReviews® 1–27 (2019).
23. Guidelines for consultation of muscular dystrophy. Nankodo, Japan. (2014).
24. Namba E. Genetic diagnosis of rare diseases and medical treatment of pediatric neurology. Brain Dev. 2018;50:183–8.
25. Sekizawa A, et al. Perinatal counseling manual. Japan: Chugai Medical Co.; 2015. p. 82–4.
26. Piyamongkol W. Detailed investigation of factors influencing amplication efficiency and allele drop-out in single cell PCR: implications for preimplantation genetic diagnosis. Mol Hum Reprod. 2003;9:411–20.
27. Watanabe M, et al. Founder SVA retrotransposal insertion in Fukuyama-type congenital muscular dystrophy and its origin in Japanese and Northeast Asian populations. Am J Med Genet. 2005;138 A:344–8.
28. Kobayashi K, et al. Deep-intronic variant of fukutin is the most prevalent point mutation of Fukuyama congenital muscular dystrophy in Japan. J Hum Genet. 2017;62:945–8.
29. Taniguchi-Ikeda M, et al. Mechanistic aspects of the formation of α-dystroglycan and therapeutic research for the treatment of α-dystroglycanopathy: a review. Mol Asp Med. 2016;51:115–24.
30. Sparks SE, et al. Congenital muscular dystrophy overview – ARCHIVED CHAPTER, FOR HISTORICAL REFERENCE ONLY. GeneReviews® (2012).
31. Finkel RS, et al. Treatment of infantile-onset spinal muscular atrophy with nusinersen: a phase 2, open-label, dose-escalation study. Lancet. 2016;388:3017–26.
32. Mendell JR, et al. Single-dose gene-replacement therapy for spinal muscular atrophy. N Engl J Med. 2017;377:1713–22.
33. Chien YH, et al. Presymptomatic diagnosis of spinal muscular atrophy through newborn screening. J Pediatr. 2017;190:124–9.
34. Su YN, et al. Carrier screening for spinal muscular atrophy (SMA) in 107,611 pregnant women during the period 2005-2009: a prospective population-based cohort study. PLoS One. 2011;6:1–7.

Chapter 9
Skeletal Dysplasia

Jun Murotsuki

Abstract Skeletal dysplasias are a heterogeneous group of more than 400 disorders that affect bone and cartilage growth. Skeletal dysplasias occur at a rate of 1 in 4000–5000 births. Prenatal diagnosis is clinically important because most of them develop from the prenatal period. The basis for the diagnosis of skeletal dysplasia disease is usually an X-ray examination. As the prenatal diagnosis of skeletal dysplasia is based on findings with ultrasound, we need to understand the difference between radiology and ultrasonography. Ultrasound images of bone are characterized by extremely high brightness. More than half of the power of the incident ultrasonic waves is reflected at the interface between soft tissue and bone, where the acoustic characteristic impedance is greatly different, that is, the surface of bone tissue.

Keywords Skeletal dysplasia · Prenatal diagnosis · Achondroplasia · Thanatophoric dysplasia · Osteogenesis imperfecta

9.1 Introduction

Skeletal dysplasias, also known as osteochondrodysplasias, are a heterogeneous group of more than 400 disorders that affect bone and cartilage growth. Skeletal dysplasias occur at a rate of 1 in 4000–5000 births. The condition is generally caused by spontaneous gene mutations or genetic abnormalities. The basis for the diagnosis of skeletal dysplasia disease is usually an X-ray examination. Although the prenatal diagnosis of skeletal dysplasia is based on findings with ultrasound, it remains challenging as radiography and ultrasonography differ fundamentally in the way images are made. We will discuss how to detect bone abnormalities by ultrasound, and the characteristics and prenatal diagnosis of some skeletal dysplasia. When observing the skeleton of the fetus with ultrasound, we must be aware of

J. Murotsuki (✉)
Department of Maternal and Fetal Medicine, Miyagi Children's Hospital, Miyagi, Japan
e-mail: murotsuki@miyagi-children.or.jp

H. Masuzaki (ed.), *Fetal Morph Functional Diagnosis*, Comprehensive Gynecology and Obstetrics, https://doi.org/10.1007/978-981-15-8171-7_9

these limitations. Ultrasonic diagnosis of achondroplasia, thanatophoric dysplasia, osteogenesis imperfecta, asphyxia dysplasia, etc. will be explained in detail.

9.2 Ultrasonic Characteristics

Because ultrasonography has the advantages of rapidity and easy accessibility, and no radiation exposure so that it could be useful for close examination of the fetus. However, there are various limitations in observing fetal bones by ultrasonography. The presence of bones can be confirmed definitely in ultrasound images, but it is difficult to obtain information on the deeper parts. Ultrasound images of bone are characterized by extremely high brightness. More than half of the power of the incident ultrasonic waves is reflected at the interface between soft tissue and bone, where the acoustic characteristic impedance is greatly different, that is, the surface of bone tissue. Besides, since the ultrasonic waves are greatly attenuated inside the bone and it is difficult to reach deeper areas, acoustic shadows will appear.

Ultrasound images from the skin to the surface layer of the bone of the fetus, and in particular, the outline of the bone is drawn. A slight depth can be seen on the image of the bone surface echo, and at first glance, it seems to depict the thickness of the bone (diaphysis) itself. But in reality, this is only an artifact. This is considered to be the result of so-called tailing because ultrasonic vibration does not end immediately, and multiple reflections occurring between the soft tissues just above the bone. We must understand these phenomena and interpret bone images.

The tissue in which the ultrasound is strongly reflected in the fetal limbs is bone, and its contour of the surface is depicted with high brightness. The tissues that transmit and partially reflect ultrasonic waves are soft tissues and cartilage, which include periosteum, fascia, and joint capsule. The tissue that does not reflect ultrasonic waves is hyaline cartilage, which corresponds to head cartilage and trochanteric cartilage of the femur.

9.3 Detection of Bone Abnormalities

9.3.1 Observation and Measurement of Long Bones

The echo gain should be adjusted so that the femoral head cartilage becomes almost echoless. To observe the bone in as much detail as possible, use the zoom function so that the image is enlarged on the monitor. First, the long bone diaphysis is visualized so that it is perpendicular to the ultrasonic beam, that is, horizontal to the screen. To carefully observe the entire diaphysis, scan the probe so that it is as perpendicular to the beam direction as possible. After that, we move to the observation of metaphysis. The ultrasound image is drawn diagonally on the screen so that the diaphysis makes an angle with the ultrasound beam so that the ultrasound waves enter the metaphyseal part.

To evaluate whether or not there is bone shortening, it is necessary to measure all extremity long bones. In the diagnosis of fetal skeletal dysplasia, most of them are screened by shortening femur length (FL). Previous reports [1, 2] have suggested that there is a risk of fetal skeletal dysplasia when the length of long bone is −2 SD or less. However, clinically, if screening is performed at FL −2 SD or lower, the number of subjects to be examined will be too large. It is practical to set it at −4 SD or lower.

It is necessary to all the long bones of the limbs, that is, humerus, ulna, radius, femur, tibia, and fibula are measured. Although it would be difficult to distinguish the ulna and radius, and the tibia and fibula on the ultrasound, the proximal ones are distinguished as ulna and tibia by the trunk. The first step in the differential diagnosis of fetal skeletal dysplasia is to measure and record all long bones of the fetus, preferably both left and right. Several normal development curves of fetal long bones have been published [3, 4]. However, it should be noted that there are racial differences in the normal values of limb length.

9.3.2 Observation of Other Bones

We would examine the shape and the degree of ossification of the head. Cloverleaf skull is found in the cases of thanatophoric dysplasia (TD) and campomelic dysplasia (CD). If the skull has ossification deficiency, the fetal skull could be easily deformed by the ultrasonic probe pressure from the maternal abdominal wall. In such cases, Osteogenesis imperfect (OI) type II or hypophosphatasia (HPP) is suspected. In a series of diseases in which endochondral ossification is selectively affected and membranous ossification is not abnormal, characteristic findings such as a large skull, frontal boss frontal bossing, nasal recess, and mandibular protrusion are shown. These are *FGFR3*-pathy such as achondroplasia (ACH) and TD.

Thoracic hypoplasia is present in many skeletal dysplasias and is an important finding closely related to postnatal prognosis. Thoracic circumference (TC) is defined by the circumference of the thorax in which the four-chamber cross-section is depicted. Based on the morphology of the chest, it is classified as extremely small (TD), extremely short ribs (short-rib dysplasia; SRD), and multiple rib fractures and deformities (OI type II).

9.3.3 Abnormal Findings of Long Bone

1. Fractures

Osteogenesis imperfect (OI) is a typical disease that causes fractures in utero. Figure 9.1 shows the ultrasound images of the tibia, femur, and ribs of three fetal cases of OI type II. The long bone is significantly shortened and deformed by

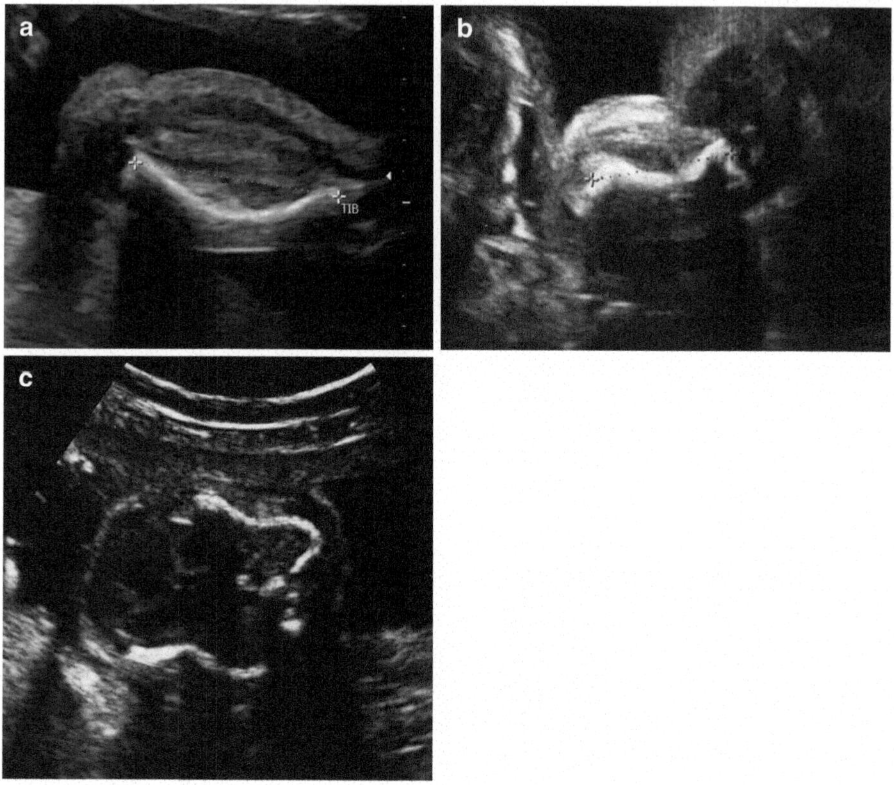

Fig. 9.1 Fetal fractures affecting long bones and ribs. (**a**) Fractured tibia at 30 weeks' gestation. (**b**) Fractured femur at 28 weeks' gestation. (**c**) Fractured ribs at 21 weeks' gestation

repeated fractures and healing in the womb (Fig. 9.1a, b). It is observed that the morphology of the long bones of the fetus changes with time throughout pregnancy. Rib fractures could also be seen (Fig. 9.1c). Intrauterine fractures occur less frequently except for OI type II.

2. Bowing or angulation

TD, CD, SRD, and HPP are among the diseases that show the bending of long bones. It has been reported that postnatal X-ray findings show femoral bowing (including those due to fractures) in 24.4% of cases of CD, 23.9% of cases of TD, 18.1% of cases of OI, 10.2% of cases of SRD, and 3.5% of cases of HPPs [5].

The long bone is remarkably curved in TD, especially in type I. A telephone-receiver deformity is a characteristic bowing of the shaft of the long bones, usually the humeri or femora, seen in TD in a frontal X-ray image. However, it is not easy to express this diagnostic finding on an ultrasound image. Since the ultrasonic image is a reflection image, the apparent image changes greatly depending on the direction of the ultrasonic wave incident on the significantly deformed femur. The curvature might be often not visible in the two-dimensional image

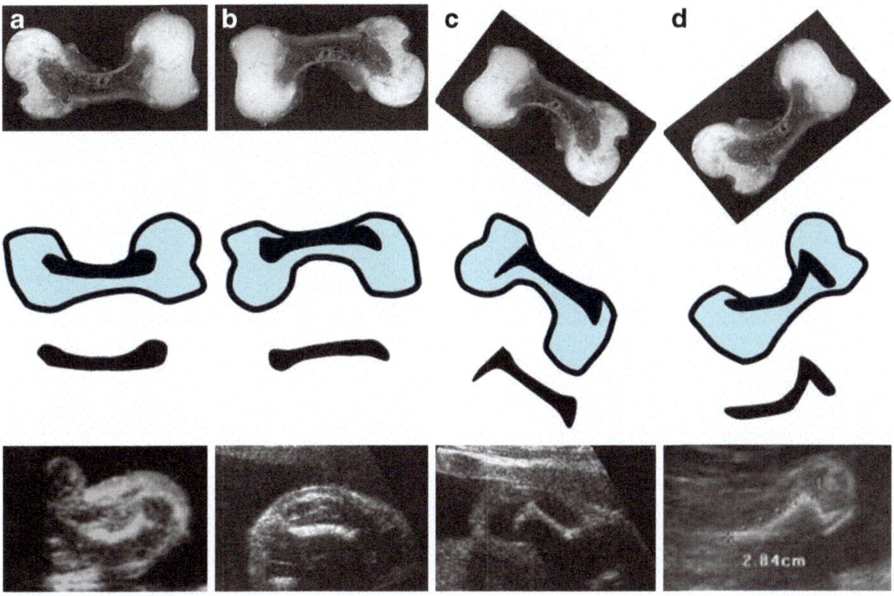

Fig. 9.2 All four ultrasound images were of the same fetus. As shown in (**a**), the ultrasound image from the medial side of the femur with large curvature looks like a telephone receiver. But when the ultrasound beam is incident from the outside, the bending of the femur is small and only the shortening is emphasized (**b**). In addition, the finding of cupping at the end of the bone trunk is clearly visible when ultrasound is injected from an oblique angle (**c**, **d**)

obtained by the usual ultrasound. If you look at the donut from its side, it looks like a club.

All four ultrasound pictures in Fig. 9.2 are femur images of the same fetus. As shown in Fig. 9.2a, the ultrasound image from the inside of the femur with large curvature looks like a telephone receiver. But when ultrasonic beams are incident from the outside, the curve is small and only the shortening is emphasized (Fig. 9.2b). Similarly, when ultrasonic beams are incident at an angle, the findings of the metaphyseal cupping appear clearly (Fig. 9.2c, d). It should be noted that the findings of the femur are completely different depending on the direction of ultrasound.

The characteristic ultrasonic findings of campomelic dysplasia (CD) are bilaterally symmetrical femoral bowing (Fig. 9.3a). However, long bone bending may be difficult to distinguish from the single fractures (Fig. 9.3b) sometimes seen in OI. Unlike the curvature that is a characteristic of the disease itself such as CD and TD, the deformity after fracture is recognized as fracture and regeneration in radiographs. That is, not only the bending but also the thickening of that part during the healing process. It is important to carefully evaluate the local area with ultrasound while imagining the X-ray findings. A curve peculiar to the disease appears to have a steep curve with the shape of V (dogleg) (Fig. 9.3c). The shape of the bone would seem to be U in the fracture of the long bone (Fig. 9.3d).

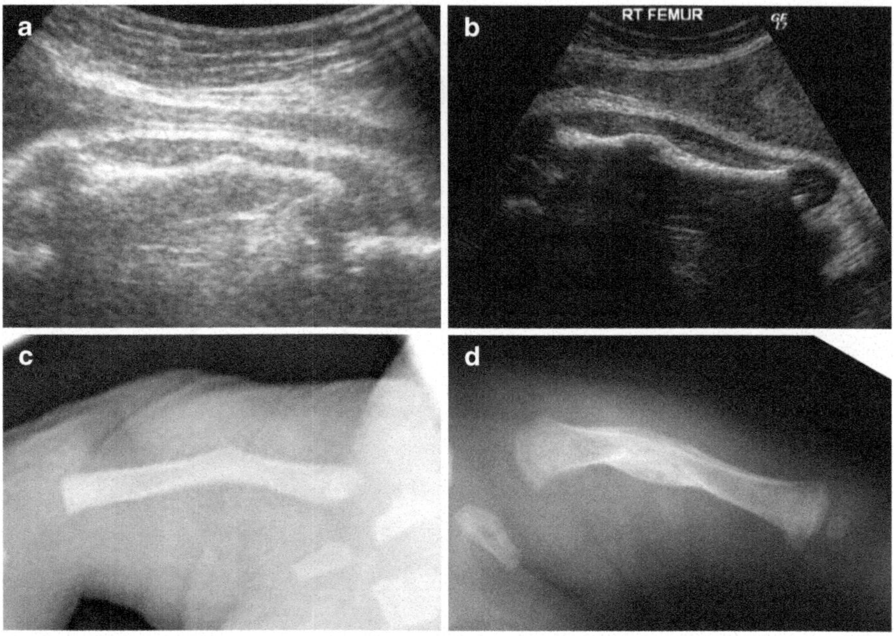

Fig. 9.3 (**a**, **c**) Bending deformities of the femur in campomelic dysplasia, (**b**, **d**) fractures of the femur in osteogenesis imperfecta. The bent portion would be slightly raised if there is a reconstructed image (**b**)

3. Poor ossification

Skeletal dysplasias showing poor ossification include OI, HP, and achondrogenesis (ACG). The evaluation of ossification would be often subjective because ultrasonography is a highly operator dependent modality. It is known that an ultrasound probe deforms when the fetal skull is pressed as a finding suggesting poor ossification (Fig. 9.4a). However, it should be noted that even normal fetuses might have shown the same finding due to mere immaturity.

Figure 9.4b is an image of the femur of a fetus with perinatal hypophosphatasia. The ultrasonic intensity at both ends of the diaphysis and metaphysis is slightly lower. Then, acoustic enhancement of ultrasonic beams occurs toward the deep part of the body [6]. This peculiar ultrasonic pattern is considered to reflect the poor ossification of the femur. The area around the center of the diaphysis is ossified to some extent and appears to have high brightness. However, ossification becomes worse at both ends of the femoral shaft, and since ultrasonic beams do not reflect much on the bone surface and pass through the bone, the bone matrix and the cartilage-massed part appear to be a soft and thick image. This is a very interesting finding.

4. Various metaphyseal changes

Metaphyseal changes are defined as cupping, splaying, or flaring. Many skeketal dysplasias present with these findings, such as ACH, TD, ACG, Kniest dysplasia,

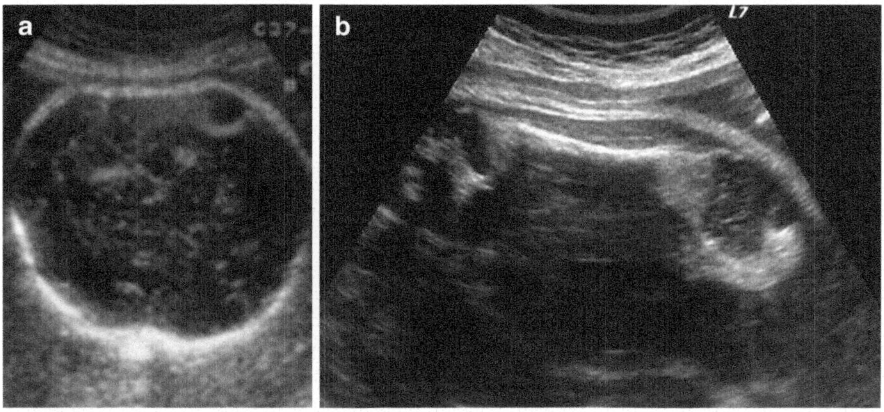

Fig. 9.4 (a) It is known that an ultrasound probe deforms when the fetal skull is pressed as a finding suggesting poor ossification in osteogenesis imperfecta. (b) is an image of the femur of a fetus with perinatal hypophosphatasia, with acoustic enhancement due to the poor ossification of both ends of the femur

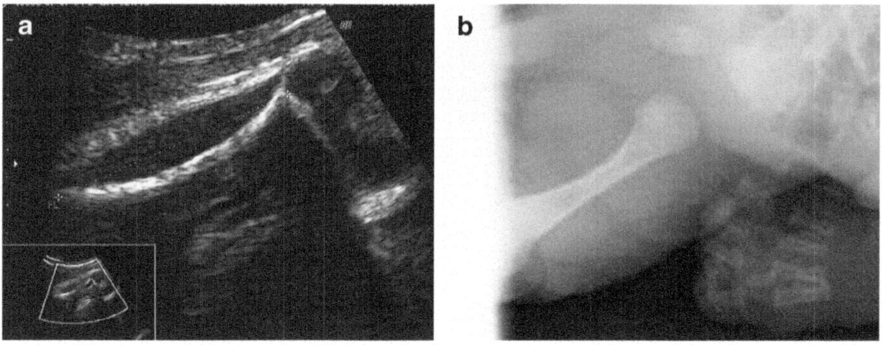

Fig. 9.5 The ultrasound image (a) and the postnatal X-ray image (b) of the femur in the case of spondyloepiphyseal dysplasia congenital (SEDC). The ultrasound probe is slightly tilted so that the ultrasound beam is injected into the metaphysis of the femur

metamorphic dysplasia, and congenital spondyloepiphyseal dysplasia congenital (SEDC).

To closely examine the long bones of the fetus, they are usually placed as perpendicular as possible to the direction of the beam. On the other hand, to observe the metaphysis, i.e., in the direction of the bone thickness, the diaphysis is intentionally moved in the direction of the ultrasound beam. Figure 9.5 compares the ultrasound image with the postnatal X-ray image of the femur in the case of SEDC. The ultrasound probe is slightly tilted so that the ultrasound beam is injected into the metaphysis of the femur.

5. Stippled epiphysis

There is a group of diseases showing punctate calcification in the epiphyseal nucleus or the soft tissue around the epiphyseal nucleus on radiographs. These are

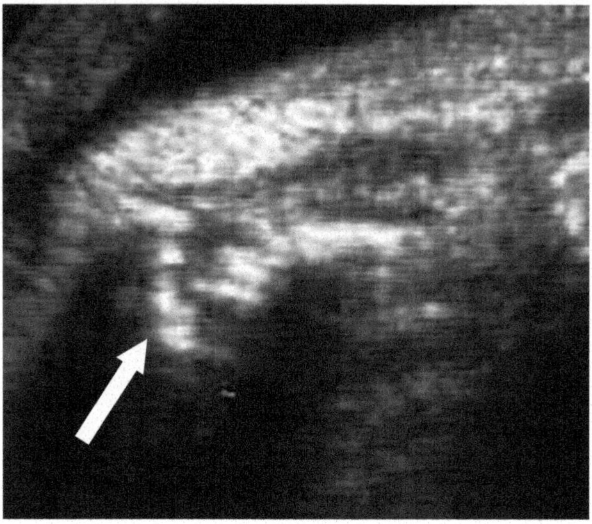

Fig. 9.6 Stippling proximal humeral epiphysis (arrow) in the case of chondrodysplasia punctata, tibial-metaphyseal type

collectively called chondrodysplasia punctata (CDP). Conradi-Hunermann type, which is relatively frequent, and rhizomelic chondrodysplasia punctata (RCDP) with marked shortening of the proximal limb, are well known.

Even punctate calcification, which can be easily observed in X-ray, may be difficult to visualize by ultrasonography. Fine calcifications like sand granuloma cannot be visualized at a size below the ultrasonic resolution, but large calcifications can be visualized (Fig. 9.6). Attention must be paid to these findings of epiphysis.

9.4 Skeletal Dysplasias

In the latest international classification [7], 463 diseases in 42 groups are registered as bone system diseases. It is known that the majority of the diseases among them develop from the fetal period. The following discussion presents a few of the most common disorders relevant to prenatal diagnosis.

9.4.1 Thanatophoric Dysplasia

Thanatophoric dysplasia (TD) is the most common skeletal dysplasia that can be differentiated at birth, with a frequency of 1 in 6000–17,000 deliveries. The prognosis for life is poor, with most deaths occurring within hours of birth due to respiratory failure. But recently, the survival of cases ranging from 1 week to several months has been reported. It has a marked limb shortening, a large head compared

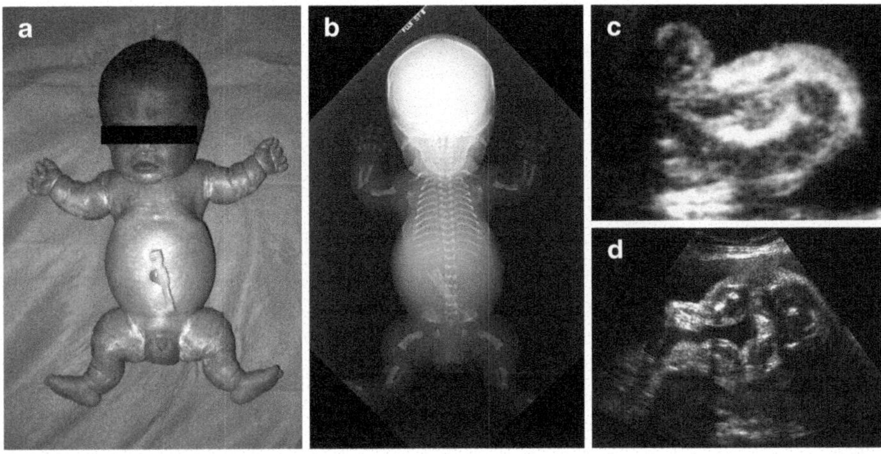

Fig. 9.7 Thanatophoric dysplasia. (**a**) Clinical photograph of a stillborn infant. Comparatively large head with frontal bossing, protuberant abdomen, and thickened soft tissues with the redundancy of the skin of extremities. (**b**) Radiograph of the fetus. Large skull, narrow thorax, and short thick bowed tubular bones of extremities. (**c**) Short femur with the appearance of a telephone receiver. (**d**) The marionette-like posture of the lower limb with thickened soft tissue

to trunk, a narrow and small chest, and distended abdomen (Fig. 9.7a). The limbs are always in an extended position, which is the so-called marionette-like posture. It is characterized by wrinkled walls due to excess skin on the extremities.

It is a group of diseases caused by heterozygous mutations in the *FGFR3* (fibroblast growth factor receptor 3) gene. Except for parental gonadal mosaicism, almost all cases occur as a mutation and are terminated in the same generation, so that so it does not affect the next pregnancy. X-rays show shortening and bending of long bones, metaphyseal cupping, and iliac hypoplasia. The vertebra is flattened and shows an inverted U or H shape. The findings of the femur are an important distinction and are called telephone-receiver deformity (Fig. 9.7b).

Prenatal ultrasound findings showed marked reductions in both femoral and humerus length, but the biparietal diameter (BPD) was larger than usual. The telephone-receiver deformity of the femur is a diagnostic finding on X-ray images, but it is not always observable on ultrasound (Fig. 9.7c). In order to diagnose TD by ultrasonography, not only the deformation of long bones but also the head, face, thorax to the abdomen, and the positions of the extremities are comprehensively judged.

Among those findings, the clover-like skull and the wrinkled wall of the skin are particularly characteristic. The clover-like skull is caused by the bulge of the temporal region due to the early closure of the cranial suture. Type II is defined as the case in which marked clover-like deformity is observed. But careful observation reveals that even type I is often mildly deformed. The wrinkled wall of the skin of the extremities is caused by a shortening of bones and excessive skin development, and the findings can be easily captured by ultrasound (Fig. 9.7d). Polyhydramnios is almost inevitable, but growth retardation is less common.

9.4.2 Achondroplasia

Achondroplasia (ACH) is a typical skeletal dysplasia with a good prognosis, with an incidence of about 1 in 10,000 births. It is caused by *FGFR3* gene abnormality similar to TD. It has an autosomal dominant inheritance pattern. When both parents have ACH, the infant has a 25% chance of homozygous achondroplasia, of which phenotype is very similar to TD with a poor prognosis.

The skull is large, the frontal part of the head protrudes, and the root of the nose is depressed. Shortening of the extremities, especially the proximal limbs, is observed. However, these characteristics are often overlooked at birth, and ACH is often pointed out for the first time at infant screening. On radiographs, the tubular bones of the extremities are thick and short, and the diaphyseal cupping is remarkable (Fig. 9.8a). The diagnostic finding is square or oval radiolucent areas in proximal femur and humerus. The iliac bones are rectangular due to a lack of iliac flaring.

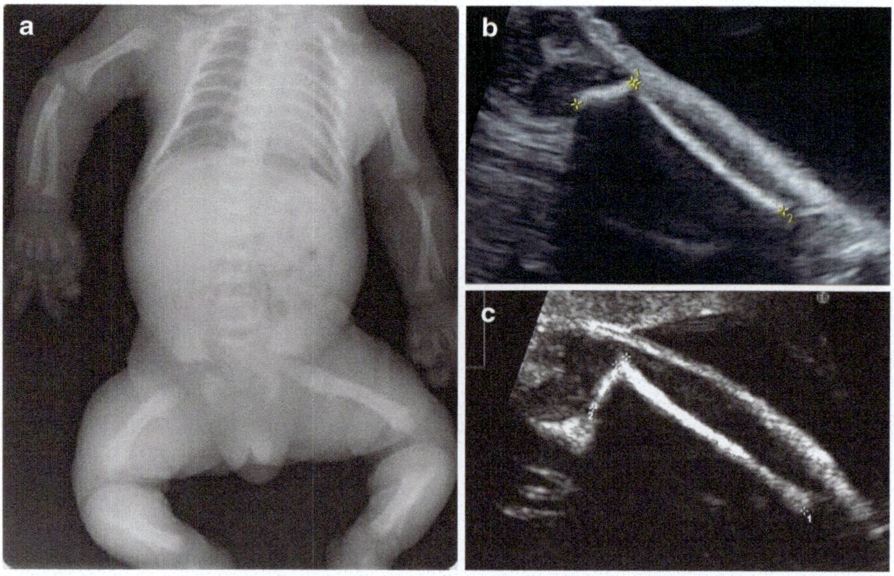

Fig. 9.8 Achondroplasia. (**a**) On radiographs, the tubular bones of the extremities are thick and short, and the diaphyseal cupping is remarkable. Note the oval transradiancy of proximal femora and sloping metaphyses. (**b**) The diaphysis and the proximal metaphysis are depicted in ultrasound. Achondroplasia is characterized by a large angle between the diaphysis and metaphysis (collar hoop sign). (**c**) The femur of a normal fetus in ultrasound

On ultrasound examination at ACH, limb shortening can occur as early as 21 weeks of gestation and as late as 27 weeks of pregnancy [8]. Although there is rhizomelic shortening with predominantly proximal long bone, ossification is normal and fractures and curves are not observed. Achondroplasia is characterized by a large angle between the diaphysis and metaphysis (collar hoop sign) (Fig. 9.8b), compared to them of a normal fetus (Fig. 9.8c), when they are depicted in ultrasound. Head circumference is slightly enlarged, but thoracic hypoplasia is not apparent. The onset of the disease is missed in the fetal period because there are few prominent findings on ultrasonography other than limb shortening. It has been reported that the trident hand recognized by ultrasound was a clue for diagnosis [9].

9.4.3 Achondrogenesis

Achondrogenesis (ACG) has a distinctive appearance of strongly shortened limbs, disproportionately large head, short neck and trunk, and abdominal distention (Fig. 9.9a). X-rays show a lack of ossification in the vertebral body, ischia, and pubis. Thorax is barrel-shaped with ribs running horizontally and its anterior end enlarged. The limbs are significantly shortened, and the metaphysis is deformed into a sawtooth shape. Rib fractures may occur.

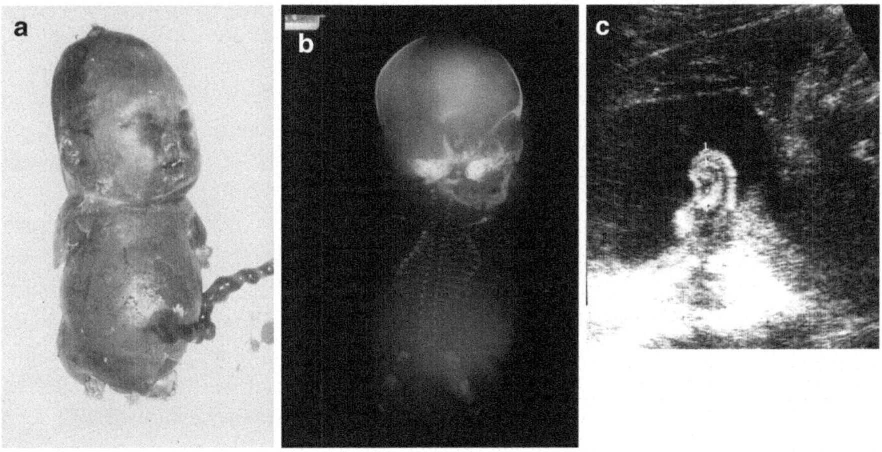

Fig. 9.9 Achondrogenesis type IB. 1220 g boy of 34 weeks gestation. (**a**) External aspect immediately after stillbirth. It presents with characteristic appearances such as strongly shortened limbs and disproportionately large head, short neck and trunk, and abdominal distention. (**b**) Whole-body radiograph. A large skull and marked shortening and deformation of the long bone are observed. Vertebral body ossification is minimal. (**c**) The femur is extremely shortened and deformed so that it is difficult to identify by ultrasound

Although the classification of ACG has changed over the years, it is now classified into type I (Fig. 9.9b), which has strong iliac and long bone deformation, and type II, which has moderate deformation. Both are extremely rare diseases, with about 1 in 75,000 births in both types combined. It is the worst skeletal dysplasia, and all are stillborn or die soon after birth. The genetic form of type I is autosomal recessive, and type II is autosomal dominant.

Ultrasonography showed extremely short limbs, and in some cases, the femur could not be visualized (Fig. 9.9c). The head is extremely large, and the skull shows mild ossification. The spine and iliac bones are also poorly visualized. There are significant growth retardation and polyhydramnios and often had fetal hydrops.

9.4.4 Osteogenesis Imperfecta Type II/III

Osteogenesis imperfecta (OI) refers to a group of genetic disorders of the systemic connective tissue, characterized by easily fractured bones, blue sclera, and deafness. It is classified into several types depending on the clinical symptoms, but type II, which develops during the fetal period and already has multiple fractures and deformities at birth, has the most severe symptoms. Special attention should be paid to perinatal management because it often causes death from the neonatal period to the infancy period. Type III shows multiple fractures in the uterus and a membranous skull and may be similar to type II, but the morphology remains the shape of long bones and can be said to be mild. However, repeated bone fractures after birth show severe limb deformity. In this section, type II and type III are explained together, and type I and type IV are taken up in the next section.

Type II and III together occur at a rate of 1 case per 25,000 births. Mutations in the type I collagen genes (*COL1A1* and *COL1A2*), which are the main components of bone and soft tissue matrix, have been attributed. Most of them are autosomal dominant, but it has been conventionally believed that sibling recurrence due to gonadal mosaicism is about 7%. Recently, however, more than 20 other causative genes for osteogenesis imperfecta besides COL1A1 and COL1A2 genes have been found, demonstrating the presence of an autosomal recessive OI.

Marked limb deformation and bell-shaped thoracic hypoplasia due to multiple fractures are observed. The skull is soft due to poor ossification and is often accompanied by the blue sclera. X-rays show multiple fractures of the long bones such as limbs and ribs, and accordion-like deformations and shortening are observed.

On ultrasound examination, there were clear fractures, flexion, shortening, and secondary thickening of the femur and humerus (Fig. 9.1). The skull is soft and membranous due to poor ossification and can be easily deformed by the pressure of the ultrasonic probe (Fig. 9.4a). Multiple fractures and deformations of the ribs cause a bell-shaped deformation of the rib cage. Mild intrauterine growth retardation is present, but polyhydramnios is not common.

9.4.5 *Osteogenesis Imperfecta Type I/IV*

OI is one of the most common skeletal dysplasia, but the frequency of type I and type IV excluding type II and type III is about 1 in 25,000. The current classification is based on the clinical picture and genetics as reported by Sillence et al. [10]. Type I shows blue sclera and comparatively mild bone changes and is often diagnosed during early childhood due to easy fracture. Long bones are thin due to over modeling and curved due to fractures. Type IV presents with the white sclera and is generally mild. However, the range of symptoms is wide, and there are a few cases with intrauterine fractures (Fig. 9.3b).

Type I is rarely diagnosed prenatally, but the echogenicity of bone may be reduced due to delayed ossification. Type IV is similar to type I and is often found postnatally, but may be noticed during fetal life because of a single fracture or slight bending of the long bone (Fig. 9.3b). Since spontaneous bone fractures are extremely rare in normal fetuses, OI should be suspected first if there is a single fracture finding.

9.4.6 *Asphyxiating Thoracic Dysplasia*

Asphyxiating thoracic dysplasia (ATD), also known as Jeune syndrome, is an autosomal recessive genetic disease that occurs in 1 in 100,000–130,000 births.

Chest hypoplasia is characteristic (Fig. 9.10a), but the prognosis ranges from those with severe respiratory failure in the neonatal period to those with almost no symptoms. In the X-ray image, it is conspicuous that a narrow thorax with bell shapes due to marked shortened ribs and short fingers and toes (Fig. 9.10b).

Chest hypoplasia and polyhydramnios were visible on ultrasound (Fig. 9.10c). The shortening of long bones is mild. When polydactyly is observed, Short-rib polydactyly syndrome (SRPS) and Ellis-van Creveld dysplasia, which are closely related diseases, are suspected. These are a series of diseases forming one skeletal dysplasia family as short-rib dysplasia group.

9.5 Conclusions

A certain diagnosis of fetal skeletal dysplasias is still a challenge. Ultrasonography is always the fundamental screening examination for fetal assessment in skeletal dysplasia. The fetal imagining through conventional ultrasound could underlie the prenatal diagnosis of fetal skeletal dysplasia. However, a certain diagnosis cannot be accurate and complete without the contribution of genetics or fetal computed tomography in the future.

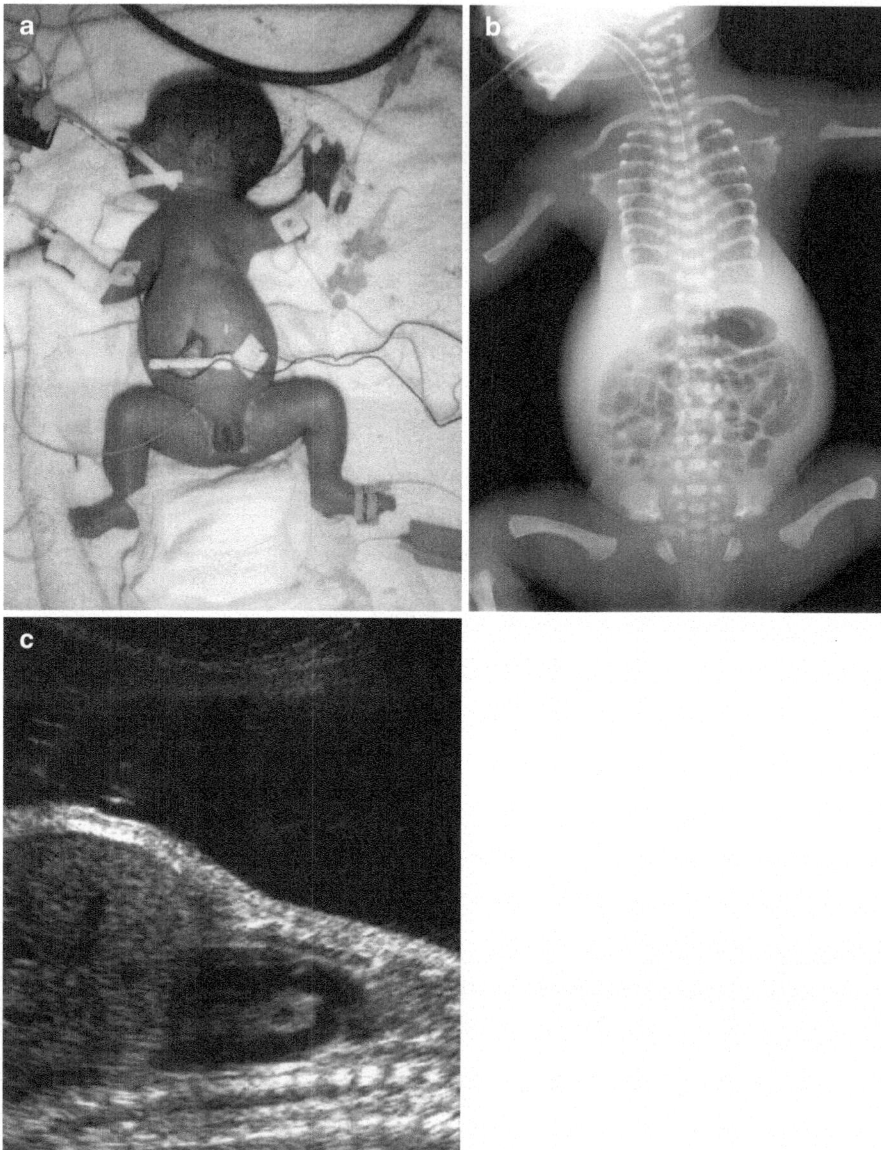

Fig. 9.10 Asphyxiating thoracic dysplasia. 1498 g girl of 33 weeks gestation. (**a**) The extremely narrow thorax and swollen abdomen are noticeable. (**b**) Extremely short, horizontal ribs show thoracic hypoplasia. (**c**) The thorax is extremely small compared to the abdomen, with long and narrow shape. Most have polyhydramnios during late pregnancy

References

1. Filly RA, Golbus MS, Carey JC, et al. Short-limed dwarfism: ultrasonographic diagnosis by mensuration of fetal femoral length. Radiology. 1981;138:653–6.
2. Kurtz AB, Needleman L, Wapner RJ, et al. Usefulness of a short femur in the in utero detection of skeletal dysplasias. Radiology. 1990;177:197–200.
3. Merz E, Kim-Kern MS, Pehl S. Ultrasonic mensuration of fetal limb bones in the second and third trimesters. J Clin Ultrasound. 1987;15:175–83.
4. Romero R, Athanassiadis AP, Jeanty P. Fetal skeletal anomalies. Radiol Clin North Am. 1990;28:75–99.
5. Alanay Y, Krakow D, Rimoin DL, et al. Angulated femurs and the skeletal dysplasias: experience of the International Skeletal Dysplasia Registry (1988-2006). Am J Med Genet Part A. 2007;143A:1159–68.
6. Brasseur-Daudruy M, Ickowicz V, Degre S, et al. Hyperechoic metaphyses in hypophosphatasia: what does it mean? Pediatr Radiol. 2008;38:340–3.
7. Mortier GR, Cohn DH, Cormier-Daire V, et al. Nosology and classification of genetic skeletal disorders: 2019 revision. Am J Genet A. 2019;179:2393–419.
8. Kurtz AB, Filly RA, Wapner RJ, et al. In utero analysis of heterozygous achondroplasia: variable time of onset as detected by femur length measurements. J Ultrasound Med. 1986;5:137–40.
9. Guzman ER, Day-Salvatore D, Westover T, et al. Prenatal ultrasonographic demonstration of the trident hand in heterozygous achondroplasia. J Ultrasound Med. 1994;13:63–6.
10. Sillence DO, Senn A, Danks DM. Genetic heterogeneity in osteogenesis imperfecta. J Med Genet. 1979;16:101–16.

Chapter 10
Genitourinary Tract Abnormalities

Takashi Kaji

Abstract Genitourinary tract abnormalities include various types of congenital diseases. Hence, this chapter concentrates on ultrasound-based fetal diagnosis of the main genitourinary tract abnormalities.

Urinary tract dilation (UTD) is one of the most common findings diagnosed prenatally. Currently, UTD is assessed based on the anteroposterior diameter of the fetal renal pelvis, the Society for Fetal Urology grading system, and the UTD classification. UTD is usually a transient physiological state; however, it can be caused by urinary tract obstruction, such as ureteropelvic junction obstruction or vesicoureteral reflux. Severe obstruction of the urinary tract damages the kidneys and may cause urinoma or obstructive renal dysplasia. In a duplicated collecting system, dilation of the upper pole and normal appearance of the lower pole moieties are key features for prenatal diagnosis. It is also important to identify the presence of ureterocele in the bladder. The pelvic kidney is located in close proximity to the bladder; however, its identification is often missed on prenatal ultrasound. Multicystic dysplastic kidney (MCDK) usually manifests as a large multicystic mass in the renal fossa. Absence of normal parenchyma and collecting system is the key to differentiating MCDK from severe UTD.

Fetal lower urinary tract obstruction is mainly caused by posterior urethral valves. The distended bladder and dilated posterior urethra (keyhole sign) with bilateral UTD are suggestive of posterior urethral valves.

The differential diagnosis of adrenal masses includes neuroblastoma and adrenal hemorrhage. Diagnosis may be difficult because neuroblastomas occasionally appear as cystic masses.

Fetal hypospadias is usually detected based on the ventral curvature and/or blunting of the penis. The uncovered tip of the penis with foreskin can lead to the suspicion of hypospadias. Gray-scale ultrasonography may locate the ventral opening of the urinary meatus by visualizing the urinary stream during fetal micturition, which leads to a definite diagnosis.

T. Kaji (✉)
Department of Obstetrics and Gynecology, Institute of Biomedical Sciences, Tokushima University Graduate School, Tokushima, Japan
e-mail: tkaji@tokushima-u.ac.jp

H. Masuzaki (ed.), *Fetal Morph Functional Diagnosis*, Comprehensive Gynecology and Obstetrics, https://doi.org/10.1007/978-981-15-8171-7_10

Fetal ovarian cysts usually manifest in the third trimester. Ovarian cysts generally appear as simple cysts, which are anechoic, unilocular, and thin-walled. The "daughter cyst" sign is reported to be pathognomonic of ovarian cysts. On the other hand, fetal ovarian cysts that exhibit internal echoic fluid, fluid-fluid levels, and septations are considered to be complicated cysts. The complicated cysts indicate torsion of the ovary.

Keywords Urinary tract dilation · Urinoma · Obstructive renal dysplasia Duplicated collecting system · Pelvic kidney · Multiple dysplastic kidney (MCDK) Posterior urethral valve · Neuroblastoma · Hypospadias · Ovarian cyst

10.1 Fetal Ultrasound Imaging of the Normal Genitourinary Tract

The fetal kidneys are visualized on both sides of the lumbar spine. They usually appear as relatively hyperechoic structures in the first trimester of pregnancy. Visualization of the renal arteries by color Doppler can facilitate their identification. Renal echogenicity decreases with advancing gestational age. Sonographic corticomedullary differentiation is more evident in the third trimester because the medulla becomes more hypoechoic than the cortex does (Fig. 10.1). The fetal bladder can be visualized in the first trimester.

The cervix of the uterus can be identified in the third trimester. The cervix appears as a hyperechoic oval structure surrounded by hypoechoic portion between

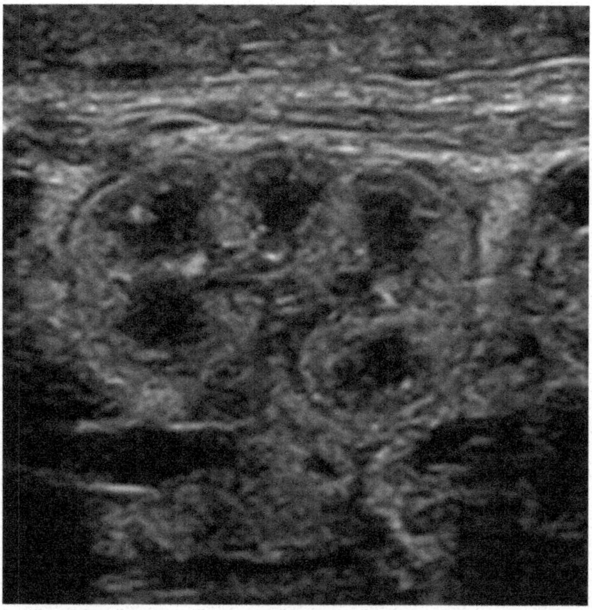

Fig. 10.1 Normal fetal kidney at 28 weeks. Corticomedullary differentiation is evident because the medulla is significantly hypoechoic in the third trimester

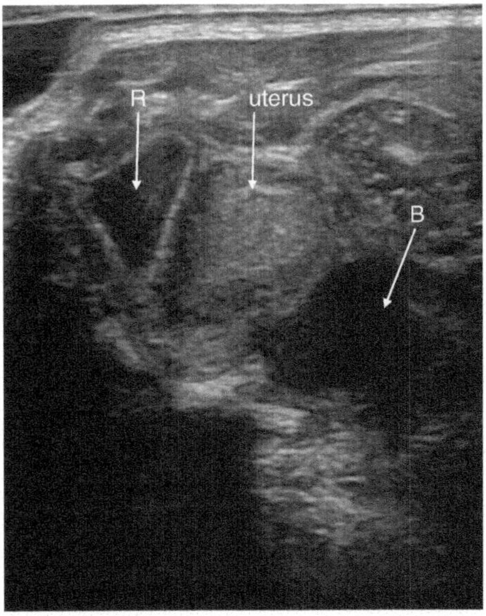

Fig. 10.2 Normal fetal uterus at 26 weeks. The cervix appears as a hyperechoic oval structure surrounded by hypoechoic portion between the bladder (B) and rectum (R) on the transverse view of the fetal pelvis

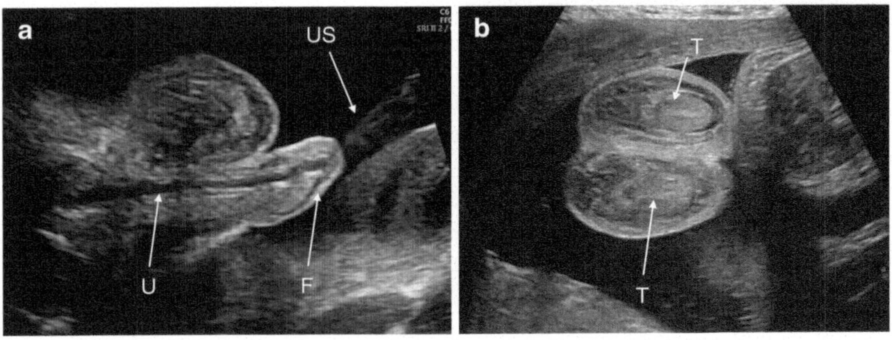

Fig. 10.3 Fetal penis and testes. (**a**) Sagittal view of fetal penis during micturition. The normal penis is straight, tapered, and completely covered with the hyperechoic foreskin (F). The urethra (U) and urinary stream (US) from the tip of the penis are visible. (**b**) The testes (T) in the scrotum are visualized as hyperechoic, homogeneous, and oval masses

the bladder and rectum on the transverse view of the fetal pelvis (Fig. 10.2). The body of the uterus is usually thinner than the cervix in the fetal period. Normal ovaries are usually not visible.

The normal penis is straight, tapered, and points cranially. During fetal micturition, the urinary stream from the tip of the penis can be visualized on gray-scale ultrasound (Fig. 10.3a). The testes in the scrotum are identifiable as hyperechoic, homogeneous, and oval masses in the third trimester (Fig. 10.3b). The testes begin to descend into the scrotum after 25 weeks of gestation, and the migration is completed at 32 weeks of gestation in 95% of fetuses [1]. Undescended testes can be detected at birth in about 4% of the newborns [2].

10.2 Fetal Ultrasound Imaging of Genitourinary Tract Abnormalities

10.2.1 Kidney

Urinary Tract Dilation

Urinary tract dilation (UTD) is a term used to describe dilation of the renal pelvis, calyces, and/or ureters. In addition, the urinary bladder may be dilated. UTD is the currently recommended term in place of hydronephrosis and pyelectasis to avoid confusion [3]. In the majority of cases, UTD is a transient physiological state; however, it can develop secondary to urinary tract obstruction or vesicoureteral reflux (VUR). Urinary tract obstruction includes ureteropelvic junction or ureterovesical junction obstructions, ureterocele, and posterior urethral valves. Several systems have been developed to diagnose and grade fetal UTD. Fetal UTD is generally detected by measurement of the maximum anteroposterior (AP) diameter of the renal pelvis on the transverse view of the fetal abdomen. Although many controversies persist, most experts agree that the threshold of AP diameter to detect fetal UTD is 4 mm during the second trimester and 7 mm during the third trimester [3, 4]. The Society for Fetal Urology system has been widely used to grade the severity of fetal UTD [4]. The system classifies the condition into four grades based on the degree of pelvic dilation, number of dilated calyces, and presence of thin renal parenchyma (Fig. 10.4). Another new system is the UTD classification [3], which has been applied in both prenatal and postnatal situations. The UTD classification system is based on six ultrasonographic features: AP diameter, calyceal dilation (central or peripheral), parenchymal thickness, parenchymal appearance (echogenicity, presence of cortical cysts, and corticomedullary differentiation), ureter visualization (transient or dilated), and urinary bladder description (wall thickness, and the presence of ureteroceles or posterior urethral valves).

Urinoma

Urinomas are encapsulated collections of urine in the perirenal fascia caused by urinary leakage from the kidney. Urinomas are usually secondary to severe urinary tract obstruction, such as ureteropelvic junction obstruction. Urinomas appear as an anechoic cystic mass on ultrasound, displacing the obstructed kidney (Fig. 10.5).

Obstructive Renal Dysplasia

Obstructive renal dysplasia is a parenchymal abnormality resulting from severe urinary tract obstruction or VUR. A decrease or loss of kidney function is observed. The kidneys are typically hyperechoic with subcortical cysts on ultrasound (Fig. 10.6). The size of the kidneys varies; however, are small in most cases and become smaller with increase in the severity due to atrophy of the renal parenchyma.

Duplicated Collecting System

A duplicated collecting system separates the upper and lower pole moieties in a single kidney. The ureter arising from the lower pole of the collecting system joins

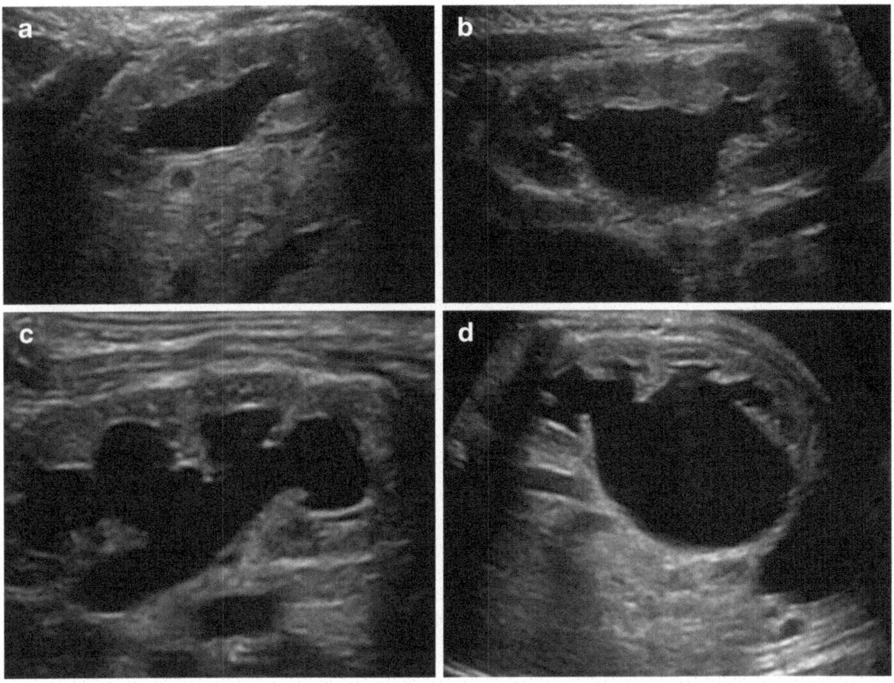

Fig. 10.4 The Society for Fetal Urology grading system. (**a**) Grade 1, mild dilation of the pelvis only. (**b**) Grade 2, moderate dilation of the pelvis and a few calyces. (**c**) Grade 3, dilation of the pelvis and all calyces, and normal renal parenchyma. (**d**) Grade 4, dilation of the pelvis and all calyces, and thinning of renal parenchyma

Fig. 10.5 Urinoma. The urinoma appears as an anechoic cystic mass displacing the obstructed kidney

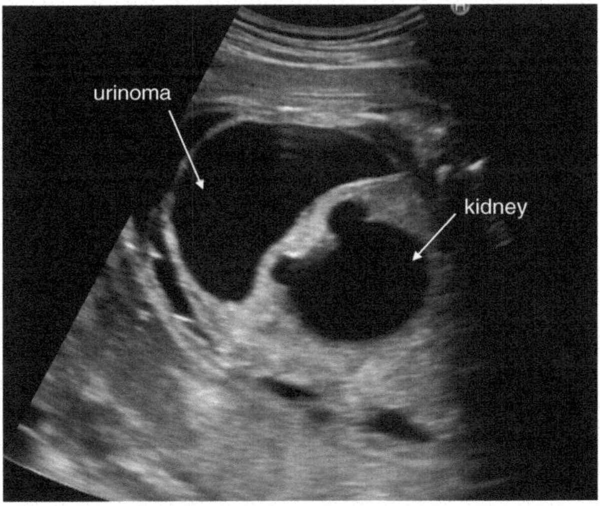

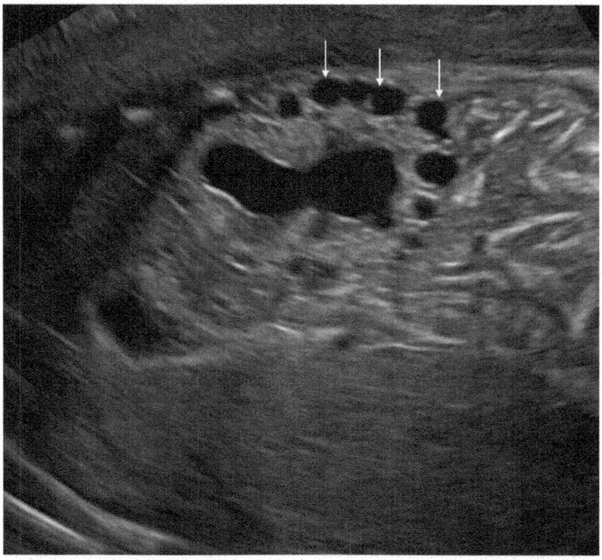

Fig. 10.6 Obstructive renal dysplasia. The renal parenchyma appears hyperechoic with subcortical cysts (arrows)

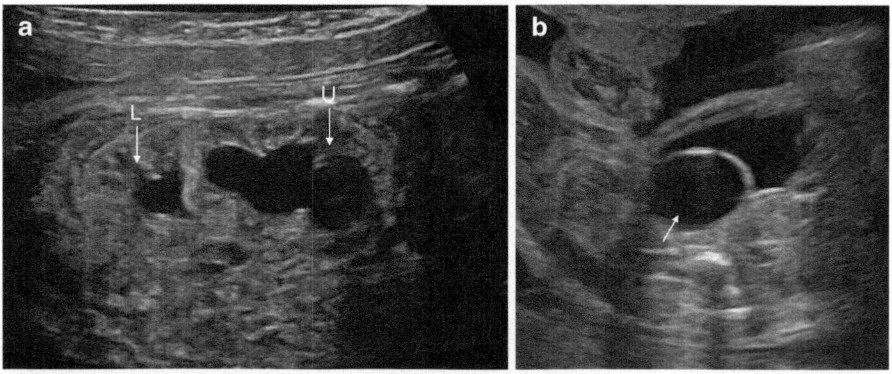

Fig. 10.7 Duplicated collecting system. (**a**) The upper pole (U) of the duplicated collecting system is significantly dilated. On the other hand, the lower pole moiety (L) is slightly dilated. (**b**) The ureter arising from the upper pole terminates in the ureterocele (arrow) in the bladder

the bladder orthotopically at one corner of the vesical trigone. On the other hand, the ureter arising from the upper pole usually joins the bladder wall inferior to the orthotopic ureteral opening and terminates in an ureterocele in the bladder. Dilation of the upper pole and normal appearance of the lower pole moieties are key features for prenatal diagnosis of duplicated collecting system (Fig. 10.7a). It is also important to identify the presence of ureterocele in the bladder. Ureterocele appears as a thin-walled cystic structure on ultrasound, projecting into the bladder (Fig. 10.7b).

Pelvic kidney

The kidney may sometimes be located in the pelvis, known as pelvic kidney, and is the most common abnormal renal position. The kidneys ascend from the pelvis into the renal fossa between the sixth and ninth weeks of gestation [5]. Abnormal renal position results from failure of the real ascent. An empty renal fossa indicates ectopic kidney as well as renal agenesis. The absence of contralateral renal hypertrophy suggests an ectopic kidney rather than unilateral renal agenesis. The pelvic kidney is usually located in close proximity to the bladder; however, its identification is often missed on prenatal ultrasound (Fig. 10.8).

Multicystic Dysplastic Kidney (MCDK)

MCDK is a severe renal dysplasia demonstrating multiple non-communicating cysts of varying sizes, atretic ureter, and absence of normal renal parenchyma. MCDK usually presents as a large multicystic mass in the renal fossa. The mass loses its reniform shape due to the constituent cysts of variable sizes (Fig. 10.9).

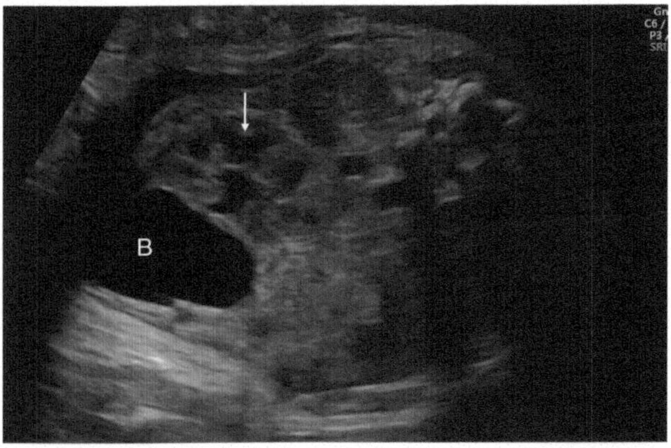

Fig. 10.8 Pelvic kidney. The kidney (arrow) is located in close proximity to the bladder in the fetal pelvis

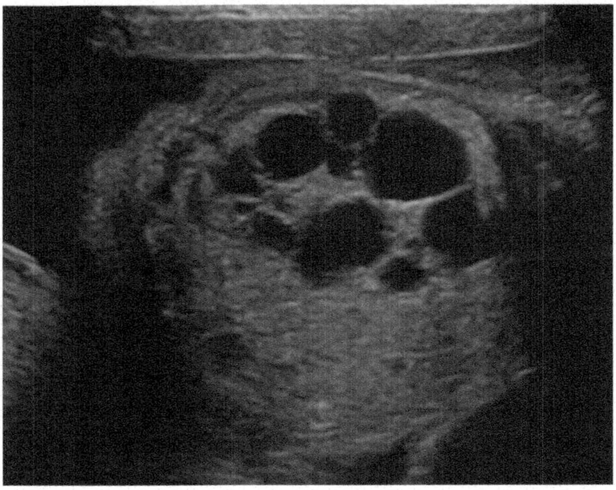

Fig. 10.9 MCDK. Many cysts of variable sizes are seen. On the other hand, no normal parenchyma or collecting system is visible

Absence of normal parenchyma and collecting system is the key to differentiating MCDK from severe UTD. Unilateral MCDK is commonly associated with contralateral renal malformation, frequently VUR and ureteropelvic junction obstruction [6]. MCDK can also be associated with chromosomal abnormalities (Trisomy 13 or 18) and fetal syndromes such as Meckel-Gruber syndrome.

10.2.2 Lower Urinary Tract

Posterior urethral valve

The posterior urethral valve (PUV) is the most common cause of congenital lower urinary tract obstruction, which occurs exclusively in male fetuses. The PUV forms a thin diaphragm and blocks the flow of urine. The distended bladder and dilated posterior urethra (keyhole sign) with bilateral urinary tract dilation are suggestive of PUV (Fig. 10.10). PUV is the likely cause of megacystis in the first trimester.

10.2.3 Adrenal Gland

Neuroblastoma

Adrenal neuroblastoma is the most common congenital malignancy. On ultrasound, the tumor appears as a well-defined, uniformly echogenic solid mass located immediately cephalad to the kidneys [7] (Fig. 10.11a). The tumor may displace the ipsilateral kidney (Fig. 10.11b). Cystic changes may develop due to hemorrhage inside the tumor and may eventually result in a complicated cystic mass. Differentiation of the cystic mass from simple adrenal hemorrhage can be difficult. The presence of normal or greater flow during Doppler evaluation helps in distinguishing neuroblastoma from simple adrenal hemorrhage [8].

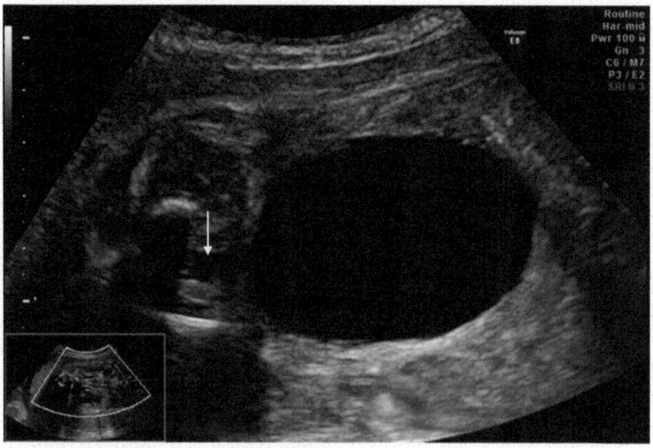

Fig. 10.10 Posterior urethral valve. The distended bladder and dilated posterior urethra (arrow) are visible, the so-called keyhole sign

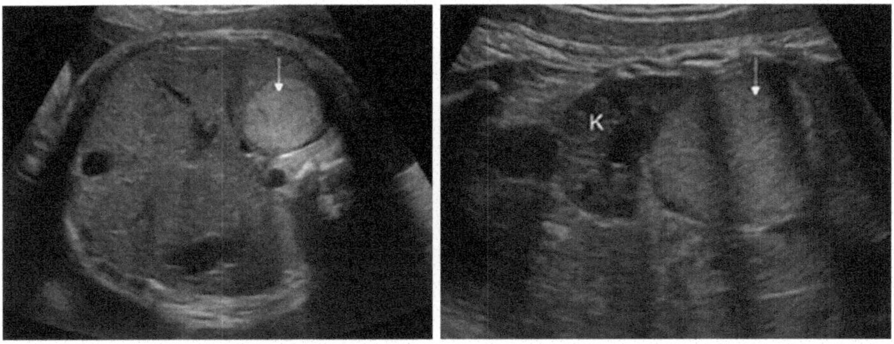

Fig. 10.11 Neuroblastoma. Adrenal neuroblastoma (arrow) appears as a well-defined and uniformly echogenic solid mass

Fig. 10.12 Adrenal hemorrhage. The septated cyst (arrow) is visible superior to the kidney

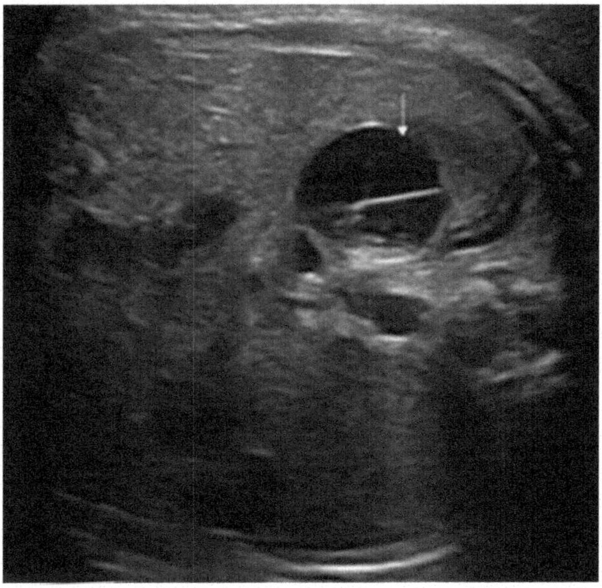

Adrenal Hemorrhage

Adrenal hemorrhage is occasionally observed in fetuses. The hemorrhage is observed on the ultrasound as a thick-walled cystic mass. Sonographic features depend on the age of bleeding. Echogenicity changes from hyperechoic to hypoechoic and finally anechoic. Septations and/or fluid-fluid level can be seen in the cyst (Fig. 10.12).

10.2.4 Genitalia

Hypospadias

Hypospadias is the most common congenital anomaly of the male external genitalia. In this condition, opening of the urethra is located on the ventral side of the penis instead of the tip. Location of the displaced urethral meatus can vary and may be present within the glans, shaft of the penis, scrotum, or perineum. Hypospadias is commonly associated with penile curvature (chordee) and incomplete closure of the foreskin around the glans. Fetal hypospadias is usually detected on ultrasound based on the ventral curvature and/or blunting of the penis (Fig. 10.13a, b). The uncovered tip of the penis with foreskin can lead to the suspicion of hypospadias (Fig. 10.13b, c). Gray-scale ultrasonography may locate the ventral opening of the

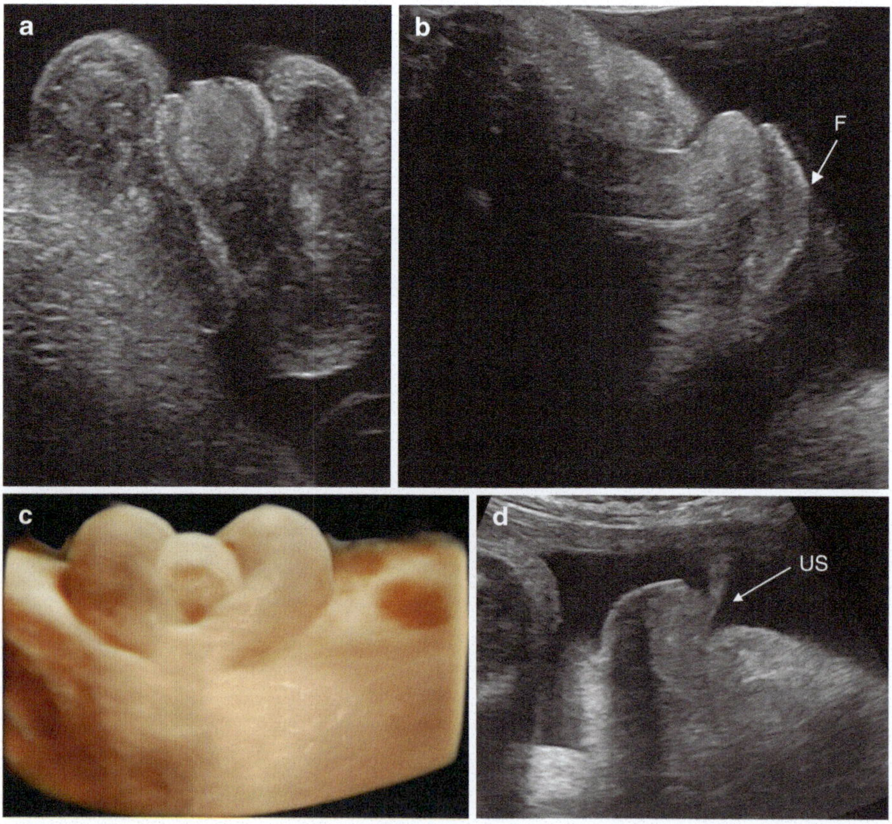

Fig. 10.13 Hypospadias. (**a**) The penis is located between the scrotums due to ventral curvature of the penis. (**b**) Sagittal view of fetal penis. The penis is ventrally curved, and the tip of penis is not covered with the foreskin (F). (**c**) Three-dimensional image of the penis and scrotums. (**d**) The urinary stream (US) originates from the ventral side of penis

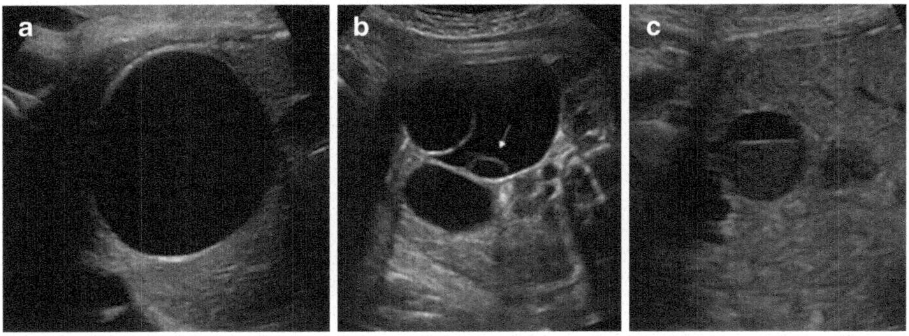

Fig. 10.14 Ovarian cysts. (**a**) Simple cyst. The cyst is anechoic, unilocular, and thin-walled. (**b**) A small cystic structure (arrow) within the ovarian cyst, the so-called daughter cyst sign. (**c**) Complicated cyst. Fluid-fluid levels are seen in the cyst

urinary meatus by visualizing the urinary stream during fetal micturition, which leads to a definite diagnosis (Fig. 10.13d). Severe hypospadias, which is often complicated by bilateral cryptorchidism, may result in disorders of sexual development.

Ovarian cysts

Fetal ovarian cysts usually manifest in the third trimester and are considered a consequence of maternal hormonal stimulation. The majority of fetal ovarian cysts resolve spontaneously after birth, likely due to hormonal changes. However, torsion can occur during the fetal or neonatal period. Ovarian cysts are located superior and lateral to the bladder. Ovarian cysts generally appear as simple cysts, which are anechoic, unilocular, and thin-walled (Fig. 10.14a). The "daughter cyst" sign refers to the presence of a small cyst along the wall of the cystic mass (Fig. 10.14b). This sign has been reported as pathognomonic of ovarian cysts [9, 10]. On the other hand, fetal ovarian cysts that exhibit internal echoic fluid, fluid-fluid levels, and septations are considered complicated cysts. The complicated cysts indicate torsion of the ovary (Fig. 10.14c). Differential diagnoses of ovarian cysts include gastrointestinal duplication cysts, urachal cysts, choledochal cysts, and hydrocolpos [11].

References

1. Achiron R, Pinhas-Hamiel O, Zalel Y, Rotstein Z, Lipitz S. Development of fetal male gender: prenatal sonographic measurement of the scrotum and evaluation of testicular descent. Ultrasound Obstet Gynecol. 1998;11:242–5.
2. Ghirri P, Ciulli C, Vuerich M, Cuttano A, Faraoni M, Guerrini L, Spinelli C, Tognetti S, Boldrini A. Incidence at birth and natural history of cryptorchidism: a study of 10,730 consecutive male infants. J Endocrinol Invest. 2002;25:709–15.
3. Nguyen HT, Benson CB, Bromley B, Campbell JB, Chow J, Coleman B, Cooper C, Crino J, Darge K, Herndon CD, Odibo AO, Somers MJ, Stein DR. Multidisciplinary consensus on the

classification of prenatal and postnatal urinary tract dilation (UTD classification system). J Pediatr Urol. 2014;10:982–98.

4. Nguyen HT, Herndon CD, Cooper C, Gatti J, Kirsch A, Kokorowski P, Lee R, Perez-Brayfield M, Metcalfe P, Yerkes E, Cendron M, Campbell JB. The Society for Fetal Urology consensus statement on the evaluation and management of antenatal hydronephrosis. J Pediatr Urol. 2010;6:212–31.
5. Kuure S, Vuolteenaho R, Vainio S. Kidney morphogenesis: cellular and molecular regulation. Mech Dev. 2000;92:31–45.
6. Schreuder MF, Westland R, van Wijk JA. Unilateral multicystic dysplastic kidney: a meta-analysis of observational studies on the incidence, associated urinary tract malformations and the contralateral kidney. Nephrol Dial Transplant. 2009;24:1810–8.
7. Hwang SM, Yoo SY, Kim JH, Jeon TY. Congenital adrenal neuroblastoma with and without cystic change: differentiating features with an emphasis on the of value of ultrasound. Am J Roentgenol. 2016;207:1105–11.
8. Mileto A, Itani M, Katz DS, Siebert JR, Dighe MK, Dubinsky TJ, Moshiri M. Fetal urinary tract anomalies: review of pathophysiology, imaging, and management. Am J Roentgenol. 2018;210:1010–21.
9. Quarello E, Gorincour G, Merrot T, Boubli L, D'Ercole C. The "daughter cyst sign": a sonographic clue to the diagnosis of fetal ovarian cyst. Ultrasound Obstet Gynecol. 2003;22:433–4.
10. Lee HJ, Woo SK, Kim JS, Suh SJ. "Daughter cyst" sign: a sonographic finding of ovarian cyst in neonates, infants, and young children. Am J Roentgenol. 2000;174:1013–5.
11. Trinh TW, Kennedy AM. Fetal ovarian cysts: review of imaging spectrum, differential diagnosis, management, and outcome. Radiographics. 2015;35:621–35.

Chapter 11
Genomic Imprinting Disorders (Including Mesenchymal Placental Dysplasia)

Hidenobu Soejima and Takashi Ohba

Abstract Genomic imprinting is an epigenetic phenomenon resulting in a parent-of-origin-dependent expression of a subset of mammalian genes. The majority of imprinted genes form clusters called imprinted domains. The expression of imprinted genes within each imprinted domain is regulated by an imprinting control region (ICR), which is characterized by differential DNA methylation between the two parental alleles. Since most imprinted genes play important roles in pre- and/or postnatal growth, placental formation, and metabolism, the aberrant expression and function of imprinted genes, due to epigenetic or genetic alterations, cause imprinting disorders (IDs). This chapter will explain the molecular regulation of imprinted gene expression and imprinted gene networks, as well as clinical characteristics and molecular mechanisms of IDs, including multi-locus imprinting disturbance (MLID). In addition, the relationship between assisted reproductive technology (ART) and IDs is also described. Furthermore, imprinting-related chorionic diseases, such as hydatidiform mole and placental mesenchymal dysplasia, are also illustrated.

Keywords Genomic imprinting · Imprinted gene · Differentially methylated region (DMR) · Imprinting control region (ICR) · Imprinting disorders (IDs) Placental mesenchymal dysplasia (PMD)

H. Soejima
Division of Molecular Genetics & Epigenetics, Department of Biomolecular Sciences, Faculty of Medicine, Saga University, Saga, Japan
e-mail: soejimah@cc.saga-u.ac.jp

T. Ohba (✉)
Department of Obstetrics and Gynecology, Faculty of Life Sciences, Kumamoto University, Kumamoto, Japan
e-mail: tkohba@kumamoto-u.ac.jp

H. Masuzaki (ed.), *Fetal Morph Functional Diagnosis*, Comprehensive Gynecology and Obstetrics, https://doi.org/10.1007/978-981-15-8171-7_11

11.1 Genomic Imprinting

11.1.1 Imprinted Genes and Differentially Methylated Regions (DMRs)

Genomic imprinting is an epigenetic phenomenon resulting in parent-of-origin-dependent expression of a subset of mammalian genes. Imprinted genes are expressed either exclusively or predominantly in a mono-allelic fashion, i.e., in one of the two parental alleles. Mono-allelic expression occurs in most tissues, but some imprinted genes are mono-allelically expressed in specific tissues or developmental windows [1–3]. Most imprinted genes play important roles in pre- and/or postnatal growth, placental formation, and metabolism [4, 5].

So far, more than 100 imprinted genes have been identified in the human genome, and the majority of imprinted genes form clusters called imprinted domains. The expression of imprinted genes within each imprinted domain is regulated by an imprinting control region (ICR). An ICR is a differentially methylated region (DMR), which is characterized by differences in DNA methylation between the two parental alleles [5–7]. Two kinds of DMRs exist, including gametic and somatic DMRs. Gametic DMRs acquire DNA methylation in the maternal and paternal germ cells, and also include ICRs. Somatic DMRs are established after fertilization, in response to nearby gametic DMRs [5, 6, 8].

To date, approximately 35 gametic DMRs have been identified in humans [5]. DNA methylation, including in gametic DMRs, is erased in primordial germ cells (PGCs). Sex-specific methylation marks are then acquired and established in developing germ cells. DNA methylation in female germ cells occurs during oocyte maturation. However, that in male germ cells occurs before entry into meiosis [5]. In mice, DNA methylation in female germ cells is accomplished mainly by the de novo DNA methyltransferase, DNMT3A, along with its regulatory cofactor DNMT3L. DNMT3A and DNMT3B, in cooperation with DNMT3L, are central players in male germ cells [9–12]. For DNA methylation occurring during oocyte maturation, transcription of ICRs is required, and may make chromatin more accessible by the DNMT3A-DNMT3L complex. However, after fertilization, transcription is dispensable [13, 14]. In male germ cells, transcription is also involved in DNA methylation [15].

Although zygotes undergo global demethylation following fertilization and until implantation, the established DNA methylation of ICRs is maintained during development. DPPA3 prevents demethylation of ICRs in both parental alleles [16, 17]. ZFP57 and its cofactors, including maintenance methyltransferase DNMT1, also protect ICRs from demethylation [18, 19].

At the implantation stage, global DNA methylation increases. DNMT3B is responsible for this methylation increase and for the establishment of somatic DMRs [20]. However, ICRs in the unmethylated allele must be protected against de novo methylation at this stage. For example, transcription factors such as CTCF and

OCT4 bind to unmethylated maternal ICR1, which is an ICR of the *IGF2/H19* imprinted domain, to protect it from de novo methylation [21, 22]. Most unmethylated ICRs, which overlap promoter CpG islands with active transcription enriched with histone H3 lysine 4 trimethylation (H3K4me3), may also be protected by H3K4me3 because H3K4me3 prevents binding of DNMT3L [23].

11.1.2 Regulation of Imprinted Gene Expression

Expression of imprinted genes within imprinted domains is regulated by ICRs. Maternally methylated ICRs are located in intragenic regions and generally correspond to promoters, often of long noncoding RNAs (lncRNAs). On the other hand, paternally methylated ICRs are intergenic, and may function as insulators or enhancers [5, 8]. Although the precise mechanisms differ among imprinted domains, there are two principal models: the lncRNA model and the insulator model [7].

One of the representative imprinted domains for the lncRNA model is the *CDKN1C/KCNQ1OT1* domain at the human chromosome 11p15 (Fig. 11.1) [7, 8]. ICR2, a maternally methylated ICR of this domain, is located in the promoter region of the lncRNA *KCNQ1OT1*. Methylated ICR2 represses *KCNQ1OT1* transcription on the maternal allele. However, unmethylated ICR2 on the paternal allele functions an active promoter to transcribe *KCNQ1OT1*. *Kcnq1ot1* RNA interacts with the H3K9 methyltransferase, G9a, and the H3K27 methyltransferase complex, PRC2 in the mouse placenta. This interaction causes repressive chromatin marks to be deposited, which repress neighboring protein-coding genes, including *Cdkc1c*, in *cis* [24–26]. *Kcnq1ot1* RNA also interacts with DNMT1 to maintain methylation of the somatic DMR of *Cdkn1c* in the mouse liver [27]. Indeed, accumulation of *KCNQ1OT1* RNA has been observed in neighboring regions containing *CDKN1C* in normal human fibroblast cell lines [28]. On the maternal allele, neighboring genes are expressed due to the lack of *Kcnq1ot1* expression.

The *IGF2/H19* domain is the best characterized imprinted domain for the insulator model (Fig. 11.1) [29, 30]. ICR1 is located upstream of *H19* and is methylated on the paternal, but not maternal, allele. For unmethylated maternal ICR1, the CTCF insulator protein can bind to ICR1 and block the access of enhancers downstream of *H19* to *IGF2* promoters, resulting in maternal *IGF2* repression. Conversely, on the paternal allele, DNA methylation prevents the binding of CTCF to ICR1. This allows enhancers to access the *IGF2* promoter, resulting in paternal *IGF2* expression [31]. CTCF is also involved in the formation of chromatin looping, and cohesin is required to stabilize the CTCF-mediated chromatin loop [32]. Previous studies of chromosome conformation capture (3C) in human cells showed that unmethylated maternal ICR1 interacts with a distal downstream region of the *H19* gene, while on the paternal allele, the distal region interacts with the *IGF2* promoter. These interactions form an allele-specific chromatin loop and may bring the enhancers into the proximity of the promoters [33, 34].

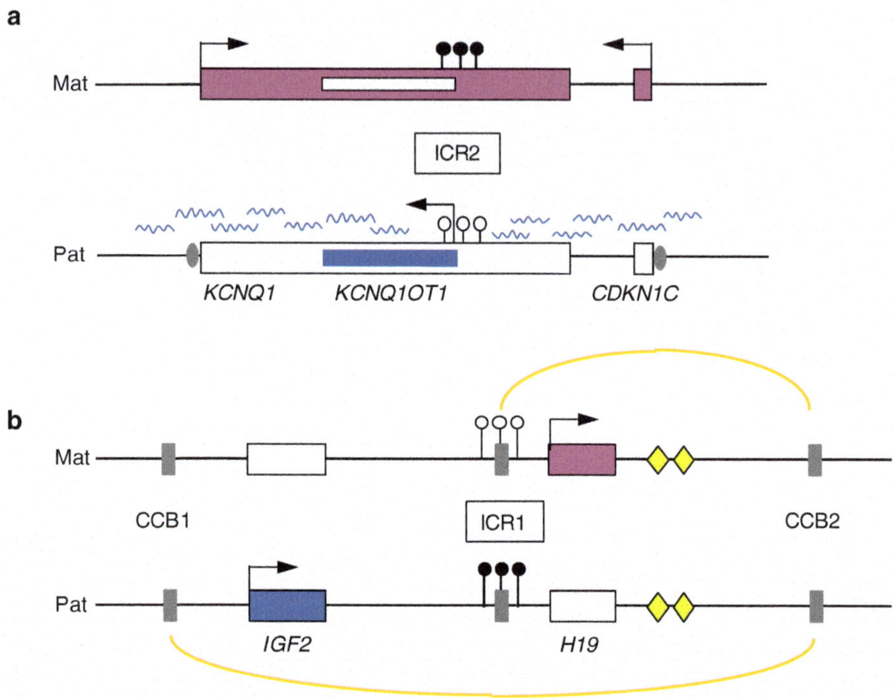

Fig. 11.1 (**a**) The *CDKN1C/KCNQ1OT1* domain for the lncRNA model. lncRNA *KCNQ1OT1* (wavy lines) transcribed from the paternal allele interacts with G9a and PRC2 to deposit repressive chromatin marks or with DNMT1 to maintain methylation of somatic DMR of neighboring genes. (**b**) The *IGF2/H19* domain for the insulator model. On the maternal allele, unmethylated ICR1 interacts with CTCF/cohesin binding site 2 (CCB2). Conversely, on the paternal allele, CCB1 interacts with CCB2, because methylated ICR1 prevents CTCF binding. The allele-specific chromatin loops, formed by these interactions, regulate the imprinted expression in this domain by bringing enhancers into the proximity of the promoters. Blue rectangle, paternally expressed gene; red rectangle, maternally expressed gene; filled lollipops, methylated ICR; open lollipops, unmethylated ICR; gray oval, repressive chromatin mark (repressive histone modifications or DNA methylation); gray rectangle, CTCF/cohesin binding site (CCB); yellow diamond, enhancer

11.1.3 Imprinted Gene Network (IGN)

Since *PLAGL1*, an imprinted gene at the transient neonatal diabetes mellitus type 1 (TNDM1) locus 6q24.2, was reported to alter the expression of other imprinted genes on other loci [35, 36], several studies have identified an imprinted gene network (IGN) consisting of numerous imprinted genes and many non-imprinted genes [37, 38]. The IGN is involved in cell proliferation, growth, cell cycle, and differentiation [39]. For example, PLAGL1, a zinc-finger transcription factor, regulates *IGF2*, *H19*, and *CDKN1C* [35, 36, 40]. Another example is the paternally expressed lncRNA *IPW* at the Prader–Willi syndrome (PWS) locus, 15q11.2. This lncRNA regulates the expression of imprinted genes at the *DLK1-DIO3* locus, 14q32.2, by recruiting G9a to IG-DMR [41]. Interactions within an IGN may influence clinical features of IDs, including several overlapping phenotypes among them.

11.2 Imprinting Disorders (IDs)

11.2.1 Clinical Characteristics of IDs

Since imprinted genes play important roles in several important life phenomena, the aberrant expression and function of imprinted genes due to epigenetic or genetic alterations often cause IDs. There have been 16 IDs reported so far (Table 11.1) [4, 5]. Most of the IDs share some features, such as aberrant pre- and/or postnatal growth; hypo- or hyperglycemia; abnormal feeding behavior in early childhood and later in development; behavioral difficulties; mental retardation; and precocious puberty [4]. Although typical clinical features of IDs have been defined, and clinical scoring systems or diagnostic guidelines are available for some IDs [42–48], the common features among IDs, and the only minor or atypical clinical features in some patients, make clinical diagnosis difficult.

11.2.2 Molecular Mechanisms of IDs

Molecular alterations underlying IDs are divided into four categories: (1) copy number variations (CNVs), i.e., deletions and duplications, of the imprinted region; (2) uniparental disomy (UPD); (3) aberrant methylation of ICRs, namely epimutations; and (4) point mutations of imprinted genes [4, 5]. CNVs, UPD, and epimutations disrupt the finely balanced expression of imprinted genes, leading to the overexpression or repression of imprinted genes, whereas point mutations directly affect the function of imprinted gene products. As for CNVs, the deletion of paternal 15q11-q13 is found in 75–80% of patients with PWS, and this deletion causes a loss of expression in paternally expressed genes, including *SNORD116*, which is a probable major gene contributing to the PWS phenotype [49, 50]. The maternal deletion of the same region is the cause of Angelman syndrome (AS) in 70–75% of patients with this syndrome, and results in the loss of the expression of maternally expressed genes, including *UBE3A* (Table 11.1).

UPD is characterized by the presence of two copies of a chromosome, or part of the chromosome derived from only one parent. Paternal UPD of chromosome 14, a major cause (in 65% of cases) of Kagami–Ogata syndrome (KOS14), causes a loss of expression in maternally expressed genes, due to a lack of the maternal copy of chromosome 14. In addition, the overexpression of the paternally expressed gene, *RTL1*, is observed [44]. In contrast with KOS14, Temple syndrome (TS14) shows maternal UPD of chromosome 14 in 29% of patients (Table 11.1).

Table 11.1 Imprinting disorders (based on [4, 5])

Imprinting disorder	OMIM	Disease locus	Molecular alteration	Frequency	Representative clinical features
Transient neonatal diabetes mellitus type1 (TNDM1)	601410	6q24	upd(6)pat (41%)dup(6q)(29%)PLAGL1-DMR-LOM (30%)	41%29%30%	IUGR, TNDM, hyperglycaemia without ketoacidosis, macroglossia, abdominal wall defects
Silver-Russell syndrome (SRS)	180860	Chr. 7, 11p15.5	upd(7)matupd(11)matdup(11p15)mat ICR1-LOM*CDKN1C* mutations*IGF2* mutations*HMGA2* mutations*PLAG1* mutations	5–10%Rare1–2%30–60%RareRareRareRare	IUGR, PNGR, relative macrocephaly at birth, body asymmetry, prominent forehead, feeding difficulties
Birk-Barel syndrome	612292	8q24.3	*KCNK9* mutations	100%	Intellectual disability, hypotonia, dysmorphism
Beckwith-Wiedemann syndrome (BWS)	130650	11p15.5	upd(11p15)patdup(11p15)patICR1-GOMICR2-LOM*CDKN1C* mutations	20%2–4%5%50%5%	Macroglossia, exomphalos, lateralized overgrowth, Wilms tumour or nephroblastomatosis, hyperinsulinism, adrenal cortex cytomegaly, placentalmesenchymaldysplasia, pancreatic adenomatosis
Kagami-Ogata syndrome (KOS14)	608149	14q32	upd(14)pat del(14q32)matIG-DMR-GOM	65%20%15%	IUGR, polyhydramnion, abdominal wall defects, bell-shaped thorax, coat-hanger ribs
Temple syndrome (TS14)	616222	14q32	upd(14)matdel(14q32)patIG-DMR-LOM	29%10%61%	IUGR, PNGR, neonatal hypotonia, feeding difficulties in infancy, truncal obesity, scoliosis, precocious puberty, small feet and hands
Prader-Willi syndrome (PWS)	176270	15q11-q13	del(15q11q13)patupd(15)matPWS-IC-GOM	75–80%20–25%~1%	PNGR, Intellectual disability, neonatal hypotonia, hypogenitalism, hypopigmentation, obesity, hyperphagia
Angelman syndrome (AS)	105830	15q11-q13	del(15q11q13)matupd(15)patPWS-IC-LOM *UBE3A* mutations	70–75% 3–7%2–3%10%	Severe intellectual disability, microcephaly, no speech, unmotivated laughing, ataxia, seizures, scoliosis

Central precocious puberty 2 (CPPB2)	615356	15q11.2	*MKRN3* mutations	100%	Early activation of the hypothalamic-pituitary-gonadal axis resulting in gonadotropin-dependent precocious puberty
Schaaf-Yang syndrome (SYS)	615547	15q11.2	*MAGEL2* mutations	100%	Delayed psychomotor development, intellectual disability, hypotonia
Pseudohypo-parathyroidism 1A (PHP1A)	103580	20q13.32	*GNAS*-inactivating variants of the mat allele	100%	Resistance to PTH and other hormones, Albright hereditary osteodystrophy, moderately reduced birth weight, obesity, cognitive impairment, decreased erythrocyte Gs activity
Pseudohypo-parathyroidism 1B (PHP1B)	603233	20q13.32	del(20q13)matGNAS-DMRs-LOMupd(20)pat	Rare>60%10–25%	Resistance to PTH and other hormones, Albright hereditary osteodystrophy, subcutaneous ossifications, feeding behaviour anomalies, abnormal growth patterns
Pseudohypo-parathyroidism 1C (PHP1C)	612462	20q13.32	*GNAS*-inactivating variants of the mat allele	100%	Resistance to PTH and other hormones, Albright hereditary osteodystrophy, moderately reduced birth weight, obesity, cognitive impairment, normal erythrocyte Gs activity
Pseudopseudohypo-parathyroidism (PPHP)	612463	20q13.32	*GNAS*-inactivating variants of the pat allele	100%	Mild resistance to PTH and other hormones, subcutaneous ossifications, birth weight and length restrictions
Progressive osseous heteroplasia (POH)	166350	20q13.32	*GNAS*-inactivating variants of the pat allele	100%	Ectopic ossifications
Mulchandani-Bhoj-Conlin syndrome (MBCS)	617352	Chr. 20	Upd(20)mat	100%	IUGR, PNGR, feeding difficulties

UPD uniparental disomy, *mat* maternal, *pat* paternal, *LOM* loss of methylation, *GOM* gain of methylation, *IUGR* intrauterine growth restriction, *PNGR* post-natal growth restriction, *PTH* parathyroid hormone

Epimutations are divided into two groups: primary epimutations and secondary epimutations [5]. Primary epimutations are aberrant methylations of ICRs without genetic alterations, and may be caused by random or environment-driven errors in the establishment or maintenance of ICR methylation. By contrast, secondary epimutations are caused by genetic alterations, such as single nucleotide variants (SNVs) and microdeletions/insertions. Such genetic alterations affect *cis*-acting elements or *trans*-acting factors. Beckwith–Wiedemann syndrome (BWS) and Silver–Russell syndrome (SRS) are frequently caused by epimutations (Table 11.1) [42, 43]. In BWS, the loss of methylation (LOM) at ICR2 occurs on the maternal chromosome as a primary epimutation. The ICR2-LOM causes *KCNQ1OT1* to be expressed aberrantly. The expressed *KCNQ1OT1* lncRNA consequently represses *CDKN1C* in *cis*, as mentioned above (Fig. 11.1). Gain of methylation (GOM) at ICR1 also occurs in BWS. The majority of ICR1-GOMs are primary epimutations, but approximately 20% are secondary epimutations caused by microdeletions, small deletions, or SNVs. Microdeletions (1.4–2.2 kb) abolish 1–3 CTCF binding sites, while small deletions and SNVs abolish the OCT4/SOX2 target site [51–54]. These genetic alterations cannot protect ICR1 from de novo methylation, leading to GOM. ICR1-GOM on the maternal allele induces *IGF2* expression, resulting in the bi-allelic expression of *IGF2* (Fig. 11.1). In addition, when an SNV of the OCT4/SOX2 target site is transmitted by the mother, DNA methylation anticipation is observed [54, 55]. It is intriguing that ICR1-LOM, which is the opposite molecular alteration to ICR1-GOM, causes SRS, a growth restriction syndrome opposite to BWS (Table 11.1).

Loss of function mutations of imprinted genes are often found in BWS and AS (Table 11.1). The maternally expressed gene, *CDKN1C* (*p57*^{Kip2}), which encodes a cyclin-dependent inhibitor, is mutated in BWS; and the maternally expressed gene, *UBE3A*, which encodes an E3 ubiquitin ligase, is mutated in AS [56, 57]. Interestingly, gain of function mutations in *CDKN1C* and loss of function mutations in *IGF2* were reported in a miniscule number of SRS patients [58, 59].

11.2.3 Multi-locus Imprinting Disturbance (MLID)

A subset of patients with IDs show multi-locus imprinting disturbances (MLIDs). MLIDs (especially LOM) are epimutations of multiple DMRs within the genome, including both gametic and somatic DMRs. Patients with MLIDs are mainly found in BWS, SRS, and TNDM1 [4, 5, 60]. In 25% of BWS patients with ICR2-LOM, 7–10% of SRS cases with ICR1-LOM, and 30% of TNDM1 cases with *PLAGL1*-DMR-LOM, MLIDs are displayed. Epigenotype–phenotype correlations in MLIDs are not always clear. Homozygous mutations in *ZFP57* have been found in TNDM1 patients with MLID [61]. In addition, maternal mutations in NLRP genes, such as *NLRP2*, *NLRP5*, and *NLRP7*, have been reported to be associated with MLIDs [62, 63].

11.2.4 Assisted Reproductive Technology (ART) and IDs

It is known that assisted reproductive technology (ART), such as in vitro fertilization (IVF) and intracytoplasmic sperm injection (ICSI), increases the risk of IDs. A systematic review revealed that the odds ratio of any ID in children conceived through ART was 3.67, in comparison with spontaneously conceived children, but did not show evidence of generalized changes in DNA methylation [64]. Another systematic review also showed that ART was associated with increased odds ratios of four IDs: 5.8 in the case of BWS; 11.3 in the case of SRS; 2.2 in the case of PWS; and 4.7 in the case of AS [65]. However, it is still unknown whether the increased risk of IDs is due to ART or to the infertility per se.

11.3 Hydatidiform Mole

Complete hydatidiform mole (CHM) is an abnormal form of pregnancy where only paternal genomes are carried (androgenetic CHM).Approximately 90% of CHMs are developed during fertilization of an enucleated oocyte by a single sperm, followed by the endoreplication of paternal chromosomes, thus leading to a 46,XX karyotype. The other 10% of CHMs show a 46,XY or 46,XX karyotype as a result of fertilization of an enucleated oocyte by two sperms (dispermy) [66, 67]. On the other hand, most partial hydatidiform moles (PHMs) are triploid (usually 69,XXY), resulting from the fertilization of a normal oocyte by two sperms [66, 67].

A fraction of CHMs can be recurrent and familial. These CHMs are characterized by a biparental genetic contribution. Homozygous or compound heterozygous maternal-effect genes, *NLRP7* and *KHDC3L*, are found in patients with recurrent CHM [68]. *NLRP7* is mutated in 48–80% of patients with recurrent CHM, whereas a mutation in *KHDC3L* is found in 10–14% of patients not having a mutation in *NLRP7* [68]. From the aspect of imprinting, the paternalization of all DMRs, which is a GOM at paternally methylated DMRs and LOM at maternally methylated DMRs, is found in androgenetic CHM, whereas the methylation defects in biparental recurrent CHM are restricted to lack of methylation at maternally methylated DMRs [69]. These observations strongly suggest that mutations in *NLRP7* and *KHDC3L* cause a failure to establish maternal imprints during oocyte maturation.

11.4 Placental Mesenchymal Dysplasia (PMD)

11.4.1 Definition of PMD

PMD is a rare, benign, morphological condition relating to human placental vascular anomaly. It is characterized by placentomegaly, and multicystic vesicles that may resemble a molar pregnancy by ultrasound and gross pathologic examination.

PMD was initially described by Moscoso et al. in 1991 and termed as *diffuse stem villous hyperplasia* [70]. In previous literature, it has also been referred to as *placentomegaly with massive hydrops of placental stem villi* [71]; *angiomatous malformation of placental chorionic stem vessels* [72]; *placental vascular malformation with mesenchymal hyperplasia and a localized chorioangioma* [73]; *diffuse cystic placental change* [74]; and *pseudopartial mole* [75]. To date, PMD is the preferred terminology.

Presumably, the reason why obstetricians started to pay attention to PMD in the 1990s was that PMD closely mimicked molar pregnancy based on ultrasound examination. These two conditions showed distinctly different clinicopathological courses. However, recent studies have clarified that imprinted genes are related to the pathogenesis of both hydatidiform mole and PMD [76].

11.4.2 Fetomaternal Complications of PMD

The number of reported cases of PMD has gradually increased since the 2000s. Its incidence has been estimated at 0.02% in examined placentas [77]. However, the true incidence is not well known, because PMD is often underdiagnosed and underreported, as not all clinicians and pathologists are aware of such a clinical entity.

PMD is related to perinatal complications including premature delivery, hypertensive disorders of pregnancy (HDP), fetal growth restriction (FGR), and fetal demise (FD). Though these clinical presentations are nonspecific, their adverse outcomes are explained by chronic fetal hypoxia, secondary to fetal vascular obstructive pathology characterized by chorionic vessel thrombosis.

PMD has been reported to be more common in women with HDP (9.0–18.7%) than in the general population [78–80]. The prevalence of HDP was higher in cases of PMD in fetuses with BWS than without BWS and in PMD with male infants compared to female infants. BWS is a representative ID, featured with macroglossia, gastroschisis, and hemihypertorophy [43, 81]. If the fetus has BWS, regardless of PMD, the incidence of maternal HDP is known to be high (17.7% of pregnancy hypertension and 8.7% of preeclampsia) [82]. Approximately 30–50% of BWS cases are thought to be due to a decreased expression of *CDKN1C* (*p57*^{Kip2}) due to ICR2-LOM of the *CDKN1C*/*KCNQ1OT1* domain. *CDKN1C* mutations in human children or mice models with preeclampsia/HELLP syndrome suggest the involvement of an imprinted gene in the pathophysiology of preeclampsia [83, 84]. How fetal BWS and male sexuality in PMD are involved in the development of maternal HDP remains to be studied.

In the earliest reliable review by Pham T et al. in 2006, FD occurred in 35.6% of fetuses, from 16 to 36 weeks of gestation [80]. In a European multicenter study, it was reported to occur in 18.0% (4/22) of fetuses [85]. We collected the PMD cases in Japan from 2000 to 2016 and analyzed the detailed clinical information from histopathological findings and the genetic/epigenetic changes of the placental tissues. In our case series, the distribution of the onset of FD, from 20 to 36 weeks, was similar to the previous review, but the incidence was lower. 33.3% (13/39) of live births were terminated by obstetrical indications due to a non-reassuring fetal status, or maternal complications including HDP; as well as threatened premature labor; or placenta previa after 24 weeks of gestation (unpublished data). The terminated pregnancy was strongly related to FGR. Though a PMD-specific perinatal care protocol still remains to be clarified, these results suggest that the conventional perinatal management of FGR in developed countries could reduce the mortality rate of fetuses with PMD.

11.4.3 Imaging and Serum Markers for PMD

Common ultrasound findings in the second trimester were a thickened chorion villosum, with a multicystic lesion resembling CHM and healthy co-twin or a PHM during the first half of pregnancy (Fig. 11.2a). The future prospects of these cystic lesions varied, either gradually becoming apparent or disappearing in some cases. The major part of these cystic lesions consisted of enlarged vessels and was

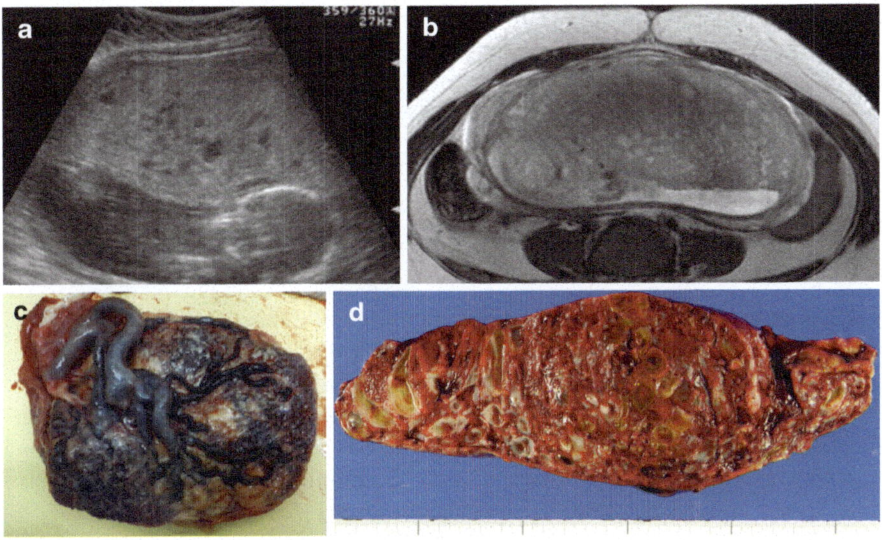

Fig. 11.2 Typical prenatal images and gross findings of PMD. (**a**) Ultrasonographic finding. 17 weeks + 5 days. (**b**) Magnetic resonance imaging (T2WI). 18 weeks + 0 day. (**c**) Macroscopic view of the fetal surface of the placenta with PMD. Fetus delivered at 38 weeks + 0 day transvaginally. Birth weight 2755 g, placental weight 1530 g. Large, tortuous vessels are observed on the fetal surface of the enlarged placenta. (**d**) Macroscopic view of the divided surface of the case described in (**c**). Cystic areas are distributed focally and are abundant on the fetal surface. (The gross finding pictures were photographed in collaboration with Prof. Yoshiki Mikami, Department of Diagnostic Pathology, Kumamoto University, Japan)

accompanied by slow blood flow, which was distinguished from a molar gestation using color Doppler imaging [86].

Magnetic resonance imaging (MRI) showed multiple cystic lesions with high intensity (T2 weighted image [T2WI]), which were often uniformly distributed in a leaf of thickened placenta (Fig. 11.2b).

Some reports have suggested that among PMD cases, the serum levels of the maternal serum alpha-fetoprotein (MSAFP) were high and the maternal serum human chorionic gonadotropin (MShCG) were normal or slightly elevated [87, 88].

Stem villi and blood vessels of PMD were negative against AFP immunohistochemical reactions, observed by microscopic analysis [70]; and elevated levels of MSAFP were seen in women with PMD, even in the presence of normal AFP levels in the amniotic fluid [89]. These findings suggest that AFP moved extraordinarily from the fetal circulation to the maternal circulation due to an increasing permeability of placental vessels derived from vascular abnormalities.

In CHM, MShCG should be elevated, while MSAFP remains in the normal range. On the contrary, the levels of both MSAFP and MShCG are sometimes elevated in triploid partial mole and hydatidiform mole with coexistent fetus [90]. Elevated MSAFP levels with normal levels of MShCG are useful for the differential diagnosis of PMD from molar pregnancies.

Ishikawa et al. (2016) reported that elevated MSAFP levels are correlated with the degree of placental vasodilation, and that these are also related with adverse outcomes, including fetal anemia or FD [91]. The authors speculated that fetal anemia could occur even in the absence of vessel rupture, because fetal erythropoiesis was insufficient for the acute increase of a vascular bed in PMD.

11.4.4 Gross, Histopathological, and Immunohistochemical Findings of PMD

PMD is characterized by both gross and relative placentomegaly. The average fixed placental weight was 933 ± 401 g (range: 210–2330 g) and the birth weight to placental weight ratio was 0.63 ± 0.57 in the cases we accumulated. The enlarged PMD placenta displayed large, tortuous vessels on the fetal surface (Fig. 11.2c). Cut surfaces showed heterogeneous areas with the cysts, including gelatinous liquid and normal red-brown or spongy villous tissues. The cystic areas were distributed predominantly on the fetal surface of the placenta (Fig. 11.2d).

Typical histopathological findings for PMD were enlarged edematous stem villi, dilated thick-walled chorionic plate vessels with fibromuscular hyperplasia, and fresh or organized thrombi. Placental villi with diffuse vascular proliferation were also observed. Abnormal trophoblastic proliferation and trophoblastic inclusions were not observed in the examination of any section.

As previously mentioned, *p57*^{Kip2} (*CDKN1C*), located at 11p15.5, is predominantly expressed on the maternal allele and encodes a cyclin-dependent kinase inhibitor. p57^{Kip2} has been used as a diagnostic marker to distinguish normal placental tissue; spontaneous abortion with hydropic changes; and partial moles from complete molar pregnancies. p57^{Kip2} protein is also implicated in some human IDs, such as BWS. Since PMD is strongly associated with BWS, the underlying 11p15 abnormality might be confined to the placenta, and the loss of activity of the *p57*^{Kip2} gene may cause a loss of cell-cycle inhibition and overgrowth [87]. p57^{Kip2} is strongly expressed in cytotrophoblasts and villous mesenchyme in the normal placenta. In PMD, p57^{Kip2} expression in villous mesenchyme is absent.

The histopathological examination of our study subjects clarified that the normal and affected lesions were concomitantly observed in most of the placental specimens of PMD. 3/36 specimens contained histopathologically normal placental tissues, and 1/11 specimens showed normal p57^{Kip2} expression. Our study suggests that the diagnosis of PMD has the potential to be affected by the sampling site and number of specimens. Establishment of a diagnostic criteria for PMD might be unable to disregard this heterology.

11.4.5 Molecular Pathogenesis of PMD

In contrast to PHMs which are 70–80% triploid, normal karyotypes have often been found in PMD [79]. Chromosomal aneuploidy or specific genetic mutations have not been described for PMD. It is already known, however, that PMD is associated with female fetuses and BWS [43]. These findings suggest that a genetic relationship may exist, including IDs.

Recent genotyping studies have shown that the phenotypic and immunohistochemical features of PMD are associated with androgenetic biparental mosaicism (ABM). ABM in PMD is characterized by a mosaicism of two cells lines: an androgenetic cell line in the chorionic mesenchyme, as well as a biparental cell line found in the villous cytotrophoblast and amnion [92]. Advanced maternal age and ART were not associated with PMD in the reported cases in Japan; however, there are many publications suggesting an association between ART and BWS [6, 93, 94]. This suggests that ART contributes in a different manner to the development of PMD and BWS.

Because PMD is a high-risk disease for both the mother and the child, prenatal diagnosis, perinatal management in a perinatal medical center, and accurate postpartum histopathological diagnosis are essential. For a prenatal diagnosis, measurements of AFP should be repeated. Elevated MSAFP and normal MShCG levels in the second to third trimester may indicate PMD. Cysts may worsen or disappear during pregnancy, and some specimens may look histopathologically normal, so multiple pathological specimens must be examined.

References

1. Rougeulle C, Glatt H, Lalande M. The Angelman syndrome candidate gene, UBE3A/E6-AP, is imprinted in brain. Nat Genet. 1997;17(1):14–5. https://doi.org/10.1038/ng0997-14.
2. Vu TH, Hoffman AR. Imprinting of the Angelman syndrome gene, UBE3A, is restricted to brain. Nat Genet. 1997;17(1):12–3. https://doi.org/10.1038/ng0997-12.
3. Yatsuki H, Watanabe H, Hattori M, Joh K, Soejima H, Komoda H, Xin Z, Zhu X, Higashimoto K, Nishimura M, Kuratomi S, Sasaki H, Sakaki Y, Mukai T. Sequence-based structural features between Kvlqt1 and Tapa1 on mouse chromosome 7F4/F5 corresponding to the Beckwith-Wiedemann syndrome region on human 11p15.5: long-stretches of unusually well conserved intronic sequences of kvlqt1 between mouse and human. DNA Res. 2000;7(3):195–206. https://doi.org/10.1093/dnares/7.3.195.
4. Soellner L, Begemann M, Mackay DJ, Gronskov K, Tumer Z, Maher ER, Temple IK, Monk D, Riccio A, Linglart A, Netchine I, Eggermann T. Recent advances in imprinting disorders. Clin Genet. 2017;91(1):3–13. https://doi.org/10.1111/cge.12827.
5. Monk D, Mackay DJG, Eggermann T, Maher ER, Riccio A. Genomic imprinting disorders: lessons on how genome, epigenome and environment interact. Nat Rev Genet. 2019;20(4):235–48. https://doi.org/10.1038/s41576-018-0092-0.
6. Soejima H, Higashimoto K. Epigenetic and genetic alterations of the imprinting disorder Beckwith-Wiedemann syndrome and related disorders. J Hum Genet. 2013;58(7):402–9. https://doi.org/10.1038/jhg.2013.51.
7. Peters J. The role of genomic imprinting in biology and disease: an expanding view. Nat Rev Genet. 2014;15(8):517–30. https://doi.org/10.1038/nrg3766.
8. Ferguson-Smith AC. Genomic imprinting: the emergence of an epigenetic paradigm. Nat Rev Genet. 2011;12(8):565–75. https://doi.org/10.1038/nrg3032.
9. Bourc'his D, Xu GL, Lin CS, Bollman B, Bestor TH. Dnmt3L and the establishment of maternal genomic imprints. Science. 2001;294(5551):2536–9. https://doi.org/10.1126/science.1065848.
10. Kaneda M, Okano M, Hata K, Sado T, Tsujimoto N, Li E, Sasaki H. Essential role for de novo DNA methyltransferase Dnmt3a in paternal and maternal imprinting. Nature. 2004;429(6994):900–3. https://doi.org/10.1038/nature02633.
11. Kato Y, Kaneda M, Hata K, Kumaki K, Hisano M, Kohara Y, Okano M, Li E, Nozaki M, Sasaki H. Role of the Dnmt3 family in de novo methylation of imprinted and repetitive sequences during male germ cell development in the mouse. Hum Mol Genet. 2007;16(19):2272–80. https://doi.org/10.1093/hmg/ddm179.
12. Smallwood SA, Tomizawa S, Krueger F, Ruf N, Carli N, Segonds-Pichon A, Sato S, Hata K, Andrews SR, Kelsey G. Dynamic CpG island methylation landscape in oocytes and preimplantation embryos. Nat Genet. 2011;43(8):811–4. https://doi.org/10.1038/ng.864.
13. Chotalia M, Smallwood SA, Ruf N, Dawson C, Lucifero D, Frontera M, James K, Dean W, Kelsey G. Transcription is required for establishment of germline methylation marks at imprinted genes. Genes Dev. 2009;23(1):105–17. https://doi.org/10.1101/gad.495809.
14. Joh K, Matsuhisa F, Kitajima S, Nishioka K, Higashimoto K, Yatsuki H, Kono T, Koseki H, Soejima H. Growing oocyte-specific transcription-dependent de novo DNA methylation at the imprinted Zrsr1-DMR. Epigenetics Chromatin. 2018;11(1):28. https://doi.org/10.1186/s13072-018-0200-6.
15. Henckel A, Chebli K, Kota SK, Arnaud P, Feil R. Transcription and histone methylation changes correlate with imprint acquisition in male germ cells. EMBO J. 2012;31(3):606–15. https://doi.org/10.1038/emboj.2011.425.
16. Nakamura T, Liu YJ, Nakashima H, Umehara H, Inoue K, Matoba S, Tachibana M, Ogura A, Shinkai Y, Nakano T. PGC7 binds histone H3K9me2 to protect against conversion of 5mC to 5hmC in early embryos. Nature. 2012;486(7403):415–9. https://doi.org/10.1038/nature11093.

17. Wossidlo M, Nakamura T, Lepikhov K, Marques CJ, Zakhartchenko V, Boiani M, Arand J, Nakano T, Reik W, Walter J. 5-Hydroxymethylcytosine in the mammalian zygote is linked with epigenetic reprogramming. Nat Commun. 2011;2:241. https://doi.org/10.1038/ncomms1240.
18. Li X, Ito M, Zhou F, Youngson N, Zuo X, Leder P, Ferguson-Smith AC. A maternal-zygotic effect gene, Zfp57, maintains both maternal and paternal imprints. Dev Cell. 2008;15(4):547–57. https://doi.org/10.1016/j.devcel.2008.08.014.
19. Quenneville S, Verde G, Corsinotti A, Kapopoulou A, Jakobsson J, Offner S, Baglivo I, Pedone PV, Grimaldi G, Riccio A, Trono D. In embryonic stem cells, ZFP57/KAP1 recognize a methylated hexanucleotide to affect chromatin and DNA methylation of imprinting control regions. Mol Cell. 2011;44(3):361–72. https://doi.org/10.1016/j.molcel.2011.08.032.
20. Monk D. Germline-derived DNA methylation and early embryo epigenetic reprogramming: the selected survival of imprints. Int J Biochem Cell Biol. 2015;67:128–38. https://doi.org/10.1016/j.biocel.2015.04.014.
21. Schoenherr CJ, Levorse JM, Tilghman SM. CTCF maintains differential methylation at the Igf2/H19 locus. Nat Genet. 2003;33(1):66–9. https://doi.org/10.1038/ng1057.
22. Engel N, Thorvaldsen JL, Bartolomei MS. CTCF binding sites promote transcription initiation and prevent DNA methylation on the maternal allele at the imprinted H19/Igf2 locus. Hum Mol Genet. 2006;15(19):2945–54. https://doi.org/10.1093/hmg/ddl237.
23. Ooi SK, Qiu C, Bernstein E, Li K, Jia D, Yang Z, Erdjument-Bromage H, Tempst P, Lin SP, Allis CD, Cheng X, Bestor TH. DNMT3L connects unmethylated lysine 4 of histone H3 to de novo methylation of DNA. Nature. 2007;448(7154):714–7. https://doi.org/10.1038/nature05987.
24. Pandey RR, Mondal T, Mohammad F, Enroth S, Redrup L, Komorowski J, Nagano T, Mancini-Dinardo D, Kanduri C. Kcnq1ot1 antisense noncoding RNA mediates lineage-specific transcriptional silencing through chromatin-level regulation. Mol Cell. 2008;32(2):232–46. https://doi.org/10.1016/j.molcel.2008.08.022.
25. Terranova R, Yokobayashi S, Stadler MB, Otte AP, van Lohuizen M, Orkin SH, Peters AH. Polycomb group proteins Ezh2 and Rnf2 direct genomic contraction and imprinted repression in early mouse embryos. Dev Cell. 2008;15(5):668–79. https://doi.org/10.1016/j.devcel.2008.08.015.
26. Wagschal A, Sutherland HG, Woodfine K, Henckel A, Chebli K, Schulz R, Oakey RJ, Bickmore WA, Feil R. G9a histone methyltransferase contributes to imprinting in the mouse placenta. Mol Cell Biol. 2008;28(3):1104–13. https://doi.org/10.1128/MCB.01111-07.
27. Mohammad F, Mondal T, Guseva N, Pandey GK, Kanduri C. Kcnq1ot1 noncoding RNA mediates transcriptional gene silencing by interacting with Dnmt1. Development. 2010;137(15):2493–9. https://doi.org/10.1242/dev.048181.
28. Murakami K, Oshimura M, Kugoh H. Suggestive evidence for chromosomal localization of non-coding RNA from imprinted LIT1. J Hum Genet. 2007;52(11):926–33. https://doi.org/10.1007/s10038-007-0196-4.
29. Bell AC, Felsenfeld G. Methylation of a CTCF-dependent boundary controls imprinted expression of the Igf2 gene. Nature. 2000;405(6785):482–5. https://doi.org/10.1038/35013100.
30. Hark AT, Schoenherr CJ, Katz DJ, Ingram RS, Levorse JM, Tilghman SM. CTCF mediates methylation-sensitive enhancer-blocking activity at the H19/Igf2 locus. Nature. 2000;405(6785):486–9. https://doi.org/10.1038/35013106.
31. Herold M, Bartkuhn M, Renkawitz R. CTCF: insights into insulator function during development. Development. 2012;139(6):1045–57. https://doi.org/10.1242/dev.065268.
32. Nativio R, Wendt KS, Ito Y, Huddleston JE, Uribe-Lewis S, Woodfine K, Krueger C, Reik W, Peters JM, Murrell A. Cohesin is required for higher-order chromatin conformation at the imprinted IGF2-H19 locus. PLoS Genet. 2009;5(11):e1000739. https://doi.org/10.1371/journal.pgen.1000739.
33. Tan L, Xing D, Chang CH, Li H, Xie XS. Three-dimensional genome structures of single diploid human cells. Science. 2018;361(6405):924–8. https://doi.org/10.1126/science.aat5641.

34. Rao SS, Huntley MH, Durand NC, Stamenova EK, Bochkov ID, Robinson JT, Sanborn AL, Machol I, Omer AD, Lander ES, Aiden EL. A 3D map of the human genome at kilobase resolution reveals principles of chromatin looping. Cell. 2014;159(7):1665–80. https://doi.org/10.1016/j.cell.2014.11.021.
35. Arima T, Kamikihara T, Hayashida T, Kato K, Inoue T, Shirayoshi Y, Oshimura M, Soejima H, Mukai T, Wake N. ZAC, LIT1 (KCNQ1OT1) and p57KIP2 (CDKN1C) are in an imprinted gene network that may play a role in Beckwith-Wiedemann syndrome. Nucleic Acids Res. 2005;33(8):2650–60. https://doi.org/10.1093/nar/gki555.
36. Varrault A, Gueydan C, Delalbre A, Bellmann A, Houssami S, Aknin C, Severac D, Chotard L, Kahli M, Le Digarcher A, Pavlidis P, Journot L. Zac1 regulates an imprinted gene network critically involved in the control of embryonic growth. Dev Cell. 2006;11(5):711–22. https://doi.org/10.1016/j.devcel.2006.09.003.
37. Al Adhami H, Evano B, Le Digarcher A, Gueydan C, Dubois E, Parrinello H, Dantec C, Bouschet T, Varrault A, Journot L. A systems-level approach to parental genomic imprinting: the imprinted gene network includes extracellular matrix genes and regulates cell cycle exit and differentiation. Genome Res. 2015;25(3):353–67. https://doi.org/10.1101/gr.175919.114.
38. Zacharek SJ, Fillmore CM, Lau AN, Gludish DW, Chou A, Ho JW, Zamponi R, Gazit R, Bock C, Jager N, Smith ZD, Kim TM, Saunders AH, Wong J, Lee JH, Roach RR, Rossi DJ, Meissner A, Gimelbrant AA, Park PJ, Kim CF. Lung stem cell self-renewal relies on BMI1-dependent control of expression at imprinted loci. Cell Stem Cell. 2011;9(3):272–81. https://doi.org/10.1016/j.stem.2011.07.007.
39. Patten MM, Cowley M, Oakey RJ, Feil R. Regulatory links between imprinted genes: evolutionary predictions and consequences. Proc Biol Sci. 2016;283(1824) https://doi.org/10.1098/rspb.2015.2760.
40. Iglesias-Platas I, Martin-Trujillo A, Petazzi P, Guillaumet-Adkins A, Esteller M, Monk D. Altered expression of the imprinted transcription factor PLAGL1 deregulates a network of genes in the human IUGR placenta. Hum Mol Genet. 2014;23(23):6275–85. https://doi.org/10.1093/hmg/ddu347.
41. Stelzer Y, Sagi I, Yanuka O, Eiges R, Benvenisty N. The noncoding RNA IPW regulates the imprinted DLK1-DIO3 locus in an induced pluripotent stem cell model of Prader-Willi syndrome. Nat Genet. 2014;46(6):551–7. https://doi.org/10.1038/ng.2968.
42. Wakeling EL, Brioude F, Lokulo-Sodipe O, O'Connell SM, Salem J, Bliek J, Canton AP, Chrzanowska KH, Davies JH, Dias RP, Dubern B, Elbracht M, Giabicani E, Grimberg A, Gronskov K, Hokken-Koelega AC, Jorge AA, Kagami M, Linglart A, Maghnie M, Mohnike K, Monk D, Moore GE, Murray PG, Ogata T, Petit IO, Russo S, Said E, Toumba M, Tumer Z, Binder G, Eggermann T, Harbison MD, Temple IK, Mackay DJ, Netchine I. Diagnosis and management of Silver-Russell syndrome: first international consensus statement. Nat Rev Endocrinol. 2017;13(2):105–24. https://doi.org/10.1038/nrendo.2016.138.
43. Brioude F, Kalish JM, Mussa A, Foster AC, Bliek J, Ferrero GB, Boonen SE, Cole T, Baker R, Bertoletti M, Cocchi G, Coze C, De Pellegrin M, Hussain K, Ibrahim A, Kilby MD, Krajewska-Walasek M, Kratz CP, Ladusans EJ, Lapunzina P, Le Bouc Y, Maas SM, Macdonald F, Ounap K, Peruzzi L, Rossignol S, Russo S, Shipster C, Skorka A, Tatton-Brown K, Tenorio J, Tortora C, Gronskov K, Netchine I, Hennekam RC, Prawitt D, Tumer Z, Eggermann T, Mackay DJG, Riccio A, Maher ER. Expert consensus document: clinical and molecular diagnosis, screening and management of Beckwith-Wiedemann syndrome: an international consensus statement. Nat Rev Endocrinol. 2018;14(4):229–49. https://doi.org/10.1038/nrendo.2017.166.
44. Ogata T, Kagami M. Kagami-Ogata syndrome: a clinically recognizable upd(14)pat and related disorder affecting the chromosome 14q32.2 imprinted region. J Hum Genet. 2016;61(2):87–94. https://doi.org/10.1038/jhg.2015.113.
45. Ioannides Y, Lokulo-Sodipe K, Mackay DJ, Davies JH, Temple IK. Temple syndrome: improving the recognition of an underdiagnosed chromosome 14 imprinting disorder: an analysis of 51 published cases. J Med Genet. 2014;51(8):495–501. https://doi.org/10.1136/jmedgenet-2014-102396.

46. Gunay-Aygun M, Schwartz S, Heeger S, O'Riordan MA, Cassidy SB. The changing purpose of Prader-Willi syndrome clinical diagnostic criteria and proposed revised criteria. Pediatrics. 2001;108(5):E92. https://doi.org/10.1542/peds.108.5.e92.
47. Mantovani G, Bastepe M, Monk D, de Sanctis L, Thiele S, Usardi A, Ahmed SF, Bufo R, Choplin T, De Filippo G, Devernois G, Eggermann T, Elli FM, Freson K, Garcia Ramirez A, Germain-Lee EL, Groussin L, Hamdy N, Hanna P, Hiort O, Juppner H, Kamenicky P, Knight N, Kottler ML, Le Norcy E, Lecumberri B, Levine MA, Makitie O, Martin R, Martos-Moreno GA, Minagawa M, Murray P, Pereda A, Pignolo R, Rejnmark L, Rodado R, Rothenbuhler A, Saraff V, Shoemaker AH, Shore EM, Silve C, Turan S, Woods P, Zillikens MC, Perez de Nanclares G, Linglart A. Diagnosis and management of pseudohypoparathyroidism and related disorders: first international Consensus Statement. Nat Rev Endocrinol. 2018;14(8):476–500. https://doi.org/10.1038/s41574-018-0042-0.
48. Mulchandani S, Bhoj EJ, Luo M, Powell-Hamilton N, Jenny K, Gripp KW, Elbracht M, Eggermann T, Turner CL, Temple IK, Mackay DJ, Dubbs H, Stevenson DA, Slattery L, Zackai EH, Spinner NB, Krantz ID, Conlin LK. Maternal uniparental disomy of chromosome 20: a novel imprinting disorder of growth failure. Genet Med. 2016;18(4):309–15. https://doi.org/10.1038/gim.2015.103.
49. Sahoo T, del Gaudio D, German JR, Shinawi M, Peters SU, Person RE, Garnica A, Cheung SW, Beaudet AL. Prader-Willi phenotype caused by paternal deficiency for the HBII-85 C/D box small nucleolar RNA cluster. Nat Genet. 2008;40(6):719–21. https://doi.org/10.1038/ng.158.
50. de Smith AJ, Purmann C, Walters RG, Ellis RJ, Holder SE, Van Haelst MM, Brady AF, Fairbrother UL, Dattani M, Keogh JM, Henning E, Yeo GS, O'Rahilly S, Froguel P, Farooqi IS, Blakemore AI. A deletion of the HBII-85 class of small nucleolar RNAs (snoRNAs) is associated with hyperphagia, obesity and hypogonadism. Hum Mol Genet. 2009;18(17):3257–65. https://doi.org/10.1093/hmg/ddp263.
51. Kraft F, Wesseler K, Begemann M, Kurth I, Elbracht M, Eggermann T. Novel familial distal imprinting centre 1 (11p15.5) deletion provides further insights in imprinting regulation. Clin Epigenetics. 2019;11(1):30. https://doi.org/10.1186/s13148-019-0629-x.
52. Demars J, Shmela ME, Rossignol S, Okabe J, Netchine I, Azzi S, Cabrol S, Le Caignec C, David A, Le Bouc Y, El-Osta A, Gicquel C. Analysis of the IGF2/H19 imprinting control region uncovers new genetic defects, including mutations of OCT-binding sequences, in patients with 11p15 fetal growth disorders. Hum Mol Genet. 2010;19(5):803–14. https://doi.org/10.1093/hmg/ddp549.
53. Higashimoto K, Jozaki K, Kosho T, Matsubara K, Fuke T, Yamada D, Yatsuki H, Maeda T, Ohtsuka Y, Nishioka K, Joh K, Koseki H, Ogata T, Soejima H. A novel de novo point mutation of the OCT-binding site in the IGF2/H19-imprinting control region in a Beckwith-Wiedemann syndrome patient. Clin Genet. 2014;86(6):539–44. https://doi.org/10.1111/cge.12318.
54. Sun F, Higashimoto K, Awaji A, Ohishi K, Nishizaki N, Tanoue Y, Aoki S, Watanabe H, Yatsuki H, Soejima H. The extent of DNA methylation anticipation due to a genetic defect in ICR1 in Beckwith-Wiedemann syndrome. J Hum Genet. 2019;64(9):937–43. https://doi.org/10.1038/s10038-019-0634-0.
55. Berland S, Appelbäck M, Bruland O, Beygo J, Buiting K, Mackay DJ, Karen Temple I, Houge G. Evidence for anticipation in Beckwith-Wiedemann syndrome. Eur J Hum Genet. 2013; https://doi.org/10.1038/ejhg.2013.71.
56. Hatada I, Ohashi H, Fukushima Y, Kaneko Y, Inoue M, Komoto Y, Okada A, Ohishi S, Nabetani A, Morisaki H, Nakayama M, Niikawa N, Mukai T. An imprinted gene p57KIP2 is mutated in Beckwith-Wiedemann syndrome. Nat Genet. 1996;14(2):171–3. https://doi.org/10.1038/ng1096-171.
57. Kishino T, Lalande M, Wagstaff J. UBE3A/E6-AP mutations cause Angelman syndrome. Nat Genet. 1997;15(1):70–3. https://doi.org/10.1038/ng0197-70.
58. Brioude F, Oliver-Petit I, Blaise A, Praz F, Rossignol S, Le Jule M, Thibaud N, Faussat AM, Tauber M, Le Bouc Y, Netchine I. CDKN1C mutation affecting the PCNA-binding domain as

a cause of familial Russell Silver syndrome. J Med Genet. 2013;50(12):823–30. https://doi.org/10.1136/jmedgenet-2013-101691.

59. Begemann M, Zirn B, Santen G, Wirthgen E, Soellner L, Buttel HM, Schweizer R, van Workum W, Binder G, Eggermann T. Paternally inherited IGF2 mutation and growth restriction. N Engl J Med. 2015;373(4):349–56. https://doi.org/10.1056/NEJMoa1415227.
60. Sanchez-Delgado M, Riccio A, Eggermann T, Maher ER, Lapunzina P, Mackay D, Monk D. Causes and consequences of multi-locus imprinting disturbances in humans. Trends Genet. 2016;32(7):444–55. https://doi.org/10.1016/j.tig.2016.05.001.
61. Mackay DJ, Callaway JL, Marks SM, White HE, Acerini CL, Boonen SE, Dayanikli P, Firth HV, Goodship JA, Haemers AP, Hahnemann JM, Kordonouri O, Masoud AF, Oestergaard E, Storr J, Ellard S, Hattersley AT, Robinson DO, Temple IK. Hypomethylation of multiple imprinted loci in individuals with transient neonatal diabetes is associated with mutations in ZFP57. Nat Genet. 2008;40(8):949–51. https://doi.org/10.1038/ng.187.
62. Docherty LE, Rezwan FI, Poole RL, Turner CL, Kivuva E, Maher ER, Smithson SF, Hamilton-Shield JP, Patalan M, Gizewska M, Peregud-Pogorzelski J, Beygo J, Buiting K, Horsthemke B, Soellner L, Begemann M, Eggermann T, Baple E, Mansour S, Temple IK, Mackay DJ. Mutations in NLRP5 are associated with reproductive wastage and multilocus imprinting disorders in humans. Nat Commun. 2015;6:8086. https://doi.org/10.1038/ncomms9086.
63. Begemann M, Rezwan FI, Beygo J, Docherty LE, Kolarova J, Schroeder C, Buiting K, Chokkalingam K, Degenhardt F, Wakeling EL, Kleinle S, Gonzalez Fassrainer D, Oehl-Jaschkowitz B, Turner CLS, Patalan M, Gizewska M, Binder G, Bich Ngoc CT, Chi Dung V, Mehta SG, Baynam G, Hamilton-Shield JP, Aljareh S, Lokulo-Sodipe O, Horton R, Siebert R, Elbracht M, Temple IK, Eggermann T, Mackay DJG. Maternal variants in NLRP and other maternal effect proteins are associated with multilocus imprinting disturbance in offspring. J Med Genet. 2018;55(7):497–504. https://doi.org/10.1136/jmedgenet-2017-105190.
64. Lazaraviciute G, Kauser M, Bhattacharya S, Haggarty P, Bhattacharya S. A systematic review and meta-analysis of DNA methylation levels and imprinting disorders in children conceived by IVF/ICSI compared with children conceived spontaneously. Hum Reprod Update. 2015;21(4):555–7. https://doi.org/10.1093/humupd/dmv017.
65. Cortessis VK, Azadian M, Buxbaum J, Sanogo F, Song AY, Sriprasert I, Wei PC, Yu J, Chung K, Siegmund KD. Comprehensive meta-analysis reveals association between multiple imprinting disorders and conception by assisted reproductive technology. J Assist Reprod Genet. 2018;35(6):943–52. https://doi.org/10.1007/s10815-018-1173-x.
66. Lurain JR. Gestational trophoblastic disease I: epidemiology, pathology, clinical presentation and diagnosis of gestational trophoblastic disease, and management of hydatidiform mole. Am J Obstet Gynecol. 2010;203(6):531–9. https://doi.org/10.1016/j.ajog.2010.06.073.
67. Candelier JJ. The hydatidiform mole. Cell Adhesion Migration. 2016;10(1–2):226–35. https://doi.org/10.1080/19336918.2015.1093275.
68. Kalogiannidis I, Kalinderi K, Kalinderis M, Miliaras D, Tarlatzis B, Athanasiadis A. Recurrent complete hydatidiform mole: where we are, is there a safe gestational horizon? Opinion and mini-review. J Assist Reprod Genet. 2018;35(6):967–73. https://doi.org/10.1007/s10815-018-1202-9.
69. Sanchez-Delgado M, Martin-Trujillo A, Tayama C, Vidal E, Esteller M, Iglesias-Platas I, Deo N, Barney O, Maclean K, Hata K, Nakabayashi K, Fisher R, Monk D. Absence of maternal methylation in biparental hydatidiform moles from women with NLRP7 maternal-effect mutations reveals widespread placenta-specific imprinting. PLoS Genet. 2015;11(11):e1005644. https://doi.org/10.1371/journal.pgen.1005644.
70. Moscoso G, Jauniaux E, Hustin J. Placental vascular anomaly with diffuse mesenchymal stem villous hyperplasia. A new clinico-pathological entity? Pathol Res Pract. 1991;187(2-3):324–8. https://doi.org/10.1016/s0344-0338(11)80791-0.
71. Lage JM. Placentomegaly with massive hydrops of placental stem villi, diploid DNA content, and fetal omphaloceles: possible association with Beckwith-Wiedemann syndrome. Hum Pathol. 1991;22(6):591–7. https://doi.org/10.1016/0046-8177(91)90237-j.

72. Sander CM. Angiomatous malformation of placental chorionic stem vessels and pseudo-partial molar placentas: report of five cases. Pediatr Pathol. 1993;13(5):621–33. https://doi.org/10.3109/15513819309048250.
73. Hojberg KE, Aagaard J, Henriques U, Sunde L. Placental vascular malformation with mesenchymal hyperplasia and a localized chorioangioma. A rarity simulating partial mole. Pathol Res Pract. 1994;190(8):808–13. ; discussion 814. https://doi.org/10.1016/s0344-0338(11)80429-2.
74. Uemura N, Kobayashi F, Korita D, Tanada S, Niwa H, Nanbu K, Konishi I, Sagawa N, Mori T. Diffuse cystic change of a term placenta with a normal newborn. J Obstet Gynaecol Res. 1997;23(5):433–8. https://doi.org/10.1111/j.1447-0756.1997.tb00869.x.
75. Paradinas FJ, Sebire NJ, Fisher RA, Rees HC, Foskett M, Seckl MJ, Newlands ES. Pseudo-partial moles: placental stem vessel hydrops and the association with Beckwith-Wiedemann syndrome and complete moles. Histopathology. 2001;39(5):447–54. https://doi.org/10.1046/j.1365-2559.2001.01256.x.
76. Morales C, Soler A, Badenas C, Rodriguez-Revenga L, Nadal A, Martinez JM, Mademont-Soler I, Borrell A, Mila M, Sanchez A. Reproductive consequences of genome-wide paternal uniparental disomy mosaicism: description of two cases with different mechanisms of origin and pregnancy outcomes. Fertil Steril. 2009;92(1):393 e395–9. https://doi.org/10.1016/j.fertnstert.2009.03.090.
77. Lokan J, Chan YF, Agnesta F. Placental mesenchymal dysplasia. Pathology. 2002;34(4):375–8. https://doi.org/10.1080/003130202760120571.
78. Nayeri UA, West AB, Grossetta Nardini HK, Copel JA, Sfakianaki AK. Systematic review of sonographic findings of placental mesenchymal dysplasia and subsequent pregnancy outcome. Ultrasound Obstet Gynecol. 2013;41(4):366–74. https://doi.org/10.1002/uog.12359.
79. Ohyama M, Kojyo T, Gotoda H, Sato T, Ijiri R, Tanaka Y. Mesenchymal dysplasia of the placenta. Pathol Int. 2000;50(9):759–64. https://doi.org/10.1046/j.1440-1827.2000.01100.x.
80. Pham T, Steele J, Stayboldt C, Chan L, Benirschke K. Placental mesenchymal dysplasia is associated with high rates of intrauterine growth restriction and fetal demise: a report of 11 new cases and a review of the literature. Am J Clin Pathol. 2006;126(1):67–78. https://doi.org/10.1309/rv45-hrd5-3yq2-yftp.
81. Beckwith J. Macroglossia, omphalocele, adrenal cytomegaly, gigantism and hyperplastic visceromegaly. Birth Defects: Original Article Series. 1969;5:188–96.
82. Wangler MF, Chang AS, Moley KH, Feinberg AP, Debaun MR. Factors associated with preterm delivery in mothers of children with Beckwith-Wiedemann syndrome: a case cohort study from the BWS registry. Am J Med Genet A. 2005;134a(2):187–91. https://doi.org/10.1002/ajmg.a.30595.
83. Dokras A, Hoffmann DS, Eastvold JS, Kienzle MF, Gruman LM, Kirby PA, Weiss RM, Davisson RL. Severe feto-placental abnormalities precede the onset of hypertension and proteinuria in a mouse model of preeclampsia. Biol Reprod. 2006;75(6):899–907. https://doi.org/10.1095/biolreprod.106.053603.
84. Romanelli V, Belinchon A, Campos-Barros A, Heath KE, Garcia-Minaur S, Martinez-Glez V, Palomo R, Mercado G, Gracia R, Lapunzina P. CDKN1C mutations in HELLP/preeclamptic mothers of Beckwith-Wiedemann Syndrome (BWS) patients. Placenta. 2009;30(6):551–4. https://doi.org/10.1016/j.placenta.2009.03.013.
85. Guenot C, Kingdom J, De Rham M, Osterheld M, Keating S, Vial Y, Van Mieghem T, Jastrow N, Raio L, Spinelli M, Di Meglio L, Chalouhi G, Baud D. Placental mesenchymal dysplasia: an underdiagnosed placental pathology with various clinical outcomes. Eur J Obstet Gynecol Reprod Biol. 2019;234:155–64. https://doi.org/10.1016/j.ejogrb.2019.01.014.
86. Kuwata T, Takahashi H, Matsubara S. 'Stained-glass' sign for placental mesenchymal dysplasia. Ultrasound Obstet Gynecol. 2014;43(3):355. https://doi.org/10.1002/uog.13230.
87. Parveen Z, Tongson-Ignacio JE, Fraser CR, Killeen JL, Thompson KS. Placental mesenchymal dysplasia. Archiv Pathol Lab Med. 2007;131(1):131–7. https://doi.org/10.1043/1543-2165.(2007)131[131:Pmd]2.0.Co;2

88. Mulch AD, Stallings SP, Salafia CM. Elevated maternal serum alpha-fetoprotein, umbilical vein varix, and mesenchymal dysplasia: are they related? Prenat Diagn. 2006;26(8):659–61. https://doi.org/10.1002/pd.1436.
89. Aviram R, Kidron D, Silverstein S, Lerer I, Abeliovich D, Tepper R, Dolfin Z, Markovitch O, Arnon S. Placental mesenchymal dysplasia associated with transient neonatal diabetes mellitus and paternal UPD6. Placenta. 2008;29(7):646–9. https://doi.org/10.1016/j.placenta.2008.04.004.
90. Smith DH, Picker RH, Saunders DM, Sinosich M, Grudzinskas JG. Hydatidiform mole with coexistent viable fetus detected by routine AFP screening. Br Med J. 1980;280(6225):1213. https://doi.org/10.1136/bmj.280.6225.1213.
91. Ishikawa S, Morikawa M, Umazume T, Yamada T, Kanno H, Takakuwa E, Minakami H. Anemia in a neonate with placental mesenchymal dysplasia. Clin Case Rep. 2016;4(5):463–5. https://doi.org/10.1002/ccr3.543.
92. Kaiser-Rogers KA, McFadden DE, Livasy CA, Dansereau J, Jiang R, Knops JF, Lefebvre L, Rao KW, Robinson WP. Androgenetic/biparental mosaicism causes placental mesenchymal dysplasia. J Med Genet. 2006;43(2):187–92. https://doi.org/10.1136/jmg.2005.033571.
93. Maher ER, Brueton LA, Bowdin SC, Luharia A, Cooper W, Cole TR, Macdonald F, Sampson JR, Barratt CL, Reik W, Hawkins MM. Beckwith-Wiedemann syndrome and assisted reproduction technology (ART). J Med Genet. 2003;40(1):62–4. https://doi.org/10.1136/jmg.40.1.62.
94. Manipalviratn S, DeCherney A, Segars J. Imprinting disorders and assisted reproductive technology. Fertil Steril. 2009;91(2):305–15. https://doi.org/10.1016/j.fertnstert.2009.01.002.

Chapter 12
Genetics in Multiple Gestation

Takeshi Murakoshi

Abstract Human twinning process is rare but not uncommon. However, the human twinning process remains unclear. Twins are genetically classified into two major groups, dizygotic (DZ), which result from two different ova fertilized by two different sperms; and monozygotic (MZ), which result from a single ovum fertilized by one sperm that divides to form two embryos; therefore, it is implied that genetic constitution of MZ twins should be identical. While, clinically, twins are classified into three groups by their chorioamnionicity, (1) dichorionic-diamniotic (DCDA) in which each fetus has two independent amniotic and chorionic membranes, (2) monochorionic-diamniotic (MCDA) type consists of one chorionic membrane enclosing two amniotic membranes and fetuses, and (3) monochorionic-monoamniotic (MCMA) involving only one chorion and one amnion around the two fetuses and they have no intertwin divided membrane. Chorioamnionicity is the most influential factor for the prognosis of twin pregnancies. According to the unique pathophysiology of placentation and angioarchitecture of monochorionic placenta, MCDA and MCMA twins have risks of twin-twin transfusion syndrome, twin anemia polycythemia sequences, twin reversed arterial perfusion sequences, selective intrauterine growth restriction, and acute feto-fetal hemorrhage. To understand the nature of twinning both clinically and genetically, an understanding of zygosity, chorionicity, and amnionicity is the first step.

Keywords Zygosity · Chorionicity · Amnionicity · Monochorionic twin
Dichorionic twin · Ultrasound determination of chorioamnionicity · Vascular anastomoses

T. Murakoshi (✉)
Fetal Diagnosis and Therapy, Department of Obstetrics and Gynecology, Maternal and Perinatal Care Center, Seirei Hamamatsu General Hospital, Hamamatsu City, Japan
e-mail: t-murakoshi@sis.seirei.or.jp

H. Masuzaki (ed.), *Fetal Morph Functional Diagnosis*, Comprehensive Gynecology and Obstetrics, https://doi.org/10.1007/978-981-15-8171-7_12

12.1 Introduction

Human embryo is developed from a single zygote which continues to divide exponentially forming 2-, 4-, 8-, and 16-celled stages known as the morula. Through the processes of compaction, cell division, and blastulation, the conceptus takes the form of the blastocyst on the fifth day of development. The blastocyst can implant in the uterus after it hatches from the zona pellucida, and then, the embryonic stage of development begins.

Twining process is not completely resolved; briefly, union of two or more ova and sperms leads to multiple zygotes, and multiple ova originating from one ovum become monozygotic multiple pregnancies. The incidences of twinning vary in mammalian species. Multi-zygotic pregnancies are more common in mammals, but less common in humans, with an incidence of less than 1%. On the other hand, monozygotic multiple pregnancies are quite rare in mammals except for humans and nine-banded armadillos.

Twin pregnancies are divided into two groups by zygosity: monozygotic (MZ) twin and dizygotic (DZ) twin, and three groups by chorionicity and amnionicity: dichorionic-diamniotic (DCDA), monochorionic-diamniotic (MCDA), and monochorionic-monoamniotic (MCMA) twin pregnancies. There are a few exceptions to the relationship between zygosity and chorionicity; however, in theory "DZ twin is DCDA, and monochorionic (MC) twin is MZ."

Monochorionic placenta can virtually have some vascular anastomoses, as arterio-arterial (AA), arterio-venous (AV), and veno-venous (VV) anastomoses. Consequently, some unique pathophysiological conditions such as twin-twin transfusion syndrome (TTTS), twin reversed arterial perfusion (TRAP) sequence, twin anemia polycythemia sequence (TAPS), and selective intrauterine growth restriction (sIUGR) can occur because of hemodynamic imbalance through these vascular anastomoses and/or angioarchitecture of monochorionic placenta. In addition, MCMA twins have highest morbidity and mortality among all types of twins because of their unique angioarchitecture of MC placenta and umbilical cord entanglement.

This chapter reviews the relationship between zygosity and chorioamnionicity including some exceptions, ultrasound prenatal diagnosis of chorionicity with pitfalls, and the role of vascular anastomoses of monochorionic placenta.

12.2 Zygosity and Chorionicity

Twin pregnancy is divided into MZ twin and DZ twin on account of their zygosity. MZ twins originate from a single zygote that splits into two separate and complete zygotes in the early embryonic stage; at cleavage, morula, and/or blastocyst stage before 13 days of conception, therefore, MZ twins are genetically identical. While DZ twins are from two separate zygotes that originate from two ova and two sperms, thus, these twins are genetically non-identical and so-called fraternal twins. In higher-order multiple pregnancies such as triplet, quadruplet, and so on, the zygosity classification remains the same way as monozygotic, dizygotic, and trizygotic triplet and so on.

Human embryo and/or fetus have two separate membranes; the inner membrane is called the amniotic membrane and the outer one is called the chorionic membrane. From the perspective of these membranes, which is called chorioamnionicity, twin pregnancies can be divided into three groups: DCDA, MCDA, and MCMA twin pregnancies. In principle, DZ twins should be DCDA because they are completely separated and genetically independent. While, MZ twins can be classified into DCDA, MCDA, and MCMA twins according to the timing of zygote splitting [1] as follows: When the zygote separation occurs between the zygote and the morula stage, that is up to 72 h post-fertilization, chorioamnionicity can be DCDA (estimated 20–30%). Splitting probably occurs very early, when embryonic cells are totipotent, between the 1-cell and the 8-cell stage [2]. When the splitting occurs at the early blastocyst stage, at 4–8 days of post-fertilization, after the formation of the inner cell mass which separates from the trophoblast before day 8; chorioamnionicity is MCDA (estimated 60–75%) [3]. Splitting of the inner cell mass takes place when the amnion has become distinct, after day 8 up to day 12 of post-fertilization, chorioamnionicity becomes MCMA (estimated 1%) [4]. In rarest cases, conjoined twins result from cleavage at even later stage, 12–13 days after fertilization (estimated 1 in 200 MZ twin pairs or 1 in 40,000 births).

According to the relationship between zygosity and chorionicity, the theory that "DZ twin is DCDA, and monochorionic (MC) twin is MZ" is the norm. However, some exceptions, such as DZ-MC twins [1, 2], DZ twins after single embryo transfer [3], and DCDA twins after a single blastocyst embryo transfer [3–5], do occur rarely.

12.2.1 Dizygotic Monochorionic (DZ-MC) Twin Pregnancy

Discordant fetal sex is believed to be due to dizygosity and hence should be DCDA twins; however, some theoretical exceptions are as follows: (1) postzygotic sex chromosome abnormalities; 45, X/46, XY twin from 46, XY zygote; 45, X/47, XXY twin from 46, XY zygote, (2) malformed external genitalia, unrelated chromosomal, or genetic disorders; genital abnormalities such as hypospadias, clitomegaly, cloacal abnormality, and so on, and (3) DZ twins forming a monochorionic placenta.

Postzygotic sex chromosome abnormalities such as 45, X/46, XY twin from 46, XY zygote and 46, XX/46, XY from 47, XXY are rare phenomena due to the loss of Y- or X-chromosome during the dividing process. Furthermore, 45, X/47, XXY twin from 46, XY zygote are due to nondisjunction of the Y-chromosome.

DZ twins forming a monochorionic placenta are rare in humans. Souter et al. [2] first described this phenomenon with completely male and female fetuses with

MCDA placenta. Blood lymphocyte karyotype examination revealed chimerism of 46, XX/46, XY in both neonates, while their skin fibroblast karyotype examination showed normal karyotype corresponding to their genders. DNA zygosity test revealed dizygosity; hence, this was confirmed as a DZ-MC twin pregnancy. Subsequently, several additional cases have been reported [1] and these are more common in assisted reproductive technology pregnancies. Disruption of the zona pellucida and spatial proximity of multiple embryos may be possible causes of a DC-MZ twin mechanism.

12.2.2 DZ Twin After a Single Embryo Transfer

Twin pregnancies after a single embryo transfer (SET) are theoretically MZ twins because a single ovum splits and grows into identical twins; however, several cases of dizygotic and/or discordant sex twins were reported after SET [3, 5, 6]. The mechanism for DZ twins following SET is believed to be twin pregnancy by SET concurrent with natural conceptions. Previously reported cases of DZ twins after SET were fresh embryo transfer cases and spontaneous natural cycle with Frozen- or Vitrified- and warmed embryo transfer cycle, which highlights that spontaneous ovulation and natural conception can occur.

12.2.3 DCDA Twins After a Single Blastocyst Embryo Transfer

One of the principles of chorionicity and zygosity is that DCDA twins can occur from the morula stage of zygote, and MCDA can occur from the blastocyst stage of zygote. Therefore, twin pregnancy following SET of a blastocyst zygote can give rise to MCDA twins only. As the formation of the inner cell mass that separates the trophoblast has already been completed, the splitting process of the inner cell mass can become only monochorionic twins, but never dichorionic twins, theoretically. However, several reports suggested that DCDA twins might develop during expansion or hatching of the blastocyst [3, 6, 7], and the division of a blastocyst into two completely separate parts during in vitro culture with using time-lapse cinematography was reported [8].

The incidence of DCDA twins after a single blastocyst transfer is unclear. Konno et al. [3] reported a single-center cohort of 655 twin pregnancies, of which 43 were after a single blastocyst embryo transfer and 3 out of 43 (7%) were MZ-DCDA twins. Furthermore, another 3 out of 43 (7%) were DZ-DCDA twins: single blastocyst embryo transfer and concurrent natural conception. DCDA twins following single blastocyst transfer is not a rare phenomenon. Both MZ, which originate from the division of blastocyst into two completely separate blastocysts, and DZ, in which natural conception happens along with SET, can occur in DCDA twins.

12.3 Prenatal Ultrasound Diagnosis of Chorionicity and Amnionicity

First-trimester ultrasonography is the most standard method of determination of chorioamnionicity of twin pregnancy. Direct counting of each membrane, chorionic and amniotic membranes, is essential (Fig. 12.1). Fetal sex, number of placentas, shape of intertwin membrane insertion as T or lambda sign, thickness, and layers of intertwin membrane, and number of yolk sacs give additional information for the determination of chorioamnionicity. Diagnosis of chorioamnionicity is made sequentially in two steps by diagnosis of chorionicity followed by amnionicity.

12.3.1 Diagnosis of Chorionicity

Two separate gestational sacs and/or intertwin membrane formed from chorionic membrane are accurate markers for diagnosis of dichorionicity (Figs. 12.1 and 12.2). Discordant fetal sex or two separated placentas suggest dichorionic twin with

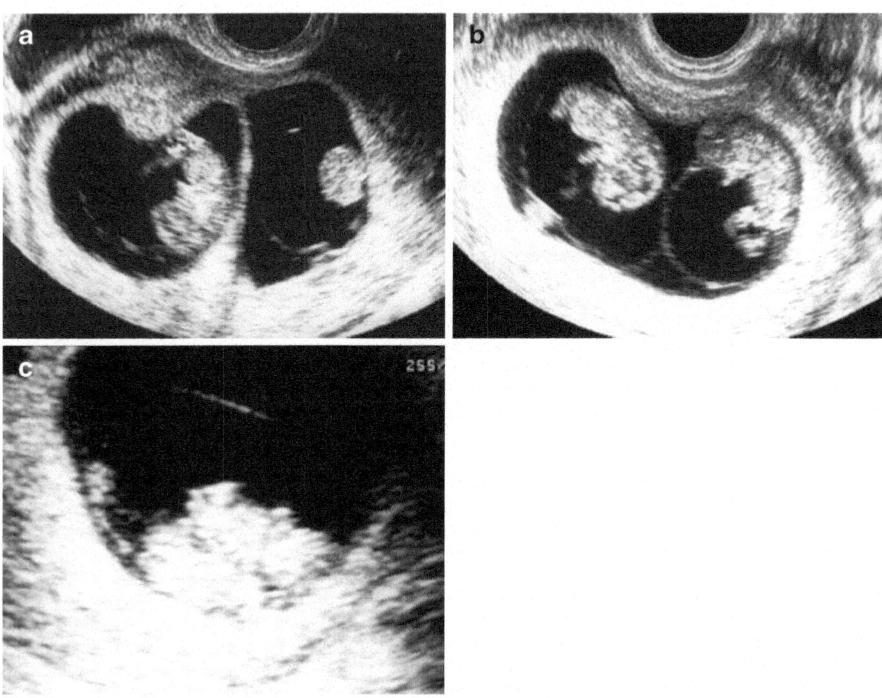

Fig. 12.1 Prenatal ultrasound diagnosis of chorionicity and amnionicity. Dichorionic-diamniotic (DCDA) twin (**a**), monochorionic-diamniotic (MCDA) twin (**b**), monochorionic-monoamniotic (MCMA) twin (**c**)

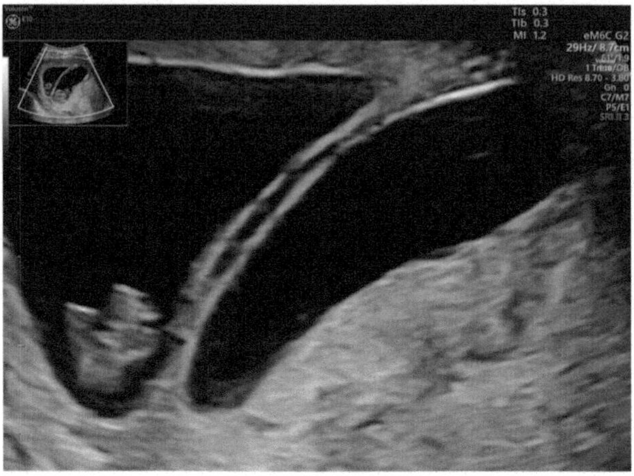

Fig. 12.2 Intertwin dividing membrane consisted of two chorionic membranes and Lambda sign

some exceptions. The shape of placental insertion of intertwin membrane is most reliable diagnostic tool (Figs. 12.1 and 12.2). The lambda sign, triangular projection of placental tissue extending into the base of intertwin membrane, indicates dichorionic twin with an accuracy as high as 99% [9]; however, false-positive [10–12] and false-negative [13] lambda signs can also exist.

12.3.2 Diagnosis of Amnionicity

After the diagnosis of monochorionic twin is made, determination of amnionicity should be performed. Visualization of intertwin amniotic membrane is essential for the diagnosis of diamniotic twin, while absence of intertwin membrane indicates monoamniotic twin. Amniotic membranes are very thin and difficult to determine by ultrasonography at early gestational age; therefore, repeated ultrasound examination is needed if intertwin membrane cannot be seen. Umbilical cord entanglement indicates monoamniotic twin pregnancy.

The number of yolk sacs used to be the diagnostic tools for determination of amnionicity as two yolk sacs indicate diamniotic and one yolk sac implies monoamniotic twin; however, there are many exceptions because the differentiation of yolk sac and amnion occurs very close, but not at the same time. Therefore, the number of yolk sacs is no longer used to determine amnionicity.

12.4 Pitfalls of Chorionicity, Amnionicity, and Zygosity

There are many pitfalls and exceptions in chorionicity, amnionicity, and zygosity. Some of the most representative pitfalls and exceptions are described below.

12.4.1 Lambda Sign Does Not Necessarily Guarantee DCDA Twin

Rarely in MCDA twins, the chorionic membrane folding grows into the intertwin dividing membrane between each amnion, like lambda sign in first or early second trimester (Fig. 12.3a). The pathology of dividing membrane exhibits partial DCDA in proximal side of placenta and partial MCDA in distal side of placenta. Some case reports described this phenomenon as "partial monochorionic/dichorionic twin" or "hybrid monochorionic/dichorionic twin"; however, they are essentially MCDA twins, and in some parts, single chorionic membrane gets prominent between the intertwin amniotic membranes as folding (Fig. 12.3b).

12.4.2 Discordant Fetal Sex Does Not Always Indicate DCDA Twin

As mentioned above, DZ twins forming monochorionic placenta are quite rare in humans; however, a few cases were reported with blood chimerism in DZ MCDA twin pregnancies [1, 2]. Our case described an MCDA twin pregnancy determined in first-trimester ultrasonography (Fig. 12.4a), and discordant fetal sex was revealed in second trimester (Fig. 12.4b, c). After gestation, a normal boy with normal male external genitalia and a normal girl with normal appearance of female genitalia were born (Fig. 12.4d, e). Placental examination of chorioamnionicity showed MCDA twin placenta with vascular anastomoses (Fig. 12.4f, g). Blood lymphocyte chromosome examination revealed 46, XX/46, XY in each infant.

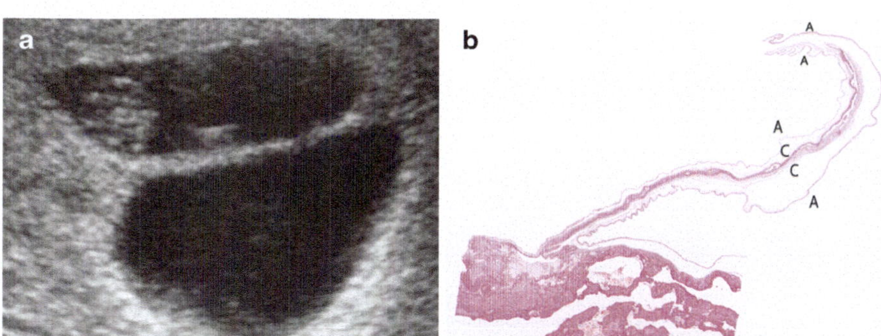

Fig. 12.3 Lambda sign is not always guaranteed DCDA twin. Two gestational sacs are detected in early first trimester (**a**). Pathological examination revealed dichorionic-diamniotic membrane at the placental proximal side (A-C-C-A) and monochorionic-diamniotic membrane at the distal side (A-A). Note the chorionic membrane was folding and continuing as monochorionic (**b**). *A* amnion, *C* chorion

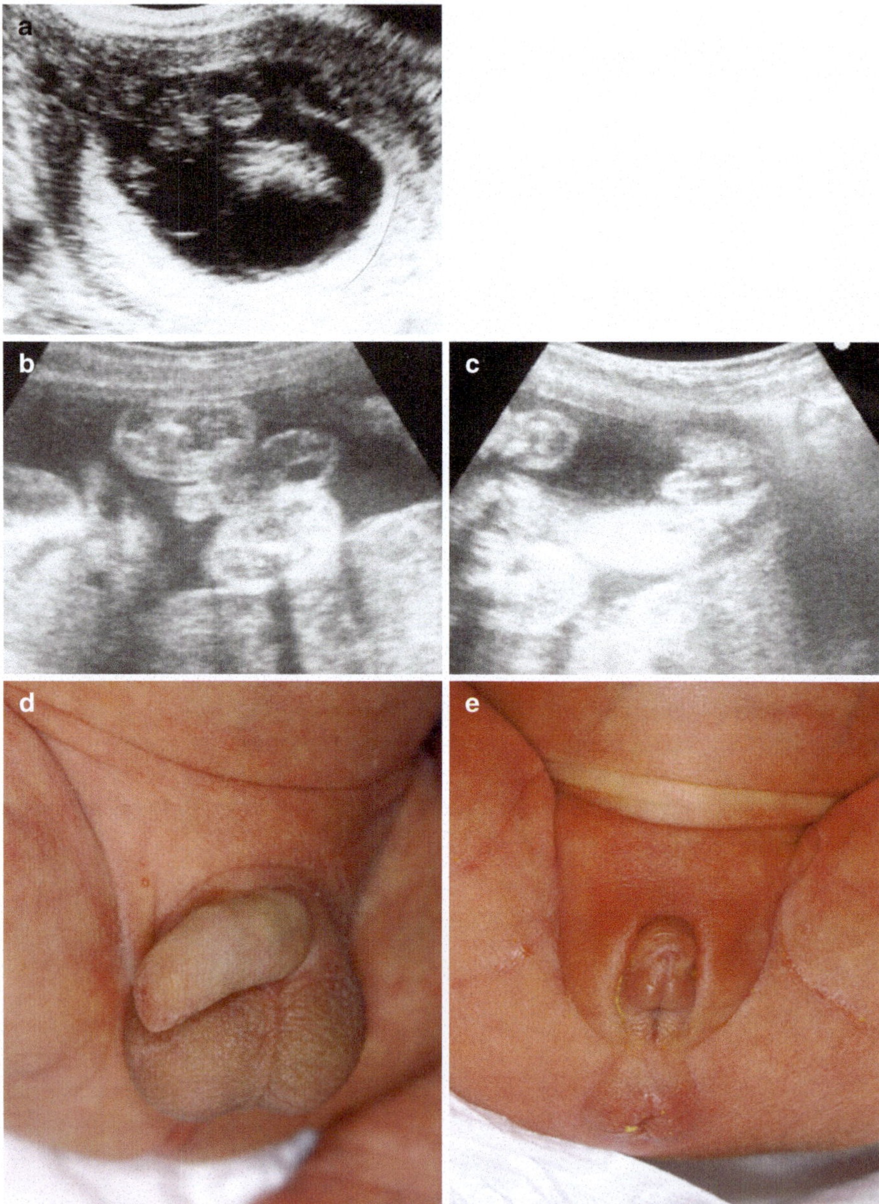

Fig. 12.4 Discordant fetal sex does not always indicate DCDA twin. First-trimester ultrasonography determined monochorionic-diamniotic twin pregnancy (**a**). Second-trimester ultrasonography revealed male (**b**) and female (**c**) genitalia. Neonatal genitalia showed normal male (**d**) and female (**e**) genitalia. Vascular anastomoses existed (**f**) and dividing membrane was monochorionic-diamniotic (**g**)

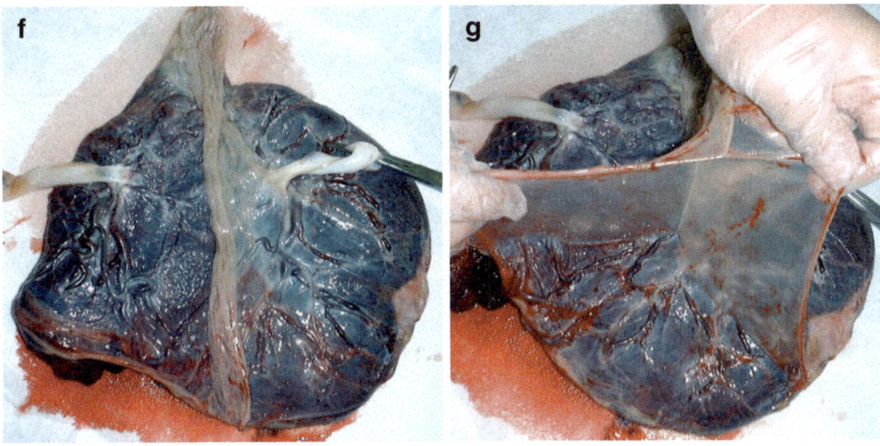

Fig. 12.4 (continued)

12.4.3 *MCDA Twin with Separate Placenta Does Exist*

MCDA twin pregnancies with separate placental mass are not rare; an incidence of around 3% of monochorionic placenta was reported [14]. There are two types of MCDA twins with separate placenta such as bipartite placenta with normal umbilical cord insertion (Fig. 12.5a), and bipartite or accessory placenta with velamentous umbilical cord insertion (Fig. 12.5b) [14–16].

12.4.4 *Two Yolk Sacs Do Not Determine MCMA Twin Any More*

The theory that two yolk sacs indicate diamniotic and single yolk sac implies monoamniotic is plausible; however, from an embryological perspective, the differentiation of yolk sac and amnion occurs almost simultaneously within 6–8 days after conception; whether the yolk sac develops prior to or following the appearance of the amnion remains unclear [17]. Therefore, many exceptions were reported as single yolk sac in MCDA twins [18] and double yolk sacs in MCMA twins [19–21]. Absence of intertwin dividing membrane and/or umbilical cord entanglement is reliable ultrasonography finding for the determination of MCMA twin pregnancies (Fig. 12.6).

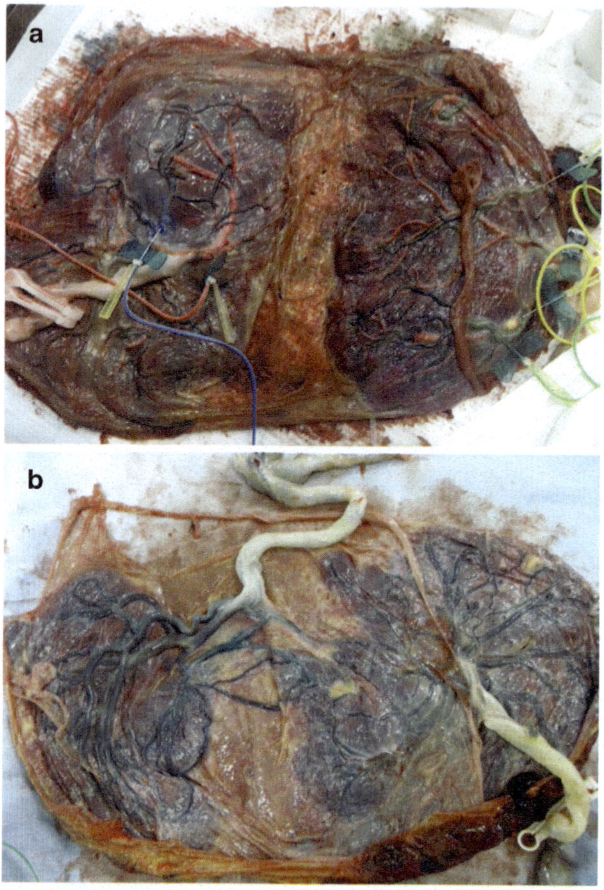

Fig. 12.5 MCDA twin with separate placenta. Bipartite placenta with normal umbilical cord insertion (**a**), accessory or bipartite placenta with velamentous umbilical cord insertion (**b**)

12.5 Role of Vascular Anastomoses in Monochorionic Placenta

In monochorionic placenta, three types of vascular anastomoses exist namely as AA, VV, and AV anastomoses. AA and VV anastomoses are also named superficial anastomoses because they have no terminal ends; AA anastomosis is described as the connection of an artery from fetus A through placental surface to the artery of fetus B with some arterial branches to the placental cotyledon, VV anastomosis is when a vein from fetus A is directly connected to a vein of fetus B with some branching like AA anastomoses, while AV anastomosis is not a direct connection between artery and vein in placental surface like AV malformation. However, they are connected via capillary vessels in placental cotyledon equally as the normal AV unit of cotyledon. In other words, the direction of feeding artery and drainage vein in cotyledon is the same fetus in normal AV unit, while the directions of artery and vein are opposite fetuses in AV anastomoses; therefore, AV anastomoses are also named deep anastomoses. Because of the simple angioarchitecture of AV

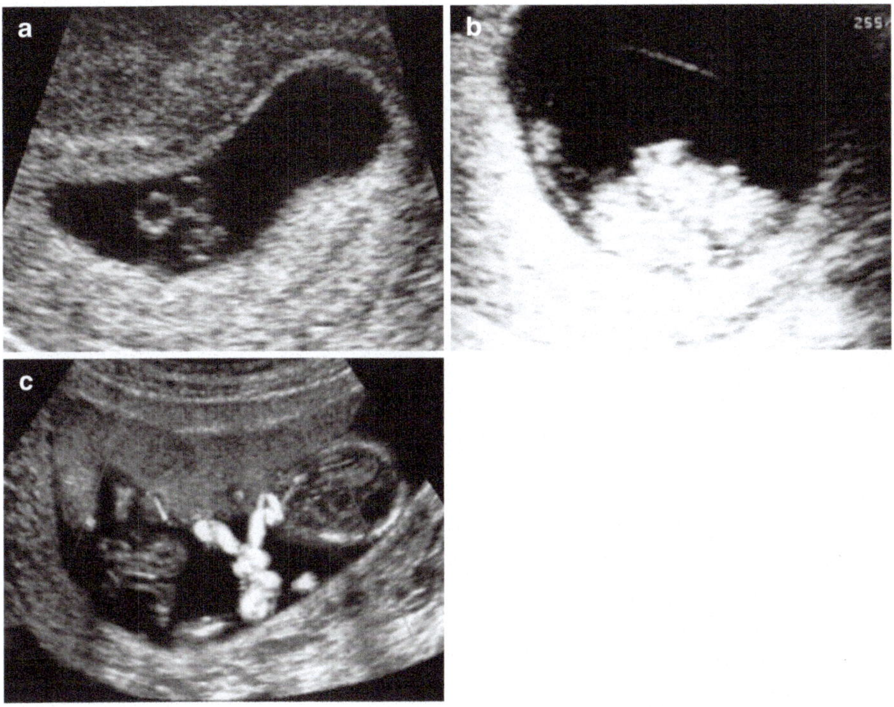

Fig. 12.6 Two yolk sacs do not determine MCMA twin any more. Two yolk sacs in monochorionic cavity (**a**), no dividing membrane can be seen (**b**), umbilical cord entanglement can be detected in early second trimester (**c**)

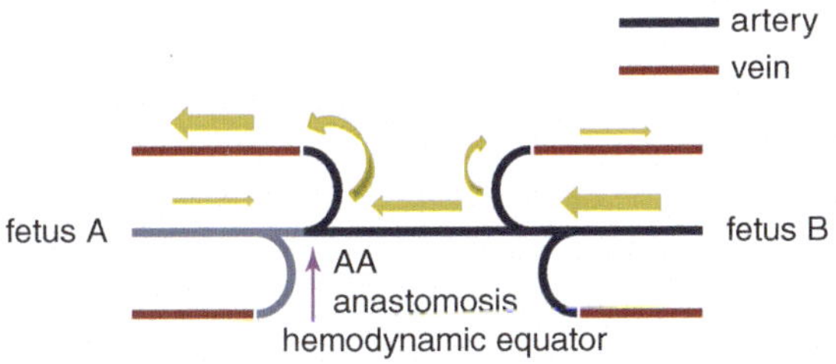

Fig. 12.7 Functional role of arterio-arterial anastomoses. Hemodynamic equator can move to fetus A when the arterial blood pressure of fetus B is higher than that of fetus A; therefore, arterio-arterial anastomoses can carry blood to fetus A from fetus B as a functional areterio-venous anastomoses

anastomoses, its role is uncomplicated and the blood volume is carried from one fetus with arterial origin to another fetus with vein.

The role of superficial anastomoses, such as AA and VV anastomoses, theoretically allows bi-directional flow via arterial or venous branches and could act as functional AV anastomoses (Figs. 12.7 and 12.8) [22–24]. AA anastomoses involve an arterial vessel without terminal end and connect directly to both twins; therefore,

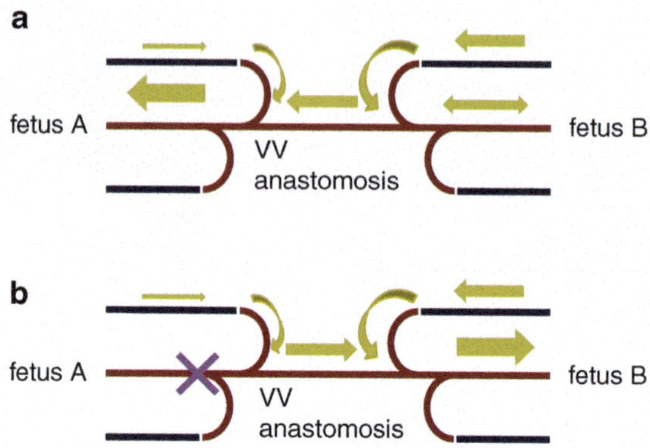

Fig. 12.8 Functional role of veno-venous anastomoses. Veno-venous (VV) anastomoses do not have hemodynamic equator. VV anastomoses can carry blood passively to fetus A from fetus B when the venous blood pressure of fetus B is higher than fetus A (**a**). VV anastomoses can carry blood to fetus B when the venous blood vessel of fetus A is compressed (X) by external impact (**b**)

hemodynamic equator, collision front of arterial blood pressure of each twin along with AA anastomosis, can exist. The direction of AA anastomoses can dynamically change depending on the blood pressure of each twin and arterial branch of AA anastomoses (Fig. 12.7). When the arterial blood pressure of fetus A is higher than fetus B, hemodynamic equator of AA anastomoses can move to fetus B and reaches an arterial branch of fetus B; therefore, AA anastomoses carry blood to fetus B from fetus A as functional AV anastomoses and vice versa. This mechanism potentially plays an etiological role to protect against TTTS because this functional AV anastomoses may rescue or reverse the transfusion of blood from one twin to the other dynamically due to an arterial blood pressure imbalance between both twins through AA anastomoses [24]. Furthermore, in TTTS with AA anastomoses, the donor may receive some blood from the recipient via AA anastomoses due to the arterial blood pressure discordance because the arterial blood pressure of the donor may be theoretically lower than that of the recipient; therefore, AA anastomoses may play a role against the advancement of TTTS [24–27].

The role of VV anastomoses, however, remains unclear and complex [22, 23, 28–30]. VV anastomoses do not have hemodynamic equator because of their venous blood origin. The direction of blood transfusion can depend on difference of venous blood pressure of each twin (Fig. 12.8) [22, 23]. When the venous blood pressure of fetus B is higher than that of fetus A, VV anastomoses carry blood passively to fetus A from fetus B according to the pressure gradient of both venous blood pressure. Transfusion blood volume may depend on the difference of venous blood pressure gradient of both twins (Fig. 12.8a). Another possible role for VV anastomoses is when the placental or umbilical vein of fetus A is compressed by an external impact, such as velamentous cord insertion and/or thin Walton jelly. In such an event, the VV anastomoses carry blood to fetus B. Almost the entire blood volume in the VV anastomoses flows to fetus B (Fig. 12.8b). Owing to these mechanisms, VV anastomoses may be involved in both the development and protection from TTTS. The role of VV anastomoses can be decided by the venous pressure gradient of both fetuses and external compression of the umbilical vein. If there is no external compression of the umbilical vein, the blood volume of umbilical vein in the recipient may be reduced through VV anastomoses, which may passively carry blood to the donor from the recipient according to the inter-twin venous pressure gradient. While, VV anastomoses may develop into TTTS because hypovolemic donor is more easily compressed than the hypervolemic recipient.

Both AA and VV anastomoses can play the role of functional AV anastomoses, which carry blood volume from one fetus to another. The direction of functional AV anastomoses of AA anastomoses depends on their arterial branch and the difference of arterial blood pressure of both fetuses, while direction of VV anastomoses depends on their venous branch and the venous pressure gradient of both twins. Furthermore, external venous compression can involve the direction of VV anastomoses.

References

1. Miura K, Niikawa N. Do monochorionic dizygotic twins increase after pregnancy by assisted reproductive technology? J Hum Genet. 2005;50(1):1–6.
2. Souter VL, Kapur RP, Nyholt DR, Skogerboe K, Myerson D, Ton CC, et al. A report of dizygous monochorionic twins. N Engl J Med. 2003;349(2):154–8.
3. Konno H, Murakoshi T, Miura K, Masuzaki H. The incidence of dichorionic diamniotic twin pregnancy after single blastocyst embryo transfer and zygosity: 8 years of single-center experience. Twin Res Hum Genet. 2020:1–4.
4. Kyono K. The precise timing of embryo splitting for monozygotic dichorionic diamniotic twins: when does embryo splitting for monozygotic dichorionic diamniotic twins occur? Evidence for splitting at the morula/blastocyst stage from studies of in vitro fertilization. Twin Res Hum Genet. 2013;16(4):827–32.
5. Kyono K, Nakajo Y, Nishinaka C, Araki Y, Doshida M, Toya M, et al. A birth of twins-one boy and one girl-from a single embryo transfer and a possible natural pregnancy. J Assist Reprod Genet. 2009;26(9–10):553–4.
6. Zou Z, Huang L, Lin S, He Z, Luo Y. Unusual twinning: additional findings during prenatal diagnosis of twin zygosity by single nucleotide polymorphism (SNP) array. Prenat Diagn. 2018;38(6):428–34.
7. Shibuya Y, Kyono K. A successful birth of healthy monozygotic dichorionic diamniotic (DD) twins of the same gender following a single vitrified-warmed blastocyst transfer. J Assist Reprod Genet. 2012;29(3):255–7.
8. Nishimura M, Tsuchiya S, Kaneko Y, Matsui Y, Iizumi A, Sato K, et al. Observation of a frozen-thawed blastocyst dividing via time-lapse cinematography and a possible mechanism for a dichorionic-diamniotic pregnancy. J Clin Embryol. 2014;17(2):191–5.
9. Maruotti GM, Saccone G, Morlando M, Martinelli P. First-trimester ultrasound determination of chorionicity in twin gestations using the lambda sign: a systematic review and meta-analysis. Eur J Obstet Gynecol Reprod Biol. 2016;202:66–70.
10. Chmait RH, Floyd R, Benirschke K. Duplicity: sonography suggested a twin gestation was dichorionic- and monochorionic. Am J Obstet Gynecol. 2011.
11. Galjaard S, Moerman P, Corveleyn A, Devlieger R, Lewi L. Partial monochorionic and monoamniotic twin pregnancies: a report of two cases. 2014;44(6):722-724.

12. Yamashita A, Ishii K, Hidaka N, Yonetani N, Hayashi S, Takeuchi M, et al. Monochorionic monozygotic twin pregnancy complicated with twin-twin transfusion syndrome presenting with an obvious lambda sign in the first trimester. Fetal Diagn Ther. 2015;37(2):154–6.
13. Wan JJ, Schrimmer D, Tache V, Quinn K, Lacoursiere DY, James G, et al. Current practices in determining amnionicity and chorionicity in multiple gestations. Prenat Diagn. 2011;31(1):125–30.
14. Lopriore E, Sueters M, Middeldorp JM, Klumper F, Oepkes D, Vandenbussche FP. Twin pregnancies with two separate placental masses can still be monochorionic and have vascular anastomoses. Am J Obstet Gynecol. 2006;194(3):804–8.
15. Konno H, Murakoshi T, Soga E, Terada S, Matsushita M, Otsuki Y. Bipartite monochorionic diamniotic placenta without intertwin vascular anastomoses. Jpn J Med Ultrasonics. 2019;46(6):555–8.
16. Lu J, Cheng YKY, Ting YH, Law KM, Leung TY. Pitfalls in assessing chorioamnionicity: novel observations and literature review. Am J Obstet Gynecol. 2018.
17. Moore KL, Persaud TVN. Formation of the bilaminar embryonic disc – The second week. The developing human, clinical oriented embryology. Philadelphia: W.B. Saunders; 1993. p. 40–52.
18. Shen O, Samueloff A, Beller U, Rabinowitz R. Number of yolk sacs does not predict amnionicity in early first-trimester monochorionic multiple gestations. Ultrasound Obstet Gynecol. 2006;27(1):53–5.
19. Bishop DK. Yolk-sac number in monoamniotic twins. Obstet Gynecol. 2010;116(Suppl 2):504–7.
20. Corbett SL, Shmorgun D. Yolk sac number does not predict reliably amnionicity in monochorionic twin pregnancies: a case of a monochorionic monoamniotic twin pregnancy with two distinct yolk sacs on early first-trimester ultrasound. Ultrasound Obstet Gynecol. 2012;39(5):607–8.
21. Murakoshi T, Ishii K, Matsushita M, Shinno T, Naruse H, Torii Y. Monochorionic monoamniotic twin pregnancies with two yolk sacs may not be a rare finding: a report of two cases. Ultrasound Obstet Gynecol. 2010;36(3):384–6.
22. Konno H, Murakoshi T, Matsushita M. The roles of superficial anastomoses in twin-twin transfusion syndrome. Placenta. 2019;82:5–9.
23. Konno H, Murakoshi T, Yamashita A, Matsushita M. Roles of venovenous anastomosis and umbilical cord insertion abnormalities in birthweight discordance in monochorionic-diamniotic twin pregnancies without twin-twin transfusion syndrome. J Obstet Gynaecol Res. 2018;44(4):623–9.
24. Murakoshi T, Quintero RA, Bornick PW, Allen MH. In vivo endoscopic assessment of arterio-arterial anastomoses: insight into their hemodynamic function. J Matern Fetal Neonatal Med. 2003;14(4):247–55.
25. Denbow ML, Cox P, Taylor M, Hammal DM, Fisk NM. Placental angioarchitecture in monochorionic twin pregnancies: relationship to fetal growth, fetofetal transfusion syndrome, and pregnancy outcome. Am J Obstet Gynecol. 2000;182(2):417–26.
26. Tan TY, Taylor MJ, Wee LY, Vanderheyden T, Wimalasundera R, Fisk NM. Doppler for artery-artery anastomosis and stage-independent survival in twin-twin transfusion. Obstet Gynecol. 2004;103(6):1174–80.
27. Denbow ML, Cox P, Talbert D, Fisk NM. Colour Doppler energy insonation of placental vasculature in monochorionic twins: absent arterio-arterial anastomoses in association with twin-to-twin transfusion syndrome. Br J Obstet Gynaecol. 1998;105(7):760–5.
28. de Villiers SF, Zhao DP, Cohen D, van Zwet EW, Duan T, Oepkes D, et al. Correlation between veno-venous anastomoses, TTTS and perinatal mortality in monochorionic twin pregnancies. Placenta. 2015;36(5):603–6.
29. Zhao DP, Cambiaso O, Otano L, Lewi L, Deprest J, Sun LM, et al. Veno-venous anastomoses in twin-twin transfusion syndrome: a multicenter study. Placenta. 2015;36(8):911–4.
30. Zhao DP, Cohen D, Middeldorp JM, Klumper FJ, Haak MC, Oepkes D, et al. The role of veno-venous anastomoses in twin-twin transfusion syndrome. Placenta. 2014;35(5):334–6.

Chapter 13
Fetal Therapy

Masayuki Endo and Haruhiko Sago

Abstract Several fetal therapies have become standard in prenatal care; however, there are no available fetal treatment options for genetic disorders. In utero stem cell transplantation (IUTx) and in utero gene therapy (IUGT) may become recognized as viable strategies for treating selective congenital genetic disorders in the near future. The advantages and disadvantages of fetal stem cell transplantation and gene therapy are discussed. The limit of the therapeutic effects after birth must be clarified, along with the safety of treatment during the fetal period for each treatment before clinical application.

Keywords Fetal therapy · Gene transfer · In utero gene therapy · In utero stem cell transplantation · Vector

With recent progress in prenatal diagnoses, advances have been made in fetal therapy to rescue fetuses facing perinatal death or devastating outcomes through the delivery of the optimal postnatal care. Some fetal therapies, such as fetoscopic laser surgery for twin-twin transfusion syndrome, thoraco-amniotic shunting for fetal hydrothorax, and radiofrequency ablation (RFA) for twin reversed arterial perfusion (TRAP) sequence, have become standard in prenatal care [1]. However, the target disorders for fetal therapy are still limited, and at present, there is no available fetal treatment option for genetic disorders.

Recent advances in the fields of regenerative medicine and gene therapy in adults and children suggest that in utero stem cell transplantation (IUTx) and in utero gene therapy (IUGT) [2] will be recognized as viable strategies for treating selective congenital genetic disorders in the near future.

M. Endo
Division of Health Science, Osaka University Graduate School of Medicine, Osaka, Japan
e-mail: endo@gyne.med.osaka-u.ac.jp

H. Sago (✉)
Center for Maternal-Fetal, Neonatal and Reproductive Medicine, National Center for Child Health and Development, Tokyo, Japan
e-mail: sagou-h@ncchd.go.jp

H. Masuzaki (ed.), *Fetal Morph Functional Diagnosis*, Comprehensive Gynecology and Obstetrics, https://doi.org/10.1007/978-981-15-8171-7_13

13.1 IUTx

Stem cells are defined as "undifferentiated cells" that combine both a "self-renewal ability" to divide and copy themselves and a "differentiation ability" to change into various cells. The treatment strategy of regenerative medicine involves regenerating damaged organs and tissues and restoring lost functions by transplanting stem cells or tissues artificially constructed from stem cells into patients. There are several types of stem cells, including (1) embryonic stem cells (ES cells), (2) somatic stem cells, and (3) induced pluripotent stem cells (iPS cells).

At present, the most common type of stem cell transplantation is hematopoietic stem cell transplantation for leukemia or lymphoma. In the fetal period, as clinical trials, hematopoietic stem cell transplantation has been performed for thalassemia and severe immunodeficiency, and mesenchymal stem cell transplantation has been performed for osteogenesis imperfecta [3]. However, in utero hematopoietic stem cell transplantation has only been successfully performed in cases of immunodeficiency. The host and maternal immune response may be limiting factors. Mesenchymal stem cell transplantation for osteogenesis imperfecta has resulted in a degree of clinical efficacy [4] and is expected to be used to treat various diseases in the future (Table 13.1).

13.2 IUGT

Gene therapy is defined as implanting therapeutic genes or genetically modified cells into a human body to treat diseases. The delivery of genes directly into the body for therapeutic purposes is called in vivo gene therapy, and the method of administering transfected cells is called ex vivo gene therapy. The carrier for

Table 13.1 Candidate diseases for IUTx

Hemoglobinopathies	α-Thalassemia
	β-thalassemia
	Sickle-cell anemia
	Rhesus isoimmunization
Immunodeficiencies	SCID
	Chronic granulomatous disease
	Bare lymphocyte syndrome
	Chediack-Higashi syndrome
	Omenn syndrome
Inborn metabolic disease	Globoid cell leukodystrophy
	Hurler's syndrome
	MPS I
	Niemann-pick disease
Musculoskeletal disease	Osteogenesis imperfecta

Table 13.2 Candidate diseases and target cells/organs of IUTG

Candidate diseases of IUGT	Target cells/organs
Cystic fibrosis	Airway and intestinal epithelial cells
Duchenne muscular dystrophy	Myocytes
Lysosomal storage disease	Hepatocytes
Spinal muscular atrophy	Motor neurons
Urea cycle defects	Hepatocytes
Hemophilia	Hepatocytes
Homozygous α-thalassemia	Erythrocyte precursors
Severe combined immunodeficiency	Hematopoietic precursors cells
Epidermolysis bullosa	Keratinocytes
Severe fetal growth restriction	Uterine arteries
Congenital diaphragmatic hernia	Alveoli

introducing genes into a cell is called the vector, and vectors for gene therapy can be viral and nonviral.

Several approaches to gene therapy have been developed, and therapeutic strategies include (1) converting a mutant gene into a normal gene, (2) inactivating or knocking out the mutant gene, and (3) introducing a new gene with a therapeutic effect.

At present, this approach has been clinically applied to cancer treatment and hereditary diseases (eye disease, hemophilia, etc.) for adults and children. However, it has not yet been clinically applied to a fetus, although there are a number of candidate diseases for IUGT [5] (Table 13.2).

13.3 Advantages of Fetal Stem Cell Transplantation and Gene Therapy

The advantages of IUTx and IUGT compared to similar therapy performed in adult or pediatric cases are generally as follows:

1. *Early intervention is possible.*

Treatment can begin while the condition is relatively mild or before the condition has progressed to an irreversible state.

2. *A fetus has a less mature immune system than an adult human.*

Since the immune system is already established in adults, an immune response is typically induced against the transplanted cells, vectors used in gene therapy, or the newly produced proteins, resulting in their consequent rejection. The amount of new protein produced decreases, as does the therapeutic effect. To combat this, adults may be given bone marrow suppression pretreatment with chemotherapy or radiation therapy to avoid triggering an immune response.

However, in the fetal period, especially before the immune system is established (said to be around 15 weeks of gestation), transplant cells, vectors, and new proteins should be recognized as self, thereby avoiding immune reactions. Bone marrow suppression before treatment is thus not required, and the long-term efficacy of treatment can be expected.

Furthermore, since atypical cells/foreign antigens recognized as self in the fetal period become immune-tolerant, rejection may be avoided if the same cell transplantation or vector administration becomes necessary after birth.

3. *Fetuses are smaller than grown humans.*

Since a fetus is smaller than an adult human, it is easy to secure the necessary number of cells for stem cell transplantation. In addition, in gene therapy, the amount of vector required is smaller for a fetus than for an adult human, so treatment costs can be reduced.

4. *There is space for the transplanted cells to survive.*

In order for the transplanted stem cells to proliferate smoothly and start differentiating, the appropriate space (niche) for engraftment in the bone marrow and the tissues is required. Such space is abundant in the fetal period compared to adults.

5. *The number of stem cells targeted for gene transfer is higher in the fetal period than as an adult.*

Theoretically, long-term efficacy can be expected when using a vector that is integrated into the genome of these stem cells, such as a lentiviral vector.

13.4 Disadvantages of Fetal Stem Cell Transplantation and Gene Therapy

However, there are also several problems associated with gene transfer during the fetal period.

1. *Transformation of cells by vector introduction (GENOTOXICITY)*

Viral vectors, such as retroviruses and lentiviruses, have the advantage of the inserted gene being expressed over a long period of time because they are integrated into the host genome. However, depending on the insertion site, oncogenesis may be induced. This is called genotoxicity.

Countermeasures that are currently being explored include the development of a vector that can insert the gene into the insertion site, the use of a vector that cannot be inserted into the genome (such as an adeno-associated virus), and the development of genome-editing gene therapy using an editing technology, such as CRISPR/Cas9, that recombines the mutated genome itself with a normal one.

2. *Gene transfer to the germline cells*

When a gene is introduced into a germline cell, the introduced gene propagates to the offspring over generations through reproductive activity. One concern is that the presence of the introduced gene could prevent the normal development and growth process which occurs from the fertilized egg to the fetus. The introduced gene can affect not only individuals, but also our entire human species. The same concern holds true for genome editing of germline cells. In 2019, a report from China described the creation of an HIV-resistant designer baby using CRISPR/Cas9 to edit the genome of human fertilized eggs. This news shocked the world. At present, it is forbidden to transplant fertilized human embryos into women anywhere in the world, including China.

3. *Unknown effects on development*

There are also concerns about the effects of the introduced genes on various organs that develop during the fetal period. In an attempt to minimize the influence on the normal development, the introduced gene should be expressed only in the target organ/tissue (targeting), or the duration and degree of gene expression should be able to be controlled (on/off system).

13.5 Academic Movement on IUTx and IUGT

The International Fetal Transplantation and Immunology Society (iFeTIS) (https://www.fetaltherapies.org) is an academic society whose goal is to apply stem cell transplantation and gene therapy to fetuses with congenital diseases. Following its first meeting in San Francisco in April 2014, the iFeTIS issued statements on IUTx and IUGT, which are shown in Table 13.3 [4].

13.6 Summary

IUTx and IUGT can be excellent treatments for fetuses suffering from selective congenital disorders. However, the limit of the therapeutic effects after birth must be clarified, along with the safety of treatment during the fetal period for each treatment before clinical application.

Table 13.3 Statements of the International Fetal Transplantation and Immunology Society 2015

• In utero transplantation is a viable strategy for treating fetuses with selective congenital disorders.
• Given recent reports that the maternal immune response can limit engraftment, the clinical strategy of in utero hematopoietic stem cell transplantation (IUHCT) should involve transplantation of autologous or maternal-derived cells. The host immune response may be a limiting factor that might be circumvented with early cell delivery.
• The fetal microenvironment plays a primary role in supporting the engraftment and expansion of transplanted cells and requires further investigation.
• Recent data from large-animal studies suggest that intravascular injection may be the delivery route of choice for achieving engraftment of hematopoietic stem cells in the fetus.
• At present, there is no proven safe method of host conditioning for fetuses. Until specific, non-toxic conditioning methods (such as antibody-mediated depletion of host HSC) are optimized in pre-clinical models, large cell doses should be used to overcome host competitive barriers.
• Experimental model data are sufficient to warrant a phase 1 clinical trial of IUHCT for select fetuses. The most suitable hematological diseases are hemoglobinopathies, such as sickle cell disease and thalassemia, given their high morbidity/mortality, the availability of reliable prenatal screening programs, and the dearth of optimum postnatal care options.
• The value of alternative cells, such as mesenchymal stromal cells (MSCs) and amniotic fluid-derived cells, for other appropriate congenital pathologies should be investigated.
• Reports of using MSCs in utero to treat osteogenesis imperfecta (OI) in a limited number of patients are promising and suggest that, after optimization, MSCs may be used to improve/treat OI.
• Treatment of fetal patients using gene therapy and gene-modified cells has great future potential and should be actively explored.

References

1. Sago H, Wada S. Fetal therapies as standard prenatal care in Japan. Obstet Gynecol Sci. 2020;63(2):108–16. https://doi.org/10.5468/ogs.2020.63.2.108.
2. Regulatory Issues: Prenatal Gene Transfer: Scientific, Medical, and Ethical Issues. A Report of the Recombinant DNA Advisory Committee. Home-Liebertpub-Com.Remote.Library.Osaka-U.Ac.Jp 2004;11(8):1211–1229. https://doi.org/10.1089/10430340050015257
3. Almeida-Porada G, Atala A, Porada CD. In utero stem cell transplantation and gene therapy: rationale, history, and recent advances toward clinical application. Mol Ther Methods Clin Dev. 2016;5:16020–17. https://doi.org/10.1038/mtm.2016.20.
4. Almeida-Porada TCMAG. Consensus statement from the first international conference for in utero stem cell transplantation and gene therapy. 2015;1–2. https://doi.org/10.3389/fphar.2015.00015/full
5. David AL, Waddington SN. Candidate diseases for prenatal gene therapy. In: Prenatal gene therapy. Totowa, NJ: Humana Press; 2012. p. 9–39. https://doi.org/10.1007/978-1-61779-873-3_2.

Part IV
Chromosomal Diseases

Chapter 14
General Remarks About Autosomal Diseases

Koh-ichiro Yoshiura

Abstract Autosomal diseases are diseases for which the responsible genetic loci are on autosomes. Chromosomal abnormalities, autosomal dominant diseases, autosomal recessive diseases, and imprinting disease are included in this category.

Keywords Autosome · Dominant · Recessive · Allele · Genetic locus

Autosomal diseases are defined as diseases for which the genetic loci are located on autosomes. Autosomes or autosomal chromosomes are chromosomes that are present in both female and male organisms. A genetic factor expressing a particular phenotype is supposed to be located at a specific genetic locus that has two or more alternative alleles. Although alleles could be considered as genes, this is not exactly correct and alleles are defined as two or more alternative forms of a genetic factor that exist in the same locus on a chromosome and define phenotype.

Human usually has two alleles on a locus that corresponds to the autosome pairs, one from the mother and one from the father, in somatic cells; the exception being the sex chromosomes. Genotype is defined as the combination of the two alleles at a genetic locus in one individual. Assuming two different genetic elements relate to a particular phenotype, "D" and "d," correspond to the alleles in one locus, then three genotypes are possible, "DD," "Dd," and "dd." "DD" and "dd" are homozygous genotypes because the same two alleles are present on the two autosomes, and "Dd" is the heterozygous genotype because two different alleles are present on the two autosomes. The terms "dominant" and "recessive" describe phenotypes that are expressed with a specific genotype. Dominant means the phenotype that is expressed in heterozygous individuals, and recessive means the phenotype that is expressed only in homozygous individuals. An autosomal dominant disease is a disease that develops in heterozygous individuals with one wild-type and one disease-related allele. An autosomal recessive disease is a disease that is found only in homozygous

K.-i. Yoshiura (✉)
Department of Human Genetics, Atomic Bomb Disease Institute, Nagasaki University, Nagasaki, Japan
e-mail: kyoshi@nagasaki-u.ac.jp

H. Masuzaki (ed.), *Fetal Morph Functional Diagnosis*, Comprehensive Gynecology and Obstetrics, https://doi.org/10.1007/978-981-15-8171-7_14

individuals with two disease-related alleles. A phenotype observed in homozygous individuals with two disease-related dominant alleles is usually severer than heterozygote in human, and the phenotype is called "incomplete dominant." Most of the dominant phenotype in human is incomplete dominant in this sense.

14.1 Chromosomal Abnormalities

Chromosomal abnormalities include aneuploidy, polyploidy, and structural abnormalities. The aneuploidy abnormalities, trisomy 13, trisomy 18, and trisomy 21 of whole chromosomes are only observed in newborn babies, and all other autosomal aneuploidies are usually spontaneously aborted at some period during pregnancy. However, various partial aneuploidies have been reported recently because newly available DNA microarray tests can detect genomic imbalances, including aneuploidy of small regions [>1 kb (kilobase pairs)] of chromosomes [1]. It should be noted that not all aneuploidies cause congenital diseases, even when the aneuploidy region contains genes. Copy number variations (CNVs) are known structural variations that involve sequence alterations that typically span >1 kb regions, and CNVs are considered as a type of aneuploidy. When an individual with (partial) aneuploidy of one of their chromosomes shows a disease phenotype, the phenotype is considered to be dominant, because the disease developed as the result of one allele abnormality. Most individuals likely have at least 4000 CNVs [2, 3], so judging the pathogenicity of CNVs or genomic copy number imbalances requires a great deal of caution. When an individual with (partial) aneuploidy in both chromosomes (homozygous state) shows a disease phenotype, the phenotype is considered to be recessive, and the CNV is defined as a recessive allele.

Special chromosome aneuploidies are one of the genetic disorders that are mediated by low copy repeat rearrangements [4, 5]. Sotos syndrome, Williams syndrome, and Langer–Giedion syndrome are examples of genomic disorders, also known as contiguous gene syndromes. These syndromes have been categorized into a definitive clinical entity by clinical geneticists over a long time. Low copy repeat-mediated chromosomal rearrangement based on genomic structure is the reason why many contiguous gene syndromes are frequently found and have been defined as a clinical entity.

14.2 Autosomal Dominant Diseases

For dominant diseases, homozygous with two disease-related (or mutation) alleles and heterozygous individuals with one wild-type allele and one disease-related allele will develop the disease. The general characteristics of autosomal dominant diseases are as follows: (1) heterozygous individuals develop the disease; (2) individuals with the disease are found in every generation in a family; (3) the patient/sex ratio is theoretically approximately 1:1; and (4) the segregation rate is 0.5. All these characteristics are based on the "dominant" definition that heterozygous individuals have one disease-related allele and will develop the disease. A dominant disease also can be caused by a de novo mutation that is found only in children, not in parents, and such diseases are dominant by definition.

Mutant alleles can either cause the encoded protein to be completely lost or to lose its function. The simplest mechanism for disease development is "loss of function" of the protein encoded by the mutated gene. Truncation-type mutations, which introduce premature termination codons in the messenger RNA (mRNA), mean functional proteins cannot be produced, so the amount of functional protein produced in individuals with this type of mutation will be half the amount produced in individuals who do not have the mutation.

The *NSD1* mutation in Sotos syndrome and the *ELN* mutation in supravalvular aortic stenosis are good examples of autosomal dominant diseases and haploinsufficiency. Haploinsufficiency is the term used to describe the condition in which the function of half of the genes is lost. In some patients with Sotos syndrome, the entire *NSD1* gene is deleted or nonsense mutations are found, so loss of one allele and haploinsufficiency leads to the development of Sotos syndrome. *ELN* loss is a usual characteristic of Williams syndrome, a contiguous gene syndrome with supravalvular aortic stenosis, and a truncation-type mutation is sometimes found in patients with solely supravalvular aortic stenosis. This evidence indicates that haploinsufficiency of *ELN* is the cause for supravalvular aortic stenosis.

Mutations can change the function of the encoded protein and can harm the functions of other proteins that interact with it. For example, a point mutation in *FGFR3* can cause achondroplasia. The encoded FGFR3 proteins (fibroblast growth factor receptor 3) form dimers that work as the complete receptor. When half of the *FGFR3* genes are mutated, only one-fourth of the dimers are completely functional. *FGFR3* also is sometimes deleted in Wolf-Hirschhorn syndrome and 4p16 deletion syndrome, but achondroplasia is not found in Wolf-Hirschhorn syndrome. This may be why only one-fourth of the FGFR3 dimers are completely functional in achondroplasia with the missense mutation, rather than half of the FGFR3 dimers in Wolf-Hirschhorn syndrome, or why the mutant FGFR4 protein can harm the functions of other proteins. The term "dominant-negative effect" defines the situation in which a mutated protein affects not only its own function but also the functions of other proteins with which it interacts.

14.3 Autosomal Recessive Diseases

For recessive diseases, homozygous and compound heterozygous individuals with two disease-related alleles (or mutation alleles) will develop the disease. Homozygous individuals have the same two mutant alleles, and compound heterozygous individuals have two different mutant alleles for one functional gene. The general characteristics of autosomal recessive diseases are (1) homozygous and compound heterozygous individuals develop the disease; (2) the disease looks occur sporadically; (3) patients can be found in siblings; (4) the patient/sex ratio is theoretically approximately 1:1; and (5) the segregation rate is 0.25. All these characteristics are based on the "recessive" definition.

When a homozygous mutation is found in a patient with a recessive disease, it may be that the mutant allele was derived from an ancestor of the patient. Parents are relatives from the historical view no matter whether they know it or not. Rare recessive diseases have been sometimes found in genetically isolated populations and, because of inbreeding, the mutant allele has been transmitted from generation to generation without any harmful effects. However, the two different mutant alleles found in compound heterozygotes are likely to have been derived from two independent ancestors, each of which had a de novo mutation in the past.

Recessive diseases develop in homozygous individuals, so all the children of homozygous parents will develop the disease. When the locus heterogeneity, two or more loci (gene) responsible for the clinical recessive disease, is exist, parents with disease may be homozygous in different loci. In this case, none of the children will develop recessive disease, because all the children will be heterozygous in both loci or in both disease-related genes; this condition is called double heterozygous. Understanding the differences among the disease-causing genes and mutations in patients is important for the prediction and prevention of recessive diseases in future generations especially in genetic counseling.

Uniparental disomy (UPD), which is a rare phenomenon, is another mechanism that causes chromosomal diseases. Instead of two alleles being transmitted, one from each parent, two alleles from only one of the parents are transmitted. Uniparental disomy could arise from trisomy rescue or monosomy rescue; however, the molecular mechanism is not well understood. Uniparental disomy has been reported, for example, in cystic fibrosis, congenital insensitivity to pain with anhidrosis, and 3M syndrome.

14.4 Imprinting Diseases

Imprinting describes the situation where one allele is expressed and other allele is inhibited in an individual depending on whether it was from the father (paternal allele) or mother (maternal allele). Imprinting diseases are caused by overexpression or loss of expression of the affected imprinted genes. The three supposed mechanisms of imprinting diseases are (1) gene mutation or partial chromosomal abnormality, including genes or imprinting control centers, that result in unbalanced gene expression; (2) uniparental disomy; and (3) abnormal methylation in differentially methylated regions. The imprinting control center is the region that controls gene expression and/or suppression and may contain differentially methylated regions. Beckwith-Wiedemann syndrome, Silver-Russell syndrome, Prader-Willi syndrome, Angelman syndrome, pseudo-hypoparathyroidism type I, Kagami-Ogata syndrome, Temple syndrome, and 6q24-related diabetes mellitus have been reported as imprinting diseases that are caused by disturbances in the expression of imprinted gene(s). Imprinted genes tend to cluster in specific regions, so clinical symptoms vary depending on the amount and kinds of affected gene products.

Imprinting diseases caused by gene mutation or partial chromosomal abnormality (mechanism 1 in the previous paragraph) have been found as familial cases in which the disease cause and phenotype are transmitted vertically. Because these diseases develop depending on the parental sex, pedigree diagrams are not typical of autosomal diseases. Imprinting diseases caused by the other two mechanisms, uniparental disomy (mechanism 2) and abnormal methylation in differentially methylated regions (mechanism 3), are not transmitted vertically or from generation to generation. However, details of the molecular mechanism of abnormal methylation are still unknown. The risk of the same disease developing in the next child of the same parents is similar to the risk of developing typical autosomal dominant or recessive diseases when disease is developed based on mechanism (1) described above. But the risk is the same as it is in the general population when the imprinting disease developed because of mechanisms (2) or (3), or recurrent risk in next child will not be increased. So the de novo methylation mutation might be a kind of replication error as de novo point mutation.

References

1. Martin CL, Warburton D. Detection of chromosomal aberrations in clinical practice from karyotype to genome sequence. Annu Rev Genomics Hum Genet. 2015;16:309–26.
2. Sudmant PH, Rausch T, Gardner EJ, Handsaker RE, Aby-zov A, Huddleston J, Zhang Y, Ye K, Jun G, Hsi-YangFritz M, et al. 1000 Genomes Project Consortium. An integrated map of structural variation in 2,504 human genomes. Nature. 2015;526:75–81.
3. Brandler WM, Antaki D, Gujral M, Noor A, Rosanio G, et al. Frequency and complexity of de novo structural mutation in autism. Am J Hum Genet. 2016;98:667–379.
4. Liu P, Carvalho CMB, Hastings PJ, Lupski JR. Mechanisms for recurrent and complex human genomic rearrangements. Curr Opin Genet Dev. 2012;22:211–20.
5. Dittwald P, Gambin T, Szafranski P, Li J, Amato S, Divon MY, et al. NAHR-mediated copy-number variants in a clinical population: mechanistic insights into both genomic disorders and Mendelizing traits. Genome Res. 2013;23:1395–409.

Chapter 15
Sex Chromosome-Linked Diseases

Haibo Li, Lulu Yan, Yuxin Zhang, Yingwen Liu, Min Xie, Ning Song, and Taosheng Li

Abstract It is widely accepted that human X and Y chromosomes are differentiated from a pair of autosomes by means of chromosomal inversions or accumulation of linked sex-determining genes. Therefore, the diseases caused by X- and Y-linked genes are not only similar to those caused by autosomes genes, but also gender specific. Some studies on the relative roles of the sex chromosome genes are likely to illuminate the reasons for the expression of some diseases within and between the sexes. Understanding the bases of these gender-based differences is also important for the development of new approaches to disease prevention, diagnosis, and treatment. In this chapter, we overview our current knowledge about the chromosomal, genomic, and single-gene diseases of the sex chromosomes, and discuss the correlation with fetal morphology.

Keywords Copy-number variation (CNV) · X chromosomal microdeletion syndrome · X chromosomal duplication syndrome · Y chromosomal microdeletion syndrome · Fetal morphology

---

H. Li (✉) · L. Yan · Y. Zhang · Y. Liu · M. Xie
Central Laboratory for Birth Defects Prevention and Control, Ningbo Women's and Children's Hospital, Zhejiang, P.R. China

N. Song
Hangzhou Diagens Biotechnology Co., Ltd, Hangzhou, Zhejiang, P.R. China

Medical School, Shanghai Jiao Tong University, Shanghai, P.R. China
e-mail: ningsong@noval-bio.com

T. Li
Department of Stem Cell Biology, Atomic Bomb Disease Institute, Nagasaki University, Nagasaki, Japan
e-mail: litaoshe@nagasaki-u.ac.jp

H. Masuzaki (ed.), *Fetal Morph Functional Diagnosis*, Comprehensive Gynecology and Obstetrics, https://doi.org/10.1007/978-981-15-8171-7_15

15.1 X Chromosome Copy-Number Variation

Genomic disorders result from copy-number variants (CNVs) or submicroscopic rearrangements of the genome rather than from single nucleotide variants (SNVs). Diverse technologies, including array comparative genomic hybridization (aCGH) and single nucleotide polymorphism (SNP) microarrays, and more recently, whole-genome sequencing and whole-exome sequencing, have enabled robust genome-wide unbiased detection of CNVs in affected individuals. There are eight expert-curated microdeletion and microduplication syndromes involved in developmental and structural disorders in DECIPHER database, but more in the literature. We summarized major information of X chromosomal microdeletion/microduplication syndrome can lead to abnormal development of the fetus in Table 15.1.

Table 15.1 The summarized major information of X chromosomal microdeletion/microduplication syndrome

Region	CNV type	Coordinates (GRCh37)	Representative gene	Phenotype
Xp22.3	Loss	chrX:585,079-8,700,228	SHOX, ARSE, STS, ANOS1	Leri–Weill syndrome, chondrodysplasia punctate 1, X-linked ichthyosis, Kallmann syndrome 1
Xp11.3	Loss	chrX:43,514,154-43,741,720	MAOA, MAOB	Intellectual disability, episodic hypotonia without EEG correlate, abnormalities in levels of catecholamines and their metabolites
Xp11.3	Loss	chrX:42359252-47459399	RP2	Mild to moderate mental retardation with severe, early-onset retinitis pigmentosa
Xq21	Loss	chrX:76020425-98354998	CHM, POU3F4	Choroideremia, hearing loss, mental retardation
Xq28	Loss	chrX:154,118,603-154,564,401	RAB39B	Embryonic/fetal lethality in males
Xp11.22p11.23	Gain	chrX:48,306,152-52,103,258	SHROOM4	Intellectual disability, speech and language delay, epilepsy and autistic behaviors
Xp11.22	Gain	chrX: 53,363,456-53,793,054	HUWE1	Nonsyndromic intellectual disability
Xq26.3	Gain	chrX:133634030-137982162	GPR101	Excessive growth, pituitary gigantism

Table 15.1 (continued)

Region	CNV type	Coordinates (GRCh37)	Representative gene	Phenotype
Xq27.3q28	Gain	chrX:142087786-155260560	FMR1	Mild mental retardation, mild facial dysmorphism, short stature, primary testicular failure
Xq28	Gain	chrX:147081520-155260560	GDI1, RAB39B, MECP2	Intellectual disability, behavioral psychiatric problems, recurrent infections, distinctive facial features, infantile hypotonia, progressive lower-limb spasticity, very poor-to-absent speech, epileptic seizures

15.1.1 X Chromosomal Microdeletion Syndrome

15.1.1.1 Xp22.3 Deletion Syndrome

Xp22.3 microdeletion syndrome is a contiguous syndrome, encompassing Leri–Weill syndrome (MIM: 127300, LWD), chondrodysplasia punctate 1 (MIM: 302950, CPDX1), X-linked ichthyosis (MIM: 308100, XLI), mental retardation, Kallmann syndrome 1 (MIM: 308700, KAL1). This interval includes several genes, especially the short stature homeobox (SHOX), arylsulfatase (ARSE), steroid sulfatase enzyme (STS), and ANOS1 genes. Depending on the size of deletion, it can be manifested as an isolated entity or as a syndrome caused by neighboring genes.

Leri–Weill Syndrome

Leri–Weill syndrome (MIM: 127300, LWD) is a pseudoautosomal dominantly inherited skeletal dysplasia characterized by short stature, mesomelic limb shortening, and a characteristic "Madelung" deformity of the forearms (bowing of the radius and restriction of pronation/supination of the forearm). Abnormalities in the growth plate may lead to short stature and skeletal deformity including Leri–Weill syndrome, which has been shown to result from deletions or mutations in the SHOX gene even its downstream regulatory domain, a homeobox gene located at the pseudoautosomal region of the X and Y chromosome [1]. SHOX protein was found in the reserve, proliferative, and hypertrophic zones of fetal growth plate from 12 week to term and childhood control and Leri Weil growth plates [2]. In some patients, the only discernible phenotype is short stature in the absence of mesomelia and Madelung deformity called idiopathic familial short stature (MIM: 300582, ISS). Although the disorder occurs in both sexes, females often have a more severe phenotype, because of sex differences in estrogen levels. Homozygous deletions of SHOX cause Langer mesomelic dysplasia (MIM: 249700, LMD) characterized by severe limb aplasia or severe hypoplasia of the ulna and fibula, or a thickened and curved radius and tibia [3].

Chondrodysplasia Punctate 1

Chondrodysplasia punctate 1 (MIM: 302950, CPDX1) is an X-linked recessive disorder characterized by chondrodysplasia punctate, brachytelephalangy, and nasomaxillary hypoplasia, which is caused by a deficiency of the Golgi enzyme arylsulfatase E (ARSE). In most patients, this condition is noted after birth due to an unusual face and respiratory problems. Most affected males have normal intellect and life span; however, some affected individuals have respiratory compromise, cervical spine stenosis, hearing loss, and intellectual disabilities. Carrier females thus far have not been affected. A hypoplastic nose with a depressed nasal bridge and contracture of wrists and fingers were clearly demonstrated by three-dimensional ultrasonography. Conventional karyotype analysis showed deletions or rearrangements of the short arm of X chromosome including *ARSE* in approximately 25% of individuals with features of CDPX1 [4, 5].

X-Linked Ichthyosis

X-linked ichthyosis (MIM: 308100, XLI) is a congenital disorder of keratinization characterized by generalized desquamation with larger polygonal scales mainly affecting the scalp, anterior aspects of the lower extremities, and other extensor surfaces. XLI is associated with a recurrent microdeletion at Xp22.31 including STS gene, ascribed to nonallelic homologous recombination. The typical size of Xp22.31 is approximately 1.5 Mb. Extracutaneous manifestations with corneal opacity present in around 50% of affected males and 25% of female carriers. The phenotype of ichthyosis usually occurs within the first year of life, and 15–20% have symptoms at birth. Female carriers do not exhibit any manifestations because the region of X chromosome encompassing STS gene does not undergo X-inactivation. The incidence of XLI is reported in 1/2500 to 1/6000 of males. Larger deletions could lead to learning disabilities with autistic spectrum problems and epilepsy, in which an adjacent X-linked mental retardation gene (such as VCX3A, PNPLA4, NLGN4) is involved [6, 7].

Kallmann Syndrome 1

Kallmann syndrome 1 (MIM: 308700, KAL1) is a genetic form of hypogonadotropic hypogonadism (HH) in association with anosmia or hyposmia. The disease is characterized by absence or incompleteness of sexual maturity by the age of 18 years, in conjunction with low levels of circulating gonadotropins and testosterone [8]. Defects in ANOS1 gene on chromosome Xp22.3 are involved in the molecular basis of KAL1. Approximately 1 in 30,000 males has the condition compared to 1 in 125,000 females [9].

15.1.1.2 Xp11.3 Deletion

Xp11.3 Deletion Includes MAOA and MAOB

The genes encoding MAOA and B are closely aligned on the Xp11.3 and have the same exon–intron structure. The absence of MAOA and MAOB appears to be associated with a phenotype that includes intellectual disability, episodic hypotonia (similar to seizures but without EEG correlate), and abnormalities in levels of catecholamines and their metabolites. Affected individuals were also reported to have varying degrees of dysmorphic characteristics and behavioral problems [10]. Deletions of MAOA and MAOB are frequently considered to be part of larger, contiguous gene deletions, and often include the adjacent NDP gene related to Norrie disease. In addition to the features of Norrie disease, individuals with deletions encompassing MAOA and MAOB are reported to have more severe neuropsychological disorders. Individuals with deletions involving only NDP and MAOB have been reported, and their features are said to be consistent with Norrie disease, but without the intellectual or behavioral issues in individuals with larger deletions including MAOA [11, 12].

Xp11.3 Deletion Includes RP2

Chromosome Xp11.3 deletion syndrome (MIM: 300578) is a contiguous gene syndrome including the RP2 gene. Affected individuals had mild to moderate mental retardation with severe, early-onset retinitis pigmentosa. The most severe retinitis pigmentosa could lead to significant visual loss before the age of 30. Some affected males also had microcephaly. Although some female carriers are manifested with visual impairment, all have normal intelligence. The absence of the RP2 gene accounts for retinal degeneration [13]. The deletion harboring several candidate genes for X-linked mental retardation (XLMR) is likely responsible for mental retardation [14].

15.1.1.3 Xq21 Deletion Includes CHM and POU3F4

Xq21 deletion syndrome (MIM: 303110) is a contiguous gene deletion syndrome including at least the CHM and POU3F4 genes. Xq21 deletion could result in choroideremia, deafness, and mental retardation syndrome. Xq21 deletion syndrome is an X-linked recessive disorder. Most female carriers are asymptomatic or show only a mild phenotype, although male carriers exhibited severe symptoms [15].

15.1.1.4 Xq28 Deletion Includes RAB39B

The absence of the Xq28 int22h1/int22h2-flanked region in males has been proposed to cause X-linked recessive embryonic/fetal lethality. Reported spontaneous abortion and lack of males identification in families with carrier females prove that such deletions may be lethal for males in utero. Female carriers are reportedly unaffected [16].

15.1.2 X Chromosomal Duplication Syndrome

15.1.2.1 Xp11.22p11.23 Recurrent Duplication Includes SHROOM4

The Xp11.22p11.23 recurrent duplication (MIM: 300801) is flanked distally and proximally by segmental duplications. The region is approximately 4.5 Mb size and both containing SSX genes and pseudogenes. Both males and females are affected. The main characteristics among patients include intellectual disability, speech and language delay, epilepsy, and autistic behaviors. Atypical breakpoints suggested phenotype/genotype correlations: FTSJ1 and SHROOM4 for intellectual disability while PQBP1 and SLC35A2 for epilepsy [17].

15.1.2.2 Xp11.22 Duplication Includes HUWE1

The Xp11.22 microduplication syndrome (MIM: 300705) causes nonsyndromic intellectual disability. The duplications are nonrecurrent and mediated by different mechanisms including the entire HUWE1 gene and at least one additional gene HSD17B10 on Xp11.22. HUWE1 is believed to be a dosage-sensitive gene responsible for the ID phenotype [18].

15.1.2.3 Xq26.3 Duplication Includes GPR101

X-linked acrogigantism (MIM: 300942, XLAG) is a recently described syndrome of pituitary gigantism, ascribed to microduplications on chromosome Xq26.3. The region encompasses the *GPR101* gene that highly upregulated in pituitary tumors.

XLAG is a unique clinical entity characterized by excessive growth, generally beginning during the first year of life in previously normal infants. Some patients with the Xq26.3 microduplication can show overgrowth at 2–3 months of age, although being normally sized newborns. Because infant overgrowth is rare and considered less important than failure to thrive, there was a delay in diagnosis in many cases. Because of this delay (most likely), unchecked growth of the pituitary hyperplasia–adenoma results in macroadenomas in most patients and expands to the level of the optic chiasm [19].

15.1.2.4 Xq27.3q28 Duplication Includes FMR1

Chromosome Xq27.3q28 duplication syndrome (MIM: 300869) is an X-linked recessive neurodevelopmental disorder characterized by mild mental retardation, mild facial dysmorphism, short stature, and primary testicular failure manifested as high-pitched voice, sparse body hair, abdominal obesity, and small testes. Female carriers may have short stature and premature ovarian failure, but may also be clinically unaffected due to nonrandom X chromosome inactivation. This disorder is caused by a copy-number increase of a 5.1 Mb region of chromosome Xq27.3q28 encompassing at least 28 genes, including FMR1 [20].

15.1.2.5 Xq28 Duplication

Xq28 Duplication Includes GDI1

A 0.3 Mb duplication of distal chromosome Xq28 (MIM: 300815) including GDI1 gene was found to correlate with X-linked intellectual disability. Vandewalle et al. considered that the increased expression of GDI1 results in impaired cognition. The duplication of the IKBKG gene, which is also in this interval, is likely to play a role in the mental retardation [21].

Xq28 Duplication Includes RAB39B

Duplication of the Xq28 int22h1/int22h2-flanked region is associated with syndromic X-linked intellectual disability, characterized in males by variable clinical features that may include: cognitive impairment, behavioral and psychiatric problems, recurrent infections and atopic diseases, obesity, and distinctive facial features. Carrier females have been reported to have a milder phenotype with learning difficulties and distinctive facies, but may also be clinically unaffected due to skewed X-inactivation [22].

Xq28 Duplication Includes MECP2

MECP2 duplication syndrome (MIM: 300260) is an X-linked neurodevelopmental disorder caused by nonrecurrent duplications of the Xq28 region involving the gene MECP2. Affected individuals are manifested with severe mental retardation (MR), infantile hypotonia, progressive lower-limb spasticity, very poor-to-absent speech, epileptic seizures, and recurrent severe infections. Only males are affected, although female carriers may have some mild neuropsychiatric features, such as anxiety [23].

15.2 X-Linked Monogenic Disorders

X-linked monogenic disorders result from mutated genes on the X chromosome. Males, who have only one X chromosome (i.e., they are hemizygous), will fully express an X-linked disorder. On the other hand, females, who have two X chromosomes, will be carriers of the defect in the majority of cases, and so they are usually asymptomatic. Although females have two X chromosomes to the male's one, products from this chromosome are quantitatively similar in both sexes because one of the two X chromosomes in females is inactivated. We summarized major information of X chromosomal monogenic disorders can lead to abnormal development of the fetus in Table 15.2.

15.2.1 X-Linked Adrenoleukodystrophy Caused by Mutations of ABCD1

X-linked adrenoleukodystrophy (MIM: 300100, X-ALD) is a rare recessive inherited disease, which is caused by the accumulation of very long chain fatty acid (VLCFA) in the central nervous system, liver, adrenal glands, and testes. Demyelinating lesions of the white matter and adrenal cortical dysfunction are the eventual affected clinical symptoms [24]. X-ALD develops in 1/17,000 births and in 1/20,000 males [25]. ABCD1 has been confirmed to be the virulence gene of X-ALD. The encoded product is peroxisomal ABC transporter protein (ALDP), which could transport the extracellular VLCFA into the cell to participate in β-oxidation. As a result, the dysfunction in ALDP could directly cause VLCFA accumulation [26, 27]. There have been more than 800 reported mutations in the ABCD1 gene, most of which are point mutations. In most conditions, single amino acid changes could induce the entire loss of the ALDP function [28].

Table 15.2 The summarized information of common X-linked monogenic disorders

Phenotype	Phenotype MIM number	Gene symbol	Cytogenetic location	Genomic coordinates (GRCh38)	Inheritance
X-linked adrenoleukodystrophy	300100	ABCD1	Xq28	X:153,724,850-153,744,754	XLR
Menkes syndrome	309400	ATP7A	Xq21.1	X:77,910,655-78,050,394	XLR
X-linked Alport syndrome	301050	COL4A5	Xq22.3	X:108,439,837-108,697,544	XLD
Duchenne/Becker muscular dystrophy	310200/300376	DMD	Xp21.2-p21.1	X:31,119,218-33,339,459	XLR
Fragile X syndrome	300624	FMR1	Xq27.3	X:147,911,918-147,951,126	XLD
Hemophilia A	306700	HEMA	Xq28	X:154,835,787-155,022,722	XLR
Lesch–Nyhan syndrome	300322	HPRT1	Xq26.2-q26.3	X:134,460,164-134,500,667	XLR
X-linked severe combined immunodeficiency	300400	IL2RG	Xq13.1	X:71,107,403-71,111,576	XLR
Oral-facial-digital syndrome type 1	311200	OFD1	Xp22.2	X:13,734,712-13,773,977	XLD
X-linked hypophosphatemia	307800	PHEX	Xp22.11	X:22,032,324-22,251,309	XLD
Immunodeficiency with hyper-IgM	308230	TNFSF5	Xq26.3	X:136,648,157-136,660,389	XLR

15.2.2 Menkes Syndrome Caused by Mutations of ATP7A

Menkes syndrome (MIM: 309400), also known as curly hair syndrome, is a rare congenital disorder of abnormal copper metabolism, which was first described by Menkes et al. in 1962 [29]. Menkes syndrome is transmitted as an X-linked recessive trait and has an incidence of 1:300,000 live births. The disease is a progressive and systemic disease, especially involving the damaged central nervous system and connective tissue. Unfortunately, most patients die before 3 years of age. Researchers have identified that Menkes syndrome is a rare congenital copper deficiency caused by the mutations of ATP7A gene, which could encode the copper transport ATPase [30]. To date, more than 350 different mutations of ATP7A gene have been reported [31]. Mechanistically, ATP7A mutations lead to double changes in the structure and function of ATPase, which cause the absorbing barrier of copper in food, resulting in a decrease in the concentration of copper ions in plasma and brain tissue, thus finally inducing the impairment of various copper-dependent enzymes [32].

15.2.3 X-Linked Alport Syndrome Caused by Mutations of COL4A5

Alport syndrome (AS) was first reported and named by Dr. Alport in 1927. Continuous studies recognize that X-linked dominant AS (MIM: 301050, XLAS) caused by COL4A5 mutations accounts for 80% of AS patients. In this crowd, the males suffered more serious clinical symptoms: the proportion of renal failure reached 90% before 40 years old [33]. In addition, approximately 15% of AS patients attribute to autosomal recessive inheritance caused by COL4A3 or COL4A4 gene mutations, and these patients would develop renal failure before the age of 30 [34].

15.2.4 Duchenne/Becker Muscular Dystrophy (DMD/BMD) Caused by Mutations of DMD

Duchenne muscular dystrophy (MIM: 310200, DMD, with an estimated incidence of 1/3500) and Becker muscular dystrophy (MIM: 300376, BMD, with an estimated incidence of 1/18,500) are the most common types of X-linked progressive muscular dystrophy, mainly affecting males, both of which attribute to the mutations in the DMD gene [35]. DMD gene on X chromosome could encode dystrophin in the normal physiological state, which would anchor elements of the internal cytoskeleton to the surface membrane and strengthen muscle cells. When the dystrophin protein is absent or nonfunctional, the clinical symptoms of sick males will be more severe, whereas BMD patients exhibit a milder symptom for a partially functional dystrophin protein [36, 37]. In general, genetic counseling and DMD genetic testing are necessary for people with a family history of DMD.

15.2.5 Fragile X Syndrome Caused by Premutation of FMR1

Fragile X syndrome (MIM: 300624, FXS) is the most common inherited form of mental retardation currently known, mainly including moderate to severe intellectual hypoplasia, large testes, often accompanied by big ears, single ears, mandibular protrusion, high palatal arch, light blue sclera membranes, language disorders, epilepsy, etc. [38]. This disorder is caused by a dynamic mutation in the FMR1 gene localized on the Xq27.3. The FMR1 product is one RNA-binding protein involved in the shearing of transcripts, RNA transport, mRNA stability, and translation level. The 5′UTR region of patient FMR1 has a genetically unstable amplification of the CGG trinucleotide repeat sequence, with abnormal methylation of the adjacent CpG island. In almost all patients, the mRNA and protein products of FMR1 are not expressed or underexpressed. Different degrees of CGG repeats amplification can cause different degrees of methylation in adjacent CpG islands, and excessive methylation of CpG islands may inhibit the normal transcription of the FMR1 gene. FXS is the ending of the excessive increase of CGG repeats and abnormal methylation of adjacent regions [39, 40].

15.2.6 Hemophilia A Caused by Mutations of HEMA

Hemophilia A (MIM: 306700) is an X-linked recessive hereditary blood disorder, mainly affecting males, along with the abnormal bleeding or prolonged oozing after injuries, surgery, or tooth extractions. Usually, after the original injury, muscle hematomas or intracranial bleeding can last 4–5 days. This disorder is induced by the deficiency of the blood clotting protein known as Factor VIII, which plays a crucial role in blood coagulation [41]. As is known, HEMA gene encodes the protein of Factor VIII, and the mutations of HEMA could cause the impaired Factor VIII, leading to the final hemophilia A [42]. Currently, gene replacement therapy for hemophilia A, including monoclonal antibody purified Factor VIII and recombinant Factor VIII, has been in progress and future clinical applications are expected [43].

15.2.7 Lesch–Nyhan Syndrome Caused by Mutations of HPRT1

Lesch–Nyhan syndrome (MIM: 300322, LNS) is a compulsive self-destructive behavior for the mentally retarded person, and an X-linked recessive inherited disease, which originates from the missing of hypoxanthine-guanine phosphoribosyltransferase (HGPRT) produced by HPRT1 gene. Unfortunately, IMP and GMP could not be converted from hypoxanthine and guanine by lack of this enzyme, which eventually leads to impaired DNA/RNA synthesis [44, 45]. Multiple different types of mutations in HPRT1 have been identified to be associated with X-linked LNS, including deletions, insertions, single-base substitutions, and frame-shift mutations [46].

15.2.8 X-Linked Severe Combined Immunodeficiency Caused by Mutations of IL2RG

Severe combined immunodeficiency (SCID) is profoundly induced by defective T cells, B cells, and natural killer cells. All forms of SCID are inherited, and approximately half of SCID cases linked to X chromosome called X-linked SCID (MIM: 300400). It is caused by a mutation in the interleukin 2 receptor gamma (IL2RG) gene, which encodes the common gamma chain subunit, a component of several IL receptors. Defective IL receptors will block the functions of T-lymphocytes and other involved cells in the immune system [47, 48].

15.2.9 Oral-Facial-Digital Syndrome Type 1 Caused by Mutations of OFD1

Oral-facial-digital syndrome type 1 (MIM: 311200, OFD1) is a rare X-linked dominant disorder, and predominantly affects females with embryonic male lethality. OFD1 is usually characterized by malformation of the oral cavity (lobulated tongue, tongue nodules, cleft of the hard or soft palate, accessory gingival frenulae, hypodontia), face (widely spaced eyes or telecanthus, hypoplasia of the alae nasi, median cleft or pseudocleft upper lip, micrognathia), and digits (brachydactyly, syndactyly, clinodactyly of the fifth finger; duplicated hallux) [49]. Abnormalities of the central nervous system (CNS) and cystic kidney disease can also be part of its symptoms. Mutations in the OFD1 gene will account for this syndrome. This gene could encode a centrosomal protein localized at the basal bodies at the origin of primary cilia, whereas the deficiency of OFD1 gene could induce the abnormal formation of cilia [50].

15.2.10 X-Linked Hypophosphatemia Caused by Mutations of PHEX

The incidence of hypophosphatemia is about 1/20,000, containing five major subtypes. The most common type is X-linked hypophosphatemia (MIM: 307800, XLH), which is mainly caused by missense mutation, nonsense mutation, or shear site mutation in the PHEX gene. As reported, mutations of PHEX could result in the increased serum levels of fibroblast growth factor-23 (FGF23), which causes phosphate wasting and hypophosphatemia [51, 52]. Clinically, children suffering from XLH are all manifested as rickets, bone deformities, and short stature. Meanwhile, adult patients may still be symptomatic with bone and joint pain, osteomalacia-related fractures, precocious osteoarthrosis, enthesopathy, or severe dental anomalies [53, 54].

15.2.11 *Immunodeficiency with Hyper-IgM Caused by Mutations of TNFSF5*

Immunodeficiency with hyper-IgM (MIM: 308230, HIM) is a rare primary immunodeficiency characterized by low serum concentrations of IgG, IgA, and IgE, but with normal or elevated serum concentrations of IgM. The main clinical manifestation of HIM patients is repeated bacterial infection, accompanied by reduced neutrophils, lymphatic hyperplasia, even individual autoimmune diseases, and tumorigenesis. This disease mainly occurs in males, and approximately 70% of them are inherited in the X-linked recessive trait [55, 56]. It is reported that the defect in TNFSF5 gene may be the main reason for X-linked HIM. This gene could normally encode a CD40 antigen ligand (CD154), a protein on T cells that binds to the CD40 receptor on B and other immune cells. The absence of CD154 could not deliver signals to B cells, thus failing to switch antibody production to IgA and IgG [57, 58]. Regular IV replacement of the missing IgG antibodies and prompt treatment of infections are the main therapeutic schedules of HIM.

15.3 Y-Linked Disorders and Genetic Mechanisms

Unlike other human chromosomes, the Y chromosome has a limited number of genes (only 54 protein-coding genes), owing to their degeneration during the whole evolution process [59, 60]. Some genetic defects including single-gene mutations/polymorphisms, CNVs, and deletions on the long arm of the Y chromosome (Yq microdeletions, see Table 15.3) may cause a series of male-specific Y-linked diseases [61]. Across these abnormal phenotypes and genetic mechanisms, male infertility induced by microdeletions of AZF loci and disorders of sex development (DSD) caused by SRY mutation/translocation can be seen as models.

15.3.1 *Male Infertility and AZF Loci Microdeletions*

AZF, called as azoospermia factor, localized in the long arm of Yq. AZF loci encompass three nonoverlapping subregions in proximal, middle, and distal of Yq11, respectively, designated "AZFa," "AZFb," and "AZFc" [62, 63]. A large number of

Table 15.3 The summarized information of AZF loci microdeletions

AZF loci	Gene symbol	Cytogenetic location	Genomic coordinates (GRCh38)
AZFa	USP9Y	Yq11.221	Y:12,701,230-12,860,838
	DBY		Y:12,903,998-12,920,477
	UTY		Y:13,231,826-13,480,669
AZFb	KDM5D	Yq11.223	Y:19,703,864-19,745,340
	RPS4Y2		Y:20,756,107-20,781,031
	XKRY	Yq11.222	Y:17,768,979-17,770,559
	HSFY		Y:18,529,677-18,588,962
	RBMY1A1	*Yq11.223*	Y:21,534,878-21,559,682
	PRY		Y:22,490,290-22,516,302
AZFc	DAZ	Yq11.223	Y:23,129,354-23,199,116
	BPY1	Yq11.221	Y:13,985,771-13,986,511
	BPY2	Yq11.223	Y:22,984,262-23,005,464
	CDY	Yq11.23	Y:25,622,094-25,625,510

genes in AZF loci have been demonstrated to be directly involved in the spermatogenesis, and the microdeletions of several functional genes are the most frequent abnormalities of Y chromosome, which could result in azoospermia or severe oligo-asthenozoospermia, thus explaining CNV-relevant male infertility [63, 64].

15.3.1.1 Genes and Deletions in AZFa

The deletions in AZFa are rare, accounting for about 1–5% of Y chromosome microdeletions. The AZFa locus is comprised of single-copy genes with X homologues that escape inactivation. In this region, three loci are identified to be possibly important for male fertility. Firstly, ubiquitin-specific peptidase 9, Y-linked (USP9Y), also known as DFFRY, located on Yq11.221, consisting of 46 exons. The protein encoded by this gene is a member of the peptidase C19 family with protease activity specific to ubiquitin [65]. USP9Y could regulate the protein turnover by preventing degradation of proteins by the proteasome through the removal of ubiquitin from protein-ubiquitin conjugates [66]. Researchers discovered that deletions of USP9Y are occurred in both infertile men and men with normal sperm count, suggesting that USP9Y deletions alone are insufficient to cause infertility [65]. DEAD box RNA helicases, Box 3, Y-linked (DBY), also known as DDX3Y, located on Yq11.221, consisting of 17 exons. Unlike USP9Y, DBY is specifically expressed in spermatogonia and plays an important role in the spermatogenic process [67, 68]. In fact, the males with DBY deletion could exhibit as Sertoli cell only syndrome (SCOS) or severe hypospermatogenesis [67, 69]. Ubiquitously transcribed tetratricopeptide repeat containing, Y-linked (UTY), located at the 5C band of AZFa, containing 50 exons. This gene encodes a male-specific histone demethylase that catalyzes trimethylated "Lys-27" (H3K27me3) demethylation [70]. Studies point out that some missense mutations of UTY have lethal effects on spermatogenesis [71]. To date, UTY deletions alone in infertile males have not been identified.

15.3.1.2 Genes and Deletions in AZFb

Single-Copy Genes

Two single-copy genes, lysine (K)-specific demethylase 5D (KDM5D) and ribosomal protein S4, Y isoform 2 (RPS4Y2), are the most relevant with male fertility. KDM5D protein is involved in male germ cell chromosome remodeling during meiosis by acting as a histone H3 lysine 4 (H3K4) demethylase [72]. In the course of spermatogenesis, the KDM5D enzyme could form a protein complex with MutS protein homolog 5 (MSH5) [73]. RPS4Y2 gene is located on Yq11.223, and the ribosomal protein encoded by this gene is specific in testis [74]. Noticeably, RPS4Y2 protein plays an important role in the posttranscriptional regulation of spermatogenesis [75].

Gene Families

Among the gene families in AZFb, four genes are emphasized to be associated with male fertility. XK, Kell blood group complex subunit-related, Y-linked (XKRY), located on Yq11.222, encodes a protein similar to XK, a putative membrane transport protein. XKRY is specifically expressed in testis, thus dysfunctions or deletions of the XKRY gene are relevant with spermatogenic failure and male infertility [76, 77]. Heat shock transcription factor, Y-linked (HSFY), also located on Yq11.222. This gene could encode two copies HSFY1 and HSFY2. The data show that both HSFY1 and HSFY2 loss due to a large 768 kb deletion around the P4 palindrome at the proximal end of the AZFb interval, which seriously injures spermatogenesis, ultimately lead to infertility [78, 79]. RNA binding motif protein, Y-linked, family 1, member A1 (RBMY1A1), another azoospermia-associated gene, located on Yq11.223, and the encoded protein is testis specific. Studies identify that RBMY1A1 CNV affects sperm motility, and its low copy number (<6) may cause asthenozoospermia [80, 81]. PTPN13-like, Y-linked (PRY), also located on Yq11.223, expressed specifically in testis. Its functional role is confirmed in spermatogenesis for regulating apoptosis [82]. Studies reveal that hypospermatogenesis is occurred by the deletions of all the genes in AZFb region, except for RBMY and PRY. However, both deletions of RBMY and PRY may induce complete meiotic arrest, which results in male infertility, suggesting their essential and positive roles in fertility [64, 83].

15.3.1.3 Genes and Deletions in AZFc

AZFc deletions account for approximately 60% of Y chromosome microdeletions [84, 85]. Analogously, deletions of four important genes are involved in male infertility. Deleted in azoospermia (DAZ), mapped at Yq11.223, is a multicopy gene family, which encodes four gene copies (DAZ1-4). DAZ controls early meiosis during spermatogenesis, and the incidence of DAZ gene deletion is higher in infertile patients compared with normal males [86]. Interestingly, DAZ was initially identified as a frequently deleted gene on the Y chromosome of infertile males [87]. DAZ deletion accounts for 10% of cases of males with dyszoospermia [88, 89]. Basic charge, Y-linked, 1 (BPY1), is also known as VCY. Its encoded protein is only existed in testicular tissue, thus called testis-specific basic protein Y 1. This position reveals its functional role in spermatogenesis [90]. Nevertheless, there is no evidence yet that deletions of BPY1 are directly correlated with male infertility. Basic protein Y2, Y-linked (BPY2), belongs to the VCX/VCY gene family as well, and also known as VCY2. BPY2A, BPY2B, and BPY2C are three copies of BPY2. It has been definitely reported that BPY2 protein is localized in the nuclei of spermatocytes, round spermatids, and spermatogonia [91]. In the Chinese and Indian populations, BPY2 deletions happen frequently in men with severe oligozoospermia or azoospermia [92]. Chromodomain Y, Y-linked (CDY), is testis-specifically expressed, and the encoded protein has histone acetyltransferase activity [93]. Researchers identify that loss of the CDY1a is positively related to male infertility ($p = 0.002$) [94].

15.3.2 DSD and Mutation/Translocation of SRY

SRY, which stands for the sex-determining region Y gene, encompasses a 35 kb region of Y-specific DNA adjacent to the pseudoautosomal boundary, which is important for testis formation [95]. Concretely, this gene encodes a testis-determining factor (TDF), which acts as a DNA-binding protein, alters DNA characteristics, and makes the undifferentiated gonad turn to testis development. As reported, all of the listed situations: point mutations, the total deletion of the SRY gene, or its translocation between the MSY region and the X chromosome, could all lead to disorders of sex development (DSD). Mutations in the SRY gene are identified in approximately 15% 46, XY females (Swyer syndrome, female habitus with gonadal dysgenesis) [96]. In this case, part of the Y chromosome is translocated to the X chromosome, which causes embryonic gonads to fail to develop into testes. Unfortunately, the gonads in these abnormal women could not develop into functional ovaries.

Permissions We confirm that this chapter has not used any excerpts from copyrighted (or previously published) works (including websites).

References

1. Ross JL, et al. The phenotype of short stature homeobox gene (SHOX) deficiency in childhood: contrasting children with Leri-Weill dyschondrosteosis and Turner syndrome. J Pediatr. 2005;147(4):499–507.

2. Munns CJ, et al. Expression of SHOX in human fetal and childhood growth plate. J Clin Endocrinol Metab. 2004;89(8):4130–5.
3. Ambrosetti F, et al. Langer mesomelic dysplasia in early fetuses: two cases and a literature review. Fetal Pediatr Pathol. 2014;33(2):71–83.
4. Nino M, et al. Clinical and molecular analysis of arylsulfatase E in patients with brachytelephalangic chondrodysplasia punctata. Am J Med Genet A. 2008;146A(8):997–1008.
5. Brunetti-Pierri N, et al. X-linked recessive chondrodysplasia punctata: spectrum of arylsulfatase E gene mutations and expanded clinical variability. Am J Med Genet A. 2003;117A(2):164–8.
6. Carrascosa-Romero MC, et al. X-chromosome-linked ichthyosis associated to epilepsy, hyperactivity, autism and mental retardation, due to the Xp22.31 microdeletion. Rev Neurol. 2012;54(4):241–8.
7. Crane JS, Wu B, Paller AS. Ichthyosis X-Linked. 2020.
8. Alnaes M, Melle KO. Kallmann syndrome. Tidsskr Nor Laegeforen. 2019;139(17).
9. de Castro F, Seal R, Maggi R. ANOS1: a unified nomenclature for Kallmann syndrome 1 gene (KAL1) and anosmin-1. Brief Funct Genomics. 2017;16(4):205–10.
10. Whibley A, et al. Deletion of MAOA and MAOB in a male patient causes severe developmental delay, intermittent hypotonia and stereotypical hand movements. Eur J Hum Genet. 2010;18(10):1095–9.
11. Suarez-Merino B, et al. Sequence analysis and transcript identification within 1.5 MB of DNA deleted together with the NDP and MAO genes in atypical Norrie disease patients presenting with a profound phenotype. Hum Mutat. 2001;17(6):523.
12. Rodriguez-Revenga L, et al. Contiguous deletion of the NDP, MAOA, MAOB, and EFHC2 genes in a patient with Norrie disease, severe psychomotor retardation and myoclonic epilepsy. Am J Med Genet A. 2007;143A(9):916–20.
13. Zhang L, et al. A microdeletion in Xp11.3 accounts for co-segregation of retinitis pigmentosa and mental retardation in a large kindred. Am J Med Genet A. 2006;140(4):349–57.
14. Lugtenberg D, et al. ZNF674: a new Kruppel-associated box-containing zinc-finger gene involved in nonsyndromic X-linked mental retardation. Am J Hum Genet. 2006;78(2):265–78.
15. Merry DE, et al. Choroideremia and deafness with stapes fixation: a contiguous gene deletion syndrome in Xq21. Am J Hum Genet. 1989;45(4):530–40.
16. El-Hattab AW, et al. Clinical characterization of int22h1/int22h2-mediated Xq28 duplication/deletion: new cases and literature review. BMC Med Genet. 2015;16:12.
17. Giorda R, et al. Complex segmental duplications mediate a recurrent dup(X)(p11.22-p11.23) associated with mental retardation, speech delay, and EEG anomalies in males and females. Am J Hum Genet. 2009;85(3):394–400.
18. Froyen G, et al. Copy-number gains of HUWE1 due to replication- and recombination-based rearrangements. Am J Hum Genet. 2012;91(2):252–64.
19. Rodd C, et al. Somatic GPR101 duplication causing X-Linked Acrogigantism (XLAG)-diagnosis and management. J Clin Endocrinol Metab. 2016;101(5):1927–30.
20. Rio M, et al. Familial interstitial Xq27.3q28 duplication encompassing the FMR1 gene but not the MECP2 gene causes a new syndromic mental retardation condition. Eur J Hum Genet. 2010;18(3):285–90.
21. Vandewalle J, et al. Dosage-dependent severity of the phenotype in patients with mental retardation due to a recurrent copy-number gain at Xq28 mediated by an unusual recombination. Am J Hum Genet. 2009;85(6):809–22.
22. El-Hattab AW, et al. Int22h-1/int22h-2-mediated Xq28 rearrangements: intellectual disability associated with duplications and in utero male lethality with deletions. J Med Genet. 2011;48(12):840–50.
23. Ramocki MB, Tavyev YJ, Peters SU. The MECP2 duplication syndrome. Am J Med Genet A. 2010;152A(5):1079–88.
24. Turk BR, et al. X-linked adrenoleukodystrophy: pathology, pathophysiology, diagnostic testing, newborn screening, and therapies. Int J Dev Neurosci. 2019;
25. Vogel BH, et al. Newborn screening for X-linked adrenoleukodystrophy in New York State: diagnostic protocol, surveillance protocol and treatment guidelines. Mol Genet Metab. 2015;114(4):599–603.

26. Montagna G, et al. Identification of seven novel mutations in ABCD1 by a DHPLC-based assay in Italian patients with X-linked adrenoleukodystrophy. Hum Mutat. 2005;25(2):222.
27. Berger J, Gartner J. X-linked adrenoleukodystrophy: clinical, biochemical and pathogenetic aspects. Biochim Biophys Acta. 2006;1763(12):1721–32.
28. Schonberger S, et al. Genotype and protein expression after bone marrow transplantation for adrenoleukodystrophy. Arch Neurol. 2007;64(5):651–7.
29. Menkes JH, et al. A sex-linked recessive disorder with retardation of growth, peculiar hair, and focal cerebral and cerebellar degeneration. Pediatrics. 1962;29:764–79.
30. Rangarh P, Kohli N. Neuroimaging findings in Menkes disease: a rare neurodegenerative disorder. BMJ Case Rep. 2018;2018
31. Tumer Z, Moller LB. Menkes disease. Eur J Hum Genet. 2010;18(5):511–8.
32. Tumer Z. An overview and update of ATP7A mutations leading to Menkes disease and occipital horn syndrome. Hum Mutat. 2013;34(3):417–29.
33. Bekheirnia MR, et al. Genotype-phenotype correlation in X-linked Alport syndrome. J Am Soc Nephrol. 2010;21(5):876–83.
34. Zhang Y, et al. Genotype-phenotype correlations in 17 Chinese patients with autosomal recessive Alport syndrome. Am J Med Genet A. 2012;158A(9):2188–93.
35. Flanigan KM. Duchenne and Becker muscular dystrophies. Neurol Clin. 2014;32(3):671–88. viii
36. Esposito G, Carsana A. Metabolic alterations in cardiomyocytes of patients with Duchenne and Becker muscular dystrophies. J Clin Med. 2019;8(12)
37. Deconinck N, Dan B. Pathophysiology of Duchenne muscular dystrophy: current hypotheses. Pediatr Neurol. 2007;36(1):1–7.
38. Razak KA, Dominick KC, Erickson CA. Developmental studies in fragile X syndrome. J Neurodev Disord. 2020;12(1):13.
39. Landowska A, et al. Fragile X syndrome and FMR1-dependent diseases – clinical presentation, epidemiology and molecular background. Dev Period Med. 2018;22(1):14–21.
40. Salcedo-Arellano MJ, et al. Fragile X syndrome and associated disorders: clinical aspects and pathology. Neurobiol Dis. 2020;136:104740.
41. Konkle BA, Huston H, Nakaya FS. Hemophilia A. 1993.
42. Mansouritorghabeh H. Clinical and laboratory approaches to hemophilia A. Iran J Med Sci. 2015;40(3):194–205.
43. Aledort L, et al. Factor VIII replacement is still the standard of care in haemophilia A. Blood Transfus. 2019;17(6):479–86.
44. Bell S, et al. Lesch-Nyhan syndrome: models, theories, and therapies. Mol Syndromol. 2016;7(6):302–11.
45. Harris JC. Lesch-Nyhan syndrome and its variants: examining the behavioral and neurocognitive phenotype. Curr Opin Psychiatry. 2018;31(2):96–102.
46. Torres RJ, Puig JG. Hypoxanthine-guanine phosphoribosyltransferase (HPRT) deficiency: Lesch-Nyhan syndrome. Orphanet J Rare Dis. 2007;2:48.
47. Diaz-Parra S, et al. X-linked severe combined immunodeficiency and hepatoblastoma: a case report and review of literature. J Pediatr Hematol Oncol. 2018;40(6):e348–9.
48. Allenspach E, Rawlings DJ, Scharenberg AM. X-linked severe combined immunodeficiency. 1993.
49. Toriello HV, et al. Oral-facial-digital syndrome type I. 1993.
50. Macca M, Franco B. The molecular basis of oral-facial-digital syndrome, type 1. Am J Med Genet C Semin Med Genet. 2009;151C(4):318–25.
51. Beck-Nielsen SS, et al. FGF23 and its role in X-linked hypophosphatemia-related morbidity. Orphanet J Rare Dis. 2019;14(1):58.
52. Kinoshita Y, Fukumoto S. X-linked hypophosphatemia and FGF23-related hypophosphatemic diseases: prospect for new treatment. Endocr Rev. 2018;39(3):274–91.
53. Lecoq AL, et al. Management of X-linked hypophosphatemia in adults. Metabolism. 2020;103S:154049.

54. Rothenbuhler A, et al. Diagnosis, treatment-monitoring and follow-up of children and adolescents with X-linked hypophosphatemia (XLH). Metabolism. 2020;103S:153892.
55. Yazdani R, et al. The hyper IgM syndromes: epidemiology, pathogenesis, clinical manifestations, diagnosis and management. Clin Immunol. 2019;198:19–30.
56. Dunn CP, de la Morena MT. X-linked hyper IgM syndrome. 1993.
57. Groeneweg M, Lankester AC, Bredius RG. From gene to disease; CD40 ligand deficiency as the cause of X-linked hyper-IgM-syndrome. Ned Tijdschr Geneeskd. 2003;147(21):1009–11.
58. Rawat A, et al. Clinical and molecular features of X-linked hyper IgM syndrome – an experience from North India. Clin Immunol. 2018;195:59–66.
59. Krausz C, Casamonti E. Spermatogenic failure and the Y chromosome. Hum Genet. 2017;136(5):637–55.
60. Quintana-Murci L, Fellous M. The human Y chromosome: the biological role of a "functional wasteland". J Biomed Biotechnol. 2001;1(1):18–24.
61. Hotaling J, Carrell DT. Clinical genetic testing for male factor infertility: current applications and future directions. Andrology. 2014;2(3):339–50.
62. Vogt PH, et al. Human Y chromosome azoospermia factors (AZF) mapped to different subregions in Yq11. Hum Mol Genet. 1996;5(7):933–43.
63. Vicdan A, et al. Genetic aspects of human male infertility: the frequency of chromosomal abnormalities and Y chromosome microdeletions in severe male factor infertility. Eur J Obstet Gynecol Reprod Biol. 2004;117(1):49–54.
64. Colaco S, Modi D. Genetics of the human Y chromosome and its association with male infertility. Reprod Biol Endocrinol. 2018;16(1):14.
65. Luddi A, et al. Spermatogenesis in a man with complete deletion of USP9Y. N Engl J Med. 2009;360(9):881–5.
66. Ginalski K, et al. Protein structure prediction for the male-specific region of the human Y chromosome. Proc Natl Acad Sci U S A. 2004;101(8):2305–10.
67. Foresta C, Ferlin A, Moro E. Deletion and expression analysis of AZFa genes on the human Y chromosome revealed a major role for DBY in male infertility. Hum Mol Genet. 2000;9(8):1161–9.
68. Ditton HJ, et al. The AZFa gene DBY (DDX3Y) is widely transcribed but the protein is limited to the male germ cells by translation control. Hum Mol Genet. 2004;13(19):2333–41.
69. Lardone MC, et al. Quantification of DDX3Y, RBMY1, DAZ and TSPY mRNAs in testes of patients with severe impairment of spermatogenesis. Mol Hum Reprod. 2007;13(10):705–12.
70. Walport LJ, et al. Human UTY(KDM6C) is a male-specific N-methyl lysyl demethylase. J Biol Chem. 2014;289(26):18302–13.
71. Nailwal M, Chauhan JB. Computational analysis of high risk missense variant in human UTY gene: a candidate gene of AZFa sub-region. J Reprod Infertil. 2017;18(3):298–306.
72. Lee MG, et al. Physical and functional association of a trimethyl H3K4 demethylase and Ring6a/MBLR, a polycomb-like protein. Cell. 2007;128(5):877–87.
73. Akimoto C, et al. Spermatogenesis-specific association of SMCY and MSH5. Genes Cells. 2008;13(6):623–33.
74. Lopes AM, et al. The human RPS4 paralogue on Yq11.223 encodes a structurally conserved ribosomal protein and is preferentially expressed during spermatogenesis. BMC Mol Biol. 2010;11:33.
75. Andres O, et al. RPS4Y gene family evolution in primates. BMC Evol Biol. 2008;8:142.
76. Lahn BT, Page DC. A human sex-chromosomal gene family expressed in male germ cells and encoding variably charged proteins. Hum Mol Genet. 2000;9(2):311–9.
77. Navarro-Costa P, Plancha CE, Goncalves J. Genetic dissection of the AZF regions of the human Y chromosome: thriller or filler for male (in)fertility? J Biomed Biotechnol. 2010;2010:936569.
78. Tessari A, et al. Characterization of HSFY, a novel AZFb gene on the Y chromosome with a possible role in human spermatogenesis. Mol Hum Reprod. 2004;10(4):253–8.
79. Vinci G, et al. A deletion of a novel heat shock gene on the Y chromosome associated with azoospermia. Mol Hum Reprod. 2005;11(4):295–8.

80. Abid S, et al. Cellular ontogeny of RBMY during human spermatogenesis and its role in sperm motility. J Biosci. 2013;38(1):85–92.
81. Yan Y, et al. Copy number variation of functional RBMY1 is associated with sperm motility: an azoospermia factor-linked candidate for asthenozoospermia. Hum Reprod. 2017;32(7):1521–31.
82. Stouffs K, et al. Expression pattern of the Y-linked PRY gene suggests a function in apoptosis but not in spermatogenesis. Mol Hum Reprod. 2004;10(1):15–21.
83. O'Flynn OK, Varghese AC, Agarwal A. The genetic causes of male factor infertility: a review. Fertil Steril. 2010;93(1):1–12.
84. Dai RL, et al. Varicocele and male infertility in Northeast China: Y chromosome microdeletion as an underlying cause. Genet Mol Res. 2015;14(2):6583–90.
85. Rodovalho RG, Arruda JT, Moura KK. Tracking microdeletions of the AZF region in a patrilineal line of infertile men. Genet Mol Res. 2008;7(3):614–22.
86. Fu XF, et al. DAZ family proteins, key players for germ cell development. Int J Biol Sci. 2015;11(10):1226–35.
87. Foresta C, et al. Y chromosome microdeletions in cryptorchidism and idiopathic infertility. J Clin Endocrinol Metab. 1999;84(10):3660–5.
88. Kuo PL, et al. Expression profiles of the DAZ gene family in human testis with and without spermatogenic failure. Fertil Steril. 2004;81(4):1034–40.
89. Sen S, et al. Susceptibility of gr/gr rearrangements to azoospermia or oligozoospermia is dependent on DAZ and CDY1 gene copy deletions. J Assist Reprod Genet. 2015;32(9):1333–41.
90. Zou SW, et al. Expression and localization of VCX/Y proteins and their possible involvement in regulation of ribosome assembly during spermatogenesis. Cell Res. 2003;13(3):171–7.
91. Tse JY, et al. Specific expression of VCY2 in human male germ cells and its involvement in the pathogenesis of male infertility. Biol Reprod. 2003;69(3):746–51.
92. Lu C, et al. Gene copy number alterations in the azoospermia-associated AZFc region and their effect on spermatogenic impairment. Mol Hum Reprod. 2014;20(9):836–43.
93. Lahn BT, et al. Previously uncharacterized histone acetyltransferases implicated in mammalian spermatogenesis. Proc Natl Acad Sci U S A. 2002;99(13):8707–12.
94. Machev N, et al. Sequence family variant loss from the AZFc interval of the human Y chromosome, but not gene copy loss, is strongly associated with male infertility. J Med Genet. 2004;41(11):814–25.
95. She ZY, Yang WX. Sry and SoxE genes: how they participate in mammalian sex determination and gonadal development? Semin Cell Dev Biol. 2017;63:13–22.
96. Quinn A, Koopman P. The molecular genetics of sex determination and sex reversal in mammals. Semin Reprod Med. 2012;30(5):351–63.

Part V
Genetic Counseling

Chapter 16
Fetal Anomaly and Genetic Counseling

Osamu Samura

Abstract Ultrasonography is widely practiced clinically to evaluate these hereditary disorders. In the diagnosis of chromosomal abnormalities, ultrasonography is considered a non-deterministic test, while ultrasonography is a definitive test in multifactorial diseases with morphological abnormalities such as congenital heart disease, cleft lip and palate, and neural tube insufficiency. Genetic counseling is essential before and after ultrasonography for these hereditary disorders. With adequate pre- and post-test counseling many of these challenges may be overcome and such counseling has to be multidisciplinary, involving clinical geneticists, genetic scientists, pediatricians, perinatal pathologists, and fetal medicine subspecialists.

Keywords Ultrasonography · Genetic counseling · Prenatal diagnosis
Chromosomal abnormalities · Monogenic disorders · multifactorial disorders

16.1 Introduction

Hereditary disorders are classified into chromosomal disorders represented by aneuploidy, monogenic disorders caused by pathological mutations in genes, and multifactorial disorders caused by multifactorial inheritance represented by congenital heart disorders.

Ultrasonography is widely practiced clinically to evaluate these hereditary disorders. In the diagnosis of chromosomal abnormalities, ultrasonography is considered a non-deterministic test, while ultrasonography is a definitive test in multifactorial diseases with morphological abnormalities such as congenital heart disease, cleft lip and palate, and neural tube insufficiency.

O. Samura (✉)
Department of Obstetrics and Gynecology, Jikei University School of Medicine, Tokyo, Japan

H. Masuzaki (ed.), *Fetal Morph Functional Diagnosis*, Comprehensive Gynecology and Obstetrics, https://doi.org/10.1007/978-981-15-8171-7_16

Even in the case of a single-gene disease, a definitive diagnosis is made by identifying a gene mutation in the final diagnosis, but for diseases with morphological characteristics such as family history, genetic background, and hereditary hydrocephalus, prenatal diagnosis by ultrasonography Diagnosis will be useful.

Genetic counseling is essential before and after ultrasonography for these hereditary disorders. Risk assessment for chromosomal aneuploidy is primarily performed in the early pregnancy. Many assessments of morphological abnormalities due to monogenic or multifactorial diseases are made in the second trimester.

Ultrasound in Genetic Assessment is a prenatal indeterminate genetic test, according to the opinion of the Japanese Society of Obstetrics and Gynecology. Because it is one of the tests, if this test is intentionally scheduled due to ethical issues, it should be conducted under a system that can provide genetic counseling by clinical geneticists and others.

This chapter outlines Fetal anomaly and genetic counseling.

16.2 Ultrasonography for Chromosomal Abnormalities and Copy Number Variation

Ultrasonography for chromosomal abnormalities is often performed early in pregnancy for risk assessment of chromosomal abnormalities for autosomal aneuploidies, such as trisomy 21. On the other hand, ultrasonography is also used during the second trimester to assess the risk of chromosomal abnormalities.

Ultrasonic soft markers in the second trimester for the purpose of assessing the risk of fetal abnormalities include the cerebellar lateral diameter, the high-intensity intestinal tract, the femoral bone shortened, the renal pelvis, the heart, the intraluminal high-intensity echo image, and a choroid plexus cyst. The presence or absence of ultrasound soft markers is determined, and the likelihood ratio of each positive/negative finding is used to determine the probability of disease.

Other than fetal chromosome aberration risk assessment, autosomal aneuploidy is often accompanied by morphological abnormalities as a disease, and ultrasonography is useful for estimating the disease. Trisomy 21 is closely associated with duodenal atresia and atrial ventricular septal defect. Trisomy 18 presents a variety of characteristic ultrasound images, including cerebellar hypoplasia, cisternal enlargement, overlapping fingers, strawberry-like skull, cardiac malformation, in utero fetal growth deficiency, hydramnios, and rocking-plantar sole. Trisomy 13 is characterized by a deep association with median facial malformations such as holoprosencephaly, cleft lip and palate, and monocular disease.

The detection of structural abnormalities in the fetus should increase the likelihood of chromosomal abnormalities or genetic molecular disease and encourage further evaluation of genetic etiology. The frequency of chromosomal abnormalities depends on the specific abnormality, the number of abnormalities, and the combination of abnormalities identified [1]. In some retrospective series of prenatally detected abnormalities with ultrasound that prompt genetic studies, isolated fetal abnormalities were associated with fetal chromosomal abnormalities in 2–18% of cases. Multiple abnormalities were associated with fetal chromosomal abnormalities in 13–35% of cases [1–6].

In cases of abnormal fetuses, mainly with ultrasonographic features that do not suggest a common trisomy, a genetic assessment with chromosomal microarray (CMA) is considered. This approach is the same whether the anomaly appears isolated or multiple structural anomalies are observed. Studies suggest that there is a higher risk of chromosomal abnormalities or genetic syndromes when multiple abnormalities are present, but consider that isolated abnormalities still require in-depth investigation if the patient wishes.

Karyotypes and microarrays—G-band karyotyping has been the standard for prenatal diagnosis, but the use of CMA is increasing. CMA detects small (10–100 kb) increases or decreases in genetic material (called copy number variants [CNV]) that is not identified by conventional karyotyping but can cause significant phenotypic abnormalities. In contrast, the resolution of G-band karyotyping is only 5–10 Mb, which is much larger. In addition, CMA does not require cell culture, reducing the time required for results.

In a 2014 systematic review of prenatal CMA, clinically significant CNV was detected in 5.6% (95% CI 4.7–6.6) fetuses, with ultrasound abnormalities in one anatomical system and normal karyotype. That was detected in 9.1% (95% CI 7.5–10.8%) of fetuses with multiple abnormalities and normal karyotype [7]. These estimates are similar to other reviews where significant CNV in fetuses with ultrasound abnormalities and normal karyotypes ranged from 5.1 to 10% [8, 9].

The depth of molecular analysis using CMA increases the likelihood of diagnosis. That is accompanied involves background variability and the identification of genetic disorders not associated with the assessed fetal abnormalities (i.e., secondary findings), which increases the complexity of prenatal counseling.

The potential and impact of variants of unknown significance (VUS) must be described. When analyzed at the CMA level, many people have DNA variability. The potential and impact of variants of unknown significance (VUS) must be described. When analyzed at the CMA level, many people have DNA variability. The curation of CMA variants from large databases, censuses, and literature reviews can determine their significance (i.e., benign or pathological properties). In others, finding a CMA variant in one of the parents can help determine its importance. For the rest, the VUS results represent results specific to the individual under test. A systematic review found VUS in 2.1% (95% CI 1.3–3.3) of cases where the indication for CMA was abnormal ultrasound findings [9]. The distress associated with VUS uncertainty is often amplified in the prenatal setting, especially if the patient is making an abortion decision. In a qualitative study of women who have undergone abnormal prenatal CMA, patients have expressed distress with uncertainty in the outcome [10]. Therefore, the authors suggested that the patient should be evaluated for tolerance to uncertainty before proceeding with the trial.

A close examination of the fetal CMA and VUS may identify genetic changes in one or both parents or identify fetal genes associated with adult-onset disease. For example, one or both parents can be found to be carriers of a genetic disease, a genetic condition that develops later in life, and a predisposition to hereditary cancer. In one study, assessment of CMA in abnormal fetal populations revealed a cancer predisposition gene in 0.92% of individuals tested [11].

Many professional organizations, including the American College of Obstetrics and Gynecology (ACOG) and the Society of Maternal and Fetal Care, recommend the use of CMA for prenatal diagnosis. The ACOG Committee's opinion states that if the fetus has one or more major structural abnormalities identified by ultrasonography, CMA rather than karyotype is recommended [12]. The ACOG also states that CMA needs to be available to all patients who choose to undergo an invasive diagnostic test.

16.3 Ultrasonography for Monogenic Diseases

Monogenic diseases include those having morphological characteristics as a phenotype. Accuracy of prenatal diagnosis of morphological abnormalities has increased along with technological innovation of ultrasonic diagnostic apparatuses, and diseases to be diagnosed have been increasing. From such a background, a definitive diagnosis of a monogenic disease is made by confirming a mutation in a gene, but an ultrasonic examination is also useful for estimating the diagnosis. Ultrasound in the second trimester is particularly useful in cases where the fetus is at high risk of having a particular disease due to family history, etc., and for diseases that show characteristic morphological abnormalities. Known examples include X-linked hereditary hydrocephalus and Meckel-Gruber syndrome, an autosomal recessive disorder, and Holt-Oram syndrome, an autosomal dominant disorder.

X-linked hereditary hydrocephalus is a disease that occurs only in boys characterized by hydrocephalus due to stenosis of the middle cerebral aqueduct, intellectual developmental disorder, inversion of the thumb, and spastic paralysis of the lower limbs. *L1CAM* is an adhesion factor and is present in EX928 [13]. On ultrasonography, a remarkable enlargement of the third ventricle and bilateral ventricles is diagnosed based on the presence of a bending finger in the thumb. The gender of the fetus can also be diagnosed by mid-gestation ultrasonography in many cases. It is relatively easy to estimate the diagnosis in male fetus from the above findings and family history. On the other hand, if sonography reveals the female fetus even if she has a family history, she may choose not to perform prenatal invasive testing.

Meckel-Gruber syndrome is associated with morphological abnormalities such as cerebral aneurysm, polydactyly, and cystic kidney [14], and Holt-Oram syndrome is accompanied by congenital heart disease and finger malformation [15]. Ultrasonography in the second trimester is useful for single-gene disease if anything is detectable by ultrasonography and the family risk is high.

Targeted gene sequencing refers to the testing of a specific gene or genes known to be associated with a genetic condition. Single-gene testing in the prenatal period often relies on a positive family history and a previously identified mutation [16]. For example, achondroplasia is caused by genetic alterations in the *FGFR3* gene.

When achondroplasia is suspected clinically, sequencing the *FGFR3* gene can confirm the diagnosis [17].

Whole-exome sequencing (WES) uses next-generation sequencer (NGS) to sequence exomes (regions of the genome that are known to encode proteins). Exomes contain about 1% of the genome, but are thought to contain 85% disease-causing mutations [18]. WES platforms vary in the sequence depth (i.e., the number of times a particular nucleotide is sequenced). The greater the depth, the more likely that the identified sequence change is truly present, and the lower the risk of a true sequence change being overlooked. WES does not sequence the rest of the DNA (99%). For this reason, sequence errors such as those that occur in the promoter region are not detected by WES.

A systematic review of 31 studies of fetal prenatal WES with abnormalities reported a diagnosis rate of 6.2–80% in more than five studies [19]. Differences in inclusion criteria and the trio versus singleton approach to sequencing were the main reasons for the wide range of diagnostic rates. Using the trio approach (fetus, mother, and father), variants identified in the fetus can be classified as "de novo" events and inherited from the parent. In the latter case, the variant is usually assumed to have no significant phenotypic contribution when present in healthy parents.

Diagnostic yields are greater in fetuses with multiple abnormalities or in preselected cases after genetic testing. Following a systematic review, two large prospective cohort studies of WES using a trio approach after nondiagnostic routine genetic testing (karyotype or microarray) were reported, including 234 [20] and 596 [21] abnormal fetuses. Diagnostic genetic variations were found in about 9–10% of all fetuses and about 15–20% of fetuses with two or more abnormalities. These findings best demonstrate the diagnostic performance of WES in abnormal fetuses after undiagnosed conventional genetic studies.

Although these results show promise for the use of this technique in the genetic evaluation of abnormal fetuses, many challenges remain for the routine clinical use of exome sequencing. Interpreting the results of exome sequencing is a very time-consuming process, and results may not be available quickly enough for patients making abortion decisions. In addition, much of the phenotypic data for a particular sequence variation is incomplete, making interpretation of the identified variants more difficult. Each of these challenges can decrease over time as time is reduced and understanding of genetic variation is improved.

Many counseling and ethical issues related to prenatal WES also need to be addressed. Key issues include the need for appropriate consent, deciding when to report secondary or incidental findings, the ongoing need to re-analyze the results, and the challenge of interpreting the results in a way that makes sense to the patient [19, 22]. An additional problem is that the cost of WES can be quite high and insurance coverage is limited.

Given the interpretation of the results, the timeliness of the results, and the complexity associated with patient/family counseling, the decision to proceed with this type of testing should be consulted with a certified genetic counselor or other specialized genetic testing provider, such as a medical geneticist.

WES is used clinically in both pediatric and adult patients who are thought to have underlying genetic symptoms [23]. The following statement reflects the key points of the 2018 Joint Statement from the International Association of Prenatal Diagnostics, the Society for Maternal and Child Medicine, and the Perinatal Quality Foundation on the use of genome-wide sequencing for fetal diagnosis [24]. The decision regarding which test to perform and the interpretation of molecular genetic results can be complex and usually should be done in consultation with a provider specializing in genetic testing, such as a certified genetic counselor or medical geneticist.

16.4 Ultrasonography for Multifactorial Diseases

Ultrasonography is the most useful for the diagnosis of multifactorial diseases because it is a disease that presents morphological abnormalities such as so-called congenital heart disease, neural tube defect, and cleft lip and palate. 3D ultrasonography is useful for external malformations such as myelomeningocele and cleft lip and palate. It often occurs in isolation and does not sporadically occur and is usually diagnosed by fetal ultrasonography through a screening test in the second trimester.

Prenatal treatment enables postnatal treatment to be performed smoothly and leads to improved prognosis. There are many diseases that have a big difference. Therefore, screening tests in the second trimester are very useful. Although the timing of screening during the second trimester and the screening check items are currently set by facilities, it is recommended that the screening would be performed systematically between 18 and 20 weeks of gestation using a checklist.

16.5 Pretest Genetic Counseling

Genetic counseling should be handled by a certified genetic counselor or clinical geneticist. This is especially important if you have malformations in the fetus. A certified genetic counselor or clinical geneticist can use the findings of fetal morphology and family history to determine what is causing this malformation and how it can be investigated for its causes. They should be close to the client's wishes and fully understand the concerns of the client and consider the options available in the future. Especially when fatal fetal malformations are anticipated, the client's emotions can sometimes be in a critical state, and care must be taken when using and communicating information. In the case of a fatal malformation, the client has the option of interrupting pregnancy, and they need to continue talking to the client with the most current information available.

Proper pretest counseling is important for patients who have decided to have a genetic test. The goal of this counseling is to help patients understand the benefits and limitations of testing, discuss possible test results, and make informed decisions that align with their goals and values [25]. Ideally, a certified genetic counselor, knowledgeable obstetrician, or medical geneticist should provide this counseling. Pretest counseling following the diagnosis of fetal abnormalities should include the following discussion:

1. All test options:
   - Invasive diagnostic tests—chorionic villus sampling or amniocentesis, percutaneous umbilical cord blood sampling.
   - Screening tests—serum screening, ultrasound, cell-free DNA.
2. Possible results:
   - Phenotypically defined aneuploidy or pathological variants.
   - Copies a number variant with a variable phenotype.
   - Variants of uncertain significance.
   - Incidental findings such as non-paternity, close marriage, adult-onset disease.
   - Normal results.
3. Patient values and goals:
   - The patient's general attitude to prenatal testing and screening.
   - Abortion views and availability.
   - Opinions on parenting, fear of addressing challenges for children with disabilities.
4. Potential psychosocial issues:
   - Certain diagnoses imply, for families, normal pregnancy and loss of baby, and significant disparities between parents and relatives.
   - Where appropriate, coping strategies, referrals, and awareness of available resources.
5. Pregnancy/Postpartum Management Options:
   - Abortion and continuation options that may change pre-, intra-, and postpartum care.
   - For patients who choose to continue pregnancy with a life-threatening diagnosis, if prenatal fetal death, fetal death during birth, or a newborn child is born, support for pregnancy and the birth of the family will be provided. Discussion of the option of perinatal palliative care that can provide guidance is expected to die. Additional resources for caregivers can be found in perinatal hospice and palliative care.
6. Interpreting the results
   - Abnormal results:
   - Importance of perinatal fetal health outcomes, including prenatal phenotypic limitations. Review patient goals and values, pregnancy management options, as described in Pre-Test Counseling.
   - Recommended follow-up after childbirth.

- Review of recurrence risk and options for future pregnancy.
- Normal results:
- Discuss that normal results are encouraging, but do not rule out the possibility of an underlying genetic condition in the fetus.
- Review options for additional postnatal assessment, including consulting with a medical geneticist if necessary.

7. Invasive procedure

    - The decision to undergo an invasive test is personal and must be based on the value and goals of the individual patient. Informed decisions by patients require prior testing counseling by a health-care provider who is suspicious of fetal diagnosis and genetic testing options. Alternatives to prenatal diagnostic tests include prenatal screening and postnatal diagnostic tests.

Depending on the age of pregnancy at diagnosis, villus sampling (CVS) or amniocentesis can be provided to obtain a fetal specimen for genetic testing. CVS is usually performed between 10 and 13 weeks of gestation. Amniocentesis is optimally completed after 15 weeks of gestation. When performed in a large and experienced facility, abortion rates for amniocentesis are 1/1000 to 1/300 (0.1–0.3%), with similar loss rates associated with CVS procedures [9].

16.6 Post-Test Counseling

Following the genetic test, it is important to give patients the opportunity to discuss the significance of the results with qualified providers. This is important for patients with both abnormal and normal results.

1. Abnormal results:

    - Importance of consequences for perinatal fetal health, including prenatal phenotypic limitations.
    - Review patient goals and values, pregnancy management options, as described in Pretest Counseling.
    - Recommended follow-up after delivery.
    - Review of options for recurrence risk and future pregnancy.

2. Normal results:

    - Discuss that normal results can be reassured but do not exclude the possibility of a potential genetic condition in the fetus.
    - Confirm options for additional postnatal assessment, including consultation with medical geneticists, if necessary.

DNA test provides additional information about the risk of aneuploidy during pregnancy and post-test counseling.

In abnormal fetuses, the frequency of chromosomal abnormalities depends on the specific abnormality, the number of abnormalities, and the combination of the abnormalities identified.

Provide an invasive procedure for genetic testing to all women whose fetal structural abnormalities have been confirmed by ultrasonography. The decision to proceed with prenatal testing is personal and must take into account the goals and values of the individual patient. Other options include noninvasive screening and postnatal testing.

For structural abnormalities consistent with common trisomy, for general aneuploidy (trisomy 21, 18, 13; sex chromosomal aneuploidy; and triploid), use interphase fluorescence in situ hybridization (FISH). If FISH is normal, chromosome microarray analysis (CMA) is performed; if FISH is abnormal, a confirmed G-band karyotype or CMA is performed. Although FISH gives quick results, it also makes sense to go directly to CMA as the cost of fetal assessment also increases. If a patient wants additional genetic testing (e.g., gene sequencing), a referral to a geneticist is recommended.

For structural abnormalities detected by FISH that do not indicate general trisomy, genetic evaluation is started by CMA. If the patient wants additional genetic testing, a referral to a geneticist is recommended.

If the patient rejects the invasive test, noninvasive screening with cell-free DNA is an option. It is important to counsel patients about the limitations of cell-free DNA screening in the context of fetal abnormalities, because normal results can be reassured by mistake and abnormal results can be falsely positive.

Diagnostic tests are recommended for patients who have no structural abnormalities in the fetus but have more than one soft marker on ultrasound and no previous cell-free DNA or biochemical marker aneuploidy screening. If patients choose this approach, they will begin with interphase fluorescence in situ hybridization (FISH) for common aneuploidy. If FISH is normal, the patient will be given the choice of CMA or conventional karyotype.

Provides a cell-free DNA screen for patients with two or more soft markers that reject invasive testing but do not have fetal structural abnormalities that are interested in further evaluation. If cell-free DNA screening does not show an increased risk of trisomy 21, 18, 13, or sex chromosomal abnormalities, provide reassurance and usually continue routine prenatal care. However, as noted above, we always emphasize that negative consequences do not rule out the possibility of fetal genetic status. Appropriate pre-test and post-test counseling is required for all patients' choice.

16.7 Conclusion

The ultrasonography performed in the second trimester is mainly for screening for individual diseases as so-called morphological abnormalities, not for the purpose of detecting hereditary diseases. Ethical considerations must be investigated for the genetic evaluation for the purpose of risk assessment of chromosome abnormalities using soft markers. The presence of morphological abnormalities in ultrasonography may be characteristic of a monogenic disorder. When the ultrasound examination was performed in the second trimester, it should be well explained that the ultrasound examination did not know what it could do beforehand, because it could also be used as a prenatal diagnosis for genetic diseases involving ethical issues. It is a good idea to check how far you want to know or do not want to know. If you want to know about hereditary diseases, you need to give genetic counseling before and after the test.

The genetic cause of how these defects occur and how that may impact a child's lifelong care is less established. Genetic testing has improved significantly in recent years, yet reviews documenting prenatal genetic counseling and testing guidelines have not been comprehensively updated.

Research is emerging on the additional prenatal diagnostic yield that exome sequencing offers when structural fetal anomalies are detected on ultrasound examination, in particular the identification of monogenic abnormalities defining prognosis and recurrence of anomalies. These are primarily technical and interpretational but also relate to service provision; cost-effectiveness; turn-around time; patient acceptability; and ethical dilemmas. With adequate pre- and post-test counseling, many of these challenges may be overcome and such counseling has to be multidisciplinary, involving clinical geneticists, genetic scientists, pediatricians, perinatal pathologists, and fetal medicine subspecialists.

References

1. Staebler M, Donner C, Van Regemorter N, Duprez L, De Maertelaer V, Devreker F, et al. Should determination of the karyotype be systematic for all malformations detected by obstetrical ultrasound? Prenat Diagn. 2005;25:567–73.
2. Nicolaides KH, Snijders RJ, Gosden CM, Berry C, Campbell S. Ultrasonographically detectable markers of fetal chromosomal abnormalities. Lancet. 1992;340:704–7.
3. Rizzo N, Pittalis MC, Pilu G, Perolo A, Banzi C, Visentin A, et al. Distribution of abnormal karyotypes among malformed fetuses detected by ultrasound throughout gestation. Prenat Diagn. 1996;16:159–63.
4. Bijok J, Massalska D, Kucińska-Chahwan A, Posiewka A, Ilnicka A, Jakiel G, et al. Complex malformations involving the fetal body wall – definition and classification issues. Prenat Diagn. 2017;37:1033–9.
5. American College of Obstetricians and Gynecologists. ACOG Practice Bulletin No. 88, December 2007. Invasive prenatal testing for aneuploidy. Obstet Gynecol. 2007;110:1459–67.
6. American College of Obstetricians and Gynecologists' Committee on Practice Bulletins—Obstetrics, Committee on Genetics, Society for Maternal–Fetal Medicine. Practice Bulletin No. 162: Prenatal diagnostic testing for genetic disorders. Obstet Gynecol. 2016;127:e108–22.
7. de Wit MC, Srebniak MI, Govaerts LC, Van Opstal D, Galjaard RJ, Go AT. Additional value of prenatal genomic array testing in fetuses with isolated structural ultrasound abnormalities and a normal karyotype: a systematic review of the literature. Ultrasound Obstet Gynecol. 2014;43:139–46.
8. Hillman SC, Pretlove S, Coomarasamy A, McMullan DJ, Davison EV, Maher ER, et al. Additional information from array comparative genomic hybridization technology over con-

ventional karyotyping in prenatal diagnosis: a systematic review and meta-analysis. Ultrasound Obstet Gynecol. 2011;37:6–14.
9. Hillman SC, McMullan DJ, Hall G, Togneri FS, James N, Maher EJ, et al. Use of prenatal chromosomal microarray: prospective cohort study and systematic review and meta-analysis. Ultrasound Obstet Gynecol. 2013;41:610–20.
10. Bernhardt BA, Soucier D, Hanson K, Savage MS, Jackson L, Wapner RJ. Women's experiences receiving abnormal prenatal chromosomal microarray testing results. Genet Med. 2013;15:139–45.
11. Innes J, Reali L, Clayton-Smith J, Hall G, Lim DH, Burghel GJ, et al. CNVs affecting cancer predisposing genes (CPGs) detected as incidental findings in routine germline diagnostic chromosomal microarray (CMA) testing. J Med Genet. 2018;55:89–96.
12. Committee on Genetics and the Society for Maternal-Fetal Medicine. Committee Opinion No.682: Microarrays and next-generation sequencing technology: the use of advanced genetic diagnostic tools in obstetrics and gynecology. Obstet Gynecol. 2016;128:e262–8. Reaffirmed 2019
13. Rosenthal A, Jouet M, Kenwrick S. Aberrant splicing of neural cell adhesion molecule L1 mRNA in family with X-linked hydrocephalus. Nat Genet. 1992;2:107–12.
14. Hartill V, Szymanska K, Sharif SM, Wheway G, Johnson CA. Meckel-Gruber syndrome: an update on diagnosis, clinical management, and research advances. Front Pediatr. 2017;5:244. https://doi.org/10.3389/fped.2017.00244. eCollection 2017
15. Vanlerberghe C, Jourdain AS, Ghoumid J, Frenois F, Mezel A, Vaksmann G, et al. Holt-Oram syndrome: clinical and molecular description of 78 patients with TBX5 variants. Eur J Hum Genet. 2019;27:360–8.
16. Krakow D, Lachman RS, Rimoin DL. Guidelines for the prenatal diagnosis of fetal skeletal dysplasias. Genet Med. 2009;11:127–33.
17. Xue Y, Sun A, Mekikian PB, Martin J, Rimoin DL, Lachman RS, et al. FGFR3 mutation frequency in 324 cases from the International Skeletal Dysplasia Registry. Mol Genet Genomic Med. 2014;2:497–503.
18. Rabbani B, Tekin M, Mahdieh N. The promise of whole-exome sequencing in medical genetics. J Hum Genet. 2014;59:5–15.
19. Best S, Wou K, Vora N, Van der Veyver IB, Wapner R, Chitty LS. Promises, pitfalls and practicalities of prenatal whole exome sequencing. Prenat Diagn. 2018;38:10–9.
20. Petrovski S, Aggarwal V, Giordano JL, Stosic M, Wou K, Bier L, et al. Whole-exome sequencing in the evaluation of fetal structural anomalies: a prospective cohort study. Lancet. 2019;393:758–67.
21. Lord J, McMullan DJ, Eberhardt RY, Rinck G, Hamilton SJ, Quinlan-Jones E, et al. Prenatal exome sequencing analysis in fetal structural anomalies detected by ultrasonography (PAGE): a cohort study. Lancet. 2019;393:747–57.
22. Horn R, Parker M. Opening Pandora's box?: Ethical issues in prenatal whole genome and exome sequencing. Prenat Diagn. 2018;38:20–5.
23. Farwell KD, Shahmirzadi L, El-Khechen D, Powis Z, Chao EC, Tippin Davis B, et al. Enhanced utility of family-centered diagnostic exome sequencing with inheritance model-based analysis: results from 500 unselected families with undiagnosed genetic conditions. Genet Med. 2015;17:578–86.
24. International Society for Prenatal Diagnosis, Society for Maternal and Fetal Medicine, Perinatal Quality Foundation. Joint Position Statement from the International Society for Prenatal Diagnosis (ISPD), the Society for Maternal Fetal Medicine (SMFM), and the Perinatal Quality Foundation (PQF) on the use of genome-wide sequencing for fetal diagnosis. Prenat Diagn. 2018;38:6–9.
25. Fonda Allen J, Stoll K, Bernhardt BA. Pre- and post-test genetic counseling for chromosomal and Mendelian disorders. Semin Perinatol. 2016;40:44–55.

Chapter 17
Soft Marker Test (NT, Nasal Bone, Etc.) and Genetic Counseling

Aiko Sasaki

Abstract Combining soft markers with maternal serum screening tests has improved the detection rate for aneuploidy (trisomy 21, 18, 13). Although many soft markers have been reported, few are suitable for clinical use in screening programs. For measuring soft markers, skill is indispensable and ultrasound practitioners must be well trained. In the NIPT era, the role of soft-marker testing is changing.

Before conducting soft-marker testing, geneticists and genetic counselors should understand each soft marker's characteristic traits (detection rate, false positive rate, and positive predictive value) as well as the prior probability of targeted fetal disease for each client.

Keywords Soft marker · Nuchal translucency · Nasal bone · Likelihood ratio Detection rate

17.1 Introduction

In the early 1970s, the only known factor related to Down syndrome (DS) was advanced maternal age (AMA). However, it was not a good screening marker for detecting DS because, reportedly, only 5% of pregnant women were of AMA and they contained about 30% of the total number of fetuses with DS [1]. This low detection rate was the primary motive for developing a more robust screening test, such as the maternal serum marker test and the combined test using soft markers, particularly among young mothers.

The use of only a single marker is associated with a low detection rate and a low positive predictive value. Combining multiple ultrasound and/or serum markers with maternal age to calculate the risk of DS increases the accuracy of the screening

A. Sasaki (✉)
Center for Maternal-Fetal, Neonatal and Reproductive Medicine, National Center for Child Health and Development, Tokyo, Japan
e-mail: sasaki-a@ncchd.go.jp

H. Masuzaki (ed.), *Fetal Morph Functional Diagnosis*, Comprehensive Gynecology and Obstetrics, https://doi.org/10.1007/978-981-15-8171-7_17

Table 17.1 Performance of different screening methods for trisomy 21

Method of screening	DR (%)	FPR (%)
MA > 35 (in the 1970s)	30	5
MA + NT	70	5
MA + NT + free β-hCG + PAPP-A (combined test)	85	5
Combined test + nasal bone or tricuspid flow or ductus venosus flow	95	2.5
NIPT	99	0.1

[1–3], modified

DR detection rate, *FPR* false-positive rate, *MA* maternal age, *NT* nuchal translucency, *β-hCG* β-human chorionic gonadotropin, *PAPP-A* pregnancy-associated plasma protein-A, *NIPT* noninvasive prenatal testing

test (Table 17.1). By combining several markers, the detection rate for DS becomes as high as >90%; however, the positive predictive value is still low at 10–20%.

Meanwhile, in recent years, with increasing maternal age, approximately half of DS cases have been associated with AMA [1]. In Japan, more than 70% of babies with DS, in the absence of TOPs, expected to be born to women of AMA [4]. Therefore, screening tests, including those based on maternal age, are not much effective now than they were earlier, especially for the population with AMA. Additionally, advancements in molecular genetics using next-generation screening (NGS) have led to a more sensitive screening method, i.e., noninvasive prenatal testing (NIPT).

Irrespective of the number of serum and ultrasound soft markers combined in a screening test, the detection rate of such a test will always be inferior to that of NIPT, which uses cell-free DNA (Table 17.1). Therefore, it can be said that we are in a transient period in prenatal diagnosis, where it is unclear which screening method should be considered to be the standard.

17.2 Soft Markers

- Measurement Skill

For measuring soft markers, the skill to handle the ultrasound transducer and the ability to obtain a reliable measurement are critical; moreover, an authorized license from the Fetal Medicine Foundation [24] or Nuchal Translucency Quality Review [25] is required. The criteria for each soft marker are shown in Fig. 17.1 and Table 17.2. Without these skills, inaccurate measurements might be obtained, leading to needless patient anxiety.

- Nuchal Translucency

A correlation between nuchal translucency (NT) and chromosomal defects was first reported in 1992 [5]. Subsequently, the association of NT with the abnormalities of the heart and great vessels [6] and with structural abnormalities and genetic

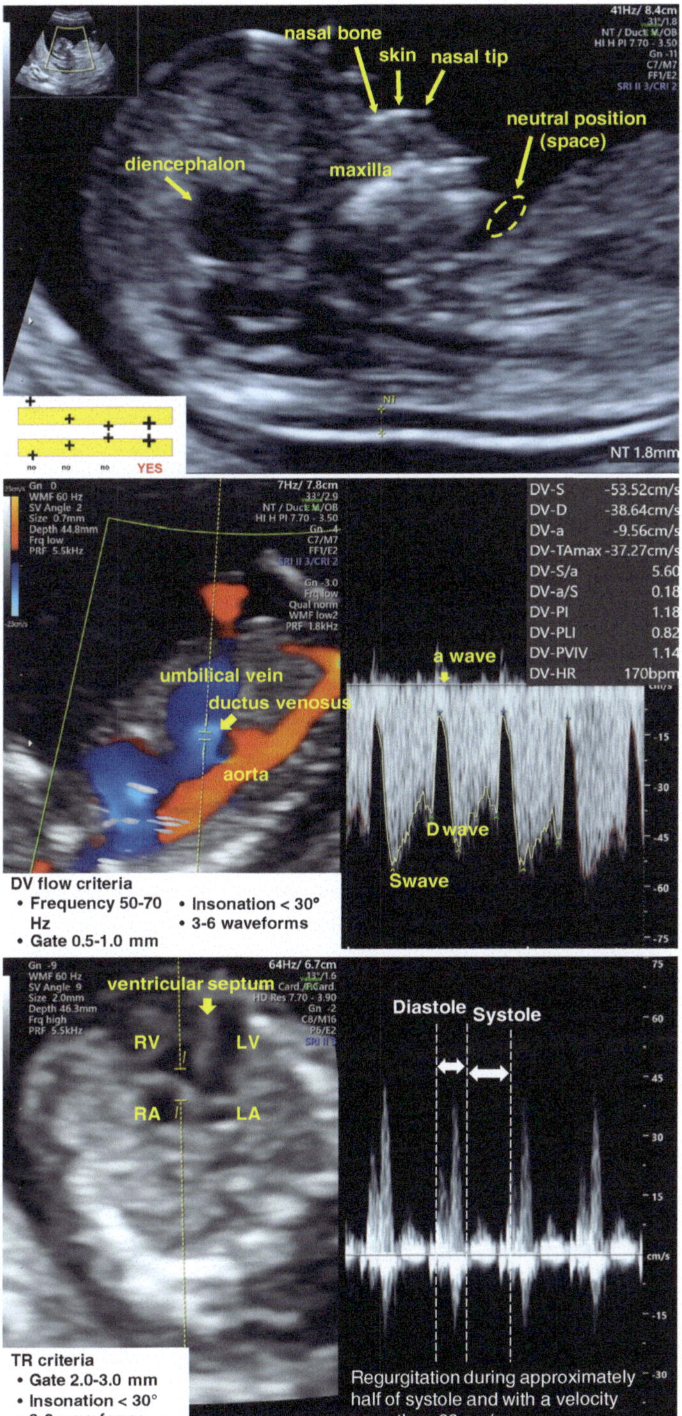

Fig. 17.1 Images of the NT, DV, and TR assesments

Table 17.2 Criteria for each soft marker

	NT	NB	DV	TR
CRL	45–84 mm	45–84 mm	45–84 mm	45–84 mm
Magnification	Fetal head and upper thorax	Fetal head and upper thorax	Fetal trunk	Fetal heart
Views	Mid-sagittal section	Mid-sagittal section	Right ventral mid-sagittal section	Apical four-chamber section
Frequency	–	–	50–70 Hz	–
Gate (sample volume)	–	–	0.5–1.0 mm	2.0–3.0 mm
Insonation angle	Transducer parallel to the skin	Transducer parallel to the nose	<30°	<30° (from the direction of the interventricular septum)
Sweep speed	–	–	High (2–3 cm/s) 3–6 waveforms	High (2–3 cm/s) 3–6 waveforms

Fetal Medicine Foundation [24], modified

CRL crown–rump length, *NT* nuchal translucency, *NB* nasal bone, *DV* ductus venosus flow, *TR* tricuspid regurgitation

syndromes [7] was also reported. The likelihood ratio (LR) for DS was 16 in fetuses with increased NT thickness.

- Nasal Bone

It is well known that individuals with DS usually have a small nose with a low nasal bridge. In utero, the nasal bone (NB) is visible via ultrasonography in 99.5% of fetuses at 11–13 weeks of gestation [8]. Since the first report in 2002 [9], several studies have demonstrated a high association between an absent NB at 11–13 weeks and trisomy 21, as well as other chromosomal abnormalities. The LR for DS was 6–146 with an absent NB [8, 10].

- Ductus Venosus flow

In the second and third trimesters of pregnancy, abnormal ductus venosus flow with an absent or reverse a-wave is a well-known sign of impending or overt cardiac failure and severe fetal growth restriction (FGR). The ductus venosus (DV) is one of the most useful vessels for assessing abnormal cardiac function during intrauterine life because it is a unique shunt that provides direct communication between the umbilical vein and the right atrium [11]. Initially, it was reported that an abnormal flow in DV with early cardiac failure could be the possible pathogenesis of increased NT in fetuses with chromosomal abnormalities [12]. The LR for DS was 7 with an abnormal DV flow [10].

- Tricuspid Regurgitation

In 2003, it was reported that tricuspid regurgitation (TR) was frequently associated with an abnormal karyotype, even in the absence of a structural cardiac

Table 17.3 Correlation between each soft marker and fetal state

		NT > 95th	NT > 99th	NB	aDV	TR
T21	DR (%)	75–80	70	60	65	55
T18	DR (%)	75	–	50	55	30
T13	DR (%)	72	–	40	55	30
CHD	DR (%)	35	21	–	27	30
Euploid	FPR (%)	4-5	1	1–3	3	1

[15–19], Fetal Medicine Foundation HP modified
DR detection rate, *NT* nuchal translucency, *NB* nasal bone, *aDV* abnormal ductus venosus flow, *TR* tricuspid regurgitation, *CHD* congenital heart defect, *FPR* false-positive rate

malformation [13]. The LR for DS was 15 when the delta NT (the difference in millimeters between the observed NT and the normal mean for the same crown–rump length) was 0 [14].

- Other Markers

The abovementioned four markers are commonly used and have proven to be effective in the detection of aneuploidy (Table 17.3). A good marker should exhibit high sensitivity and specificity and also be independent of other markers. Although there are many markers other than the four noted previously (such as facial angle, short maxilla, and cardiac echogenic foci), currently, they are all considered to have little or no ability to improve the detection of DS.

17.3 Soft Markers and the Future

In the NIPT era, the use of these soft markers is shifting toward becoming a tool for the detection of not only aneuploidy but also congenital heart defects (Table 17.3) and other congenital diseases [20]. In one study, more than half of all major heart defects were diagnosed on an 11–13 weeks' scan using a combination of three soft ultrasound markers: increased NT thickness, abnormal DV flow, and TR [17].

NT measurement is also instrumental in screening for other fetal abnormalities such as microdeletions, single gene disorders, and isolated structural abnormalities. Although NIPT is superior to the combined test in the detection of aneuploidies like trisomy 21, 34% of congenital abnormalities in fetuses with increased NT thickness may remain undetected in the first trimester (Fig. 17.2) [20].

17.4 Application of Soft Markers in Twin Pregnancies

In monochorionic diamniotic (MD) twin pregnancies, severe twin-to-twin transfusion syndrome (TTTS), with the development of polyhydramnios, usually becomes apparent in the second trimester, often as late as 16–24 weeks of gestation. NT has been reported to be a predictor of the development of TTTS as early as 11–13

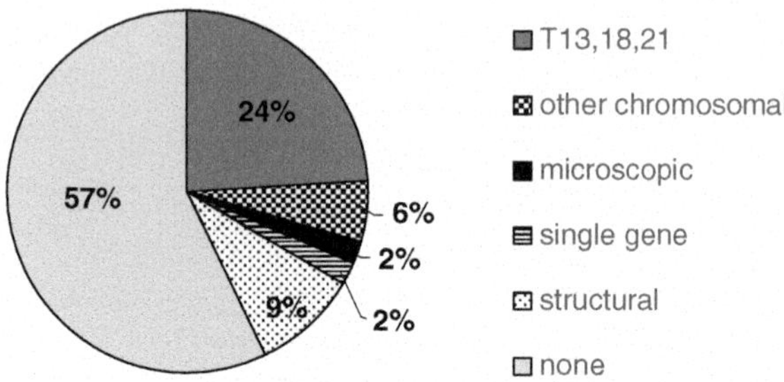

Fig. 17.2 Congenital abnormalities associated with increased NT fetuses

gestational weeks [21, 22]. Furthermore, reportedly, in MD pregnancies at 11–13 weeks, the prevalence of increased NT thickness in at least one of the fetuses among those who subsequently develop TTTS is approximately 30% compared to 10% in those who do not develop TTTS, and the LR of increased NT thickness for the prediction of TTTS is approximately 3. The intertwin NT thickness discrepancy and abnormal DV flow are also highly sensitive markers for TTTS, with sensitivities of 52.8% and 50.0%, respectively [22, 23].

Therefore, in the case of an MD twin pregnancy with increased NT thickness or abnormal DV flow, the possibility of TTTS development should be anticipated in addition to the possibility of chromosomal abnormalities and congenital heart defects.

17.5 Genetic Counseling

During genetic counseling, it is imperative to respect the patients' autonomy and to offer balanced information. Before a screening test using soft markers is performed, the patient, and her family, should be well-informed that soft markers can also be seen in some normal fetuses. Just because a soft marker is positive, it is not necessary that the fetus will have a congenital anomaly such as DS because the positive predictive value may be as low as 5–20%. In genetic counseling, it is important to realize not only what the soft marker means for the expectant mother but also the purpose of ultrasound for the medical professionals (clinicians, sonographers, and genetic counselors). Using ultrasound for detecting soft markers is just a screening for certain diseases, and it is different from a routine ultrasound checkup for fetal well-being or a targeted-diagnostic ultrasound test for fetal structural abnormalities.

The acceptance of diversity, including that of individuals with DS, has increased significantly over the past few years, suggesting that individual choice to opt for prenatal screening or diagnosis should be accepted. It is up to each individual whether or not to undergo a screening test because it is a personal choice that only the expectant mother, and her family, can make. Moreover, the patient and her family should be allowed sufficient time to discuss each of the offered screening tests with their midwife or doctor and decide whether or not it is right for them.

References

1. Nicolaides KH. Screening for fetal aneuploidies at 11 to 13 weeks. Prenat Diagn. 2011;31(1):7–15.
2. Bulletins ACoP. ACOG Practice Bulletin No. 77: Screening for fetal chromosomal abnormalities. Obstet Gynecol. 2007;109(1):217–27.
3. Taylor-Phillips S, Freeman K, Geppert J, Agbebiyi A, Uthman OA, Madan J, Clarke A, Quenby S, Clarke A. Accuracy of non-invasive prenatal testing using cell-free DNA for detection of Down, Edwards and Patau syndromes: a systematic review and meta-analysis. BMJ Open. 2016;6(1):e010002.
4. Sasaki A, Sago H. Equipoise of recent estimated Down syndrome live births in Japan. Am J Med Genet A. 2019;179(9):1815–9.
5. Nicolaides KH, Azar G, Byrne D, Mansur C, Marks K. Fetal nuchal translucency: ultrasound screening for chromosomal defects in first trimester of pregnancy. BMJ. 1992;304(6831):867–9.
6. Hyett J, Moscoso G, Papapanagiotou G, Perdu M, Nicolaides KH. Abnormalities of the heart and great arteries in chromosomally normal fetuses with increased nuchal translucency thickness at 11-13 weeks of gestation. Ultrasound Obstet Gynecol. 1996;7(4):245–50.
7. Souka AP, Snijders RJ, Novakov A, Soares W, Nicolaides KH. Defects and syndromes in chromosomally normal fetuses with increased nuchal translucency thickness at 10-14 weeks of gestation. Ultrasound Obstet Gynecol. 1998;11(6):391–400.
8. Cicero S, Curcio P, Papageorghiou A, Sonek J, Nicolaides K. Absence of nasal bone in fetuses with trisomy 21 at 11-14 weeks of gestation: an observational study. Lancet. 2001;358(9294):1665–7.
9. Sonek JD, Nicolaides KH. Prenatal ultrasonographic diagnosis of nasal bone abnormalities in three fetuses with Down syndrome. Am J Obstet Gynecol. 2002;186(1):139–41.
10. Prefumo F, Sethna F, Sairam S, Bhide A, Thilaganathan B. First-trimester ductus venosus, nasal bones, and Down syndrome in a high-risk population. Obstet Gynecol. 2005;105(6):1348–54.
11. Kiserud T. In a different vein: the ductus venosus could yield much valuable information. Ultrasound Obstet Gynecol. 1997;9(6):369–72.
12. Montenegro N, Matias A, Areias JC, Castedo S, Barros H. Increased fetal nuchal translucency: possible involvement of early cardiac failure. Ultrasound Obstet Gynecol. 1997;10(4):265–8.
13. Huggon IC, DeFigueiredo DB, Allan LD. Tricuspid regurgitation in the diagnosis of chromosomal anomalies in the fetus at 11-14 weeks of gestation. Heart. 2003;89(9):1071–3.
14. Faiola S, Tsoi E, Huggon IC, Allan LD, Nicolaides KH. Likelihood ratio for trisomy 21 in fetuses with tricuspid regurgitation at the 11 to 13 + 6-week scan. Ultrasound Obstet Gynecol. 2005;26(1):22–7.
15. Kagan KO, Cicero S, Staboulidou I, Wright D, Nicolaides KH. Fetal nasal bone in screening for trisomies 21, 18 and 13 and Turner syndrome at 11-13 weeks of gestation. Ultrasound Obstet Gynecol. 2009a;33(3):259–64.
16. Kagan KO, Valencia C, Livanos P, Wright D, Nicolaides KH. Tricuspid regurgitation in screening for trisomies 21, 18 and 13 and Turner syndrome at 11+0 to 13+6 weeks of gestation. Ultrasound Obstet Gynecol. 2009b;33(1):18–22.
17. Minnella GP, Crupano F, Syngelaki A, Zidere V, Akolekar R, Nicolaides KH. Diagnosis of major heart defects by routine first-trimester ultrasound examination: association with high nuchal translucency, tricuspid regurgitation and abnormal flow in the ductus venosus. Ultrasound Obstet Gynecol. 2019.

18. Nicolaides KH. Nuchal translucency and other first-trimester sonographic markers of chromosomal abnormalities. Am J Obstet Gynecol. 2004;191(1):45–67.
19. Snijders RJ, Noble P, Sebire N, Souka A, Nicolaides KH. UK multicentre project on assessment of risk of trisomy 21 by maternal age and fetal nuchal-translucency thickness at 10-14 weeks of gestation.Fetal Medicine Foundation First Trimester Screening Group. Lancet. 1998;352(9125):343–6.
20. Bardi F, Bosschieter P, Verheij J, Go A, Haak M, Bekker M, Sikkel E, Coumans A, Pajkrt E, Bilardo C. Is there still a role for nuchal translucency measurement in the changing paradigm of first trimester screening? Prenat Diagn. 2020;40(2):197–205.
21. Kagan KO, Gazzoni A, Sepulveda-Gonzalez G, Sotiriadis A, Nicolaides KH. Discordance in nuchal translucency thickness in the prediction of severe twin-to-twin transfusion syndrome. Ultrasound Obstet Gynecol. 2007;29(5):527–32.
22. Stagnati V, Zanardini C, Fichera A, Pagani G, Quintero RA, Bellocco R, Prefumo F. Early prediction of twin-to-twin transfusion syndrome: systematic review and meta-analysis. Ultrasound Obstet Gynecol. 2017;49(5):573–82.
23. Sebire NJ, Souka A, Skentou H, Geerts L, Nicolaides KH. Early prediction of severe twin-to-twin transfusion syndrome. Hum Reprod. 2000;15(9):2008–10.
24. Fetal medicine foundation HP. https://www.fetalmedicine.org/education/the-11-13-weeks-scan
25. Nuchal Translucency and Quality Review. https://www.ntqr.org/

Chapter 18
Noninvasive Prenatal Testing and Genetic Counseling

Junko Yotsumoto

Abstract With the advent of new fetal testing techniques such as NIPT (noninvasive prenatal testing), perinatal genetic counseling has entered a major turning point.

NIPT has drawn attention to the fact that the direct and quantitative evaluation of maternal and fetal cell-free DNA significantly reduces the rate of false positive and false negative results compared to conventional screening tests. However, it should be noted that NIPT is not a definitive diagnosis, as pointed out that it tends to be overestimated as a means of evaluating fetal chromosomal disorders. Furthermore, NIPT is a screening test and therefore still has the possibility for false test results. Pretest counseling is important, but a positive result requires further detailed genetic counseling by a specialist. In any case, NIPT should be an informed patient choice tailored to each patient's purpose and clinical situation through shared decision-making with the physician.

Keywords NIPT · Cell-free fetal DNA

18.1 Introduction

Noninvasive prenatal testing (NIPT) uses cell-free fetal DNA (cffDNA) in the maternal plasma. NIPT is a screening test that utilizes bioinformatic algorithms and the fragments of DNA in maternal plasma to determine the probability of certain chromosomal conditions in a pregnancy. Since the first report of the presence of cffDNA in maternal plasma in 1997 [1], studies on the genetic testing of many fetuses using cffDNA have been conducted. Circulating in the maternal plasma is cffDNA, which originates from trophoblasts mixed with cell-free maternal DNA. NIPT was first used in 2011 as a clinical test for detecting aneuploidies in the United States.

At present, NIPT mainly addresses fetal aneuploidy, but some tests also address sex chromosomal abnormalities and chromosomal microdeletions and duplications.

J. Yotsumoto (✉)
International University of Health and Welfare Hospital, Tokyo, Japan

H. Masuzaki (ed.), *Fetal Morph Functional Diagnosis*, Comprehensive Gynecology and Obstetrics, https://doi.org/10.1007/978-981-15-8171-7_18

Now, NIPT for fetal aneuploidies by scanning cffDNA in maternal plasma is rapidly becoming a first-tier aneuploidy screening test in clinical practice [2–4]. An increasing number of clinical studies suggest that NIPT has a high sensitivity and specificity for screening trisomy 21, 18, and 13. While several molecular methods have been developed to analyze cffDNA, recent studies have shown that the PPV (positive predictive value) range of trisomy 21 was 65–97%, T18 was 47–85%, and T13 was 12–64%. As demonstrated by these reports, PPV varies by condition, the study population, the incidence of a condition within that population (priori risk), as well as the sensitivity and specificity of the cffDNA screen [5–8] (Table 18.1) (Fig. 18.1).

Table 18.1 Positive predictive value of NIPT

	Trisomy 21	Trisomy 18	Trisomy 13	Sex chromosome aneuploidy	Micro deletion and duplication
Van der Meij KRM et al. Duch NIPT Consortium. 2019	96%	98%	53%	–	–
Hu et al. [8]	80%	60%	14.3%	45.8%	36.1%
Samura et al. [6] Japan NIPT Consortium. 2017	96.5%	82.8%	63.6%	–	–
Petersen et al. [7]	84%	75%	45%	26–86% (depending on the syndrome)	0–21%
Norton et al. [5]	80.1%	90%	50%	–	–

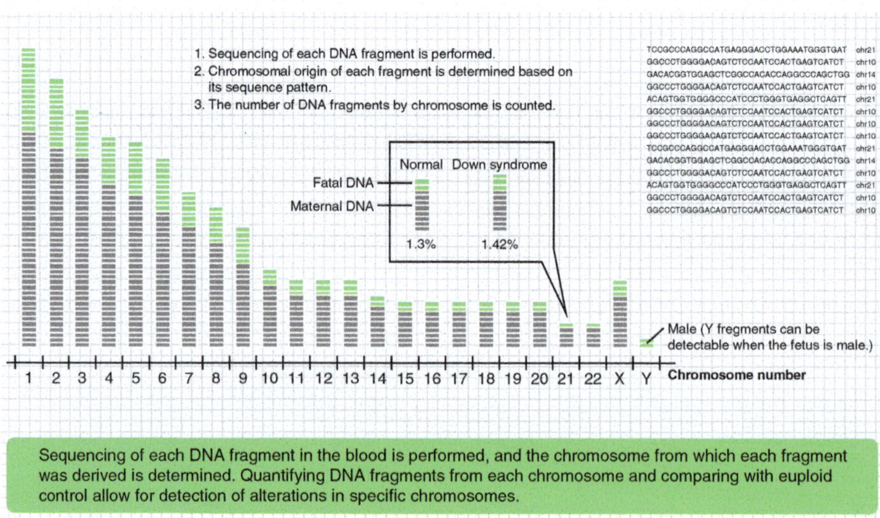

Fig. 18.1 Massively parallel Sequencing for NIPT

18.2 NIPT for Aneuploidy Screening

18.2.1 NIPT and Guidelines

The frequency of congenital diseases in newborns is around 3–5%, of which around 25% are due to chromosomal disorders. Chromosomal disorders include aneuploidy, structural abnormalities such as balanced and unbalanced translocations, and ultrastructural abnormalities. Currently, NIPT targets chromosomal aneuploidy, and the most frequent aneuploidy is Down syndrome (approximately 1/730), followed by trisomy 18 and trisomy 13. These three account for about 70% of chromosomal abnormalities among new born babies [9]. In addition to these chromosomal disorders, NIPT is able to test for sex chromosome disorders, chromosome microdeletions, and duplications in the United States and some other countries.

In 2016, The American College of Obstetricians and Gynecologists (ACOG) recommended that all women should be offered the option of aneuploidy screening, including NIPT or diagnostic testing [10]. Also, in 2018, the NHS (National Health Service) of the United Kingdom began to offer NIPT to women identified as having a high risk of an affected pregnancy. After the introduction of NIPT for aneuploidy screening, the rate of uptake of NIPT started to increase rapidly. Therefore, ACOG has made NIPT the most effective screening test for high-risk pregnancies. However, although NIPT is a test with great potential, it is currently not a substitute for villus or amniotic fluid tests, but it is a highly accurate screening test for high-risk pregnancies [10].

18.2.2 Where Does cffDNA Come from?

CffDNA, short DNA fragments of around 50–70 bp, is released into the maternal circulation primarily from placental cells undergoing apoptosis or programmed cell death and comprises, on average, 10% of the total cfDNA in maternal plasma.

Thus, cell-free DNA from both the mother and the fetus is present in the blood of pregnant women. The majority of fetal DNA in maternal plasma is derived from villous cells. Maternal blood circulating in the intervillous space of the placenta contacts the villi over a large area and performs oxygen and substance exchange between mother and infant. The villus surface is covered with villous cells, and DNA that has flowed out of the cell nucleus flows into maternal blood. Since the fetus and villi (placenta) are derived from the same fertilized egg, it is assumed that the genetic information is completely shared. However, the genetic information of the fetus and placenta, called placenta mosaic (CPM), is generally different. It should also be noted that there is around 1–2% of this.

The cffDNA present in the maternal plasma during pregnancy disappears quickly, within hours after delivery. Therefore, cffDNA in maternal plasma need not consider the effects of previous pregnancies. The cffDNA in maternal plasma

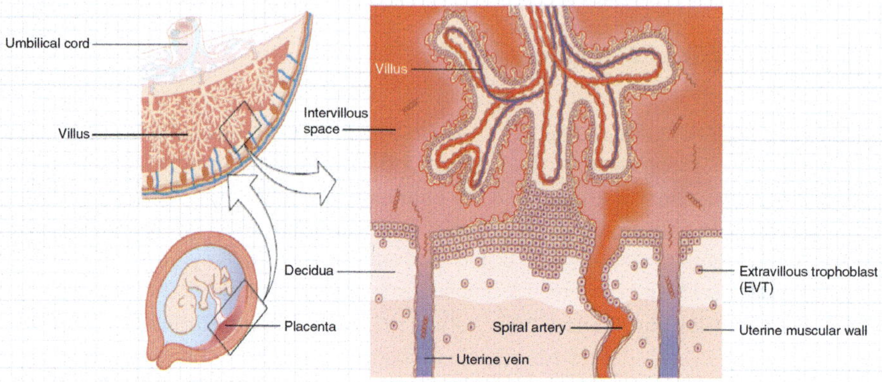

Fig. 18.2 Structure of placenta

can be confirmed from around 7 weeks of pregnancy, and it is thought that about 10–15% of cell-free DNA is derived from the fetus (Fig. 18.2). It has been confirmed that cffDNA levels increase with gestational age and are not affected by maternal age, fetal gender, race, place of residence, high-risk pregnancy, or in vitro fertilization.

18.2.3 Accuracy

When the result of NIPT is negative, the technique is superior in both sensitivity and specificity, and the negative predictive value is extremely high at 99.9% for Down syndrome, trisomy 18, and trisomy 13. Thus, it should be noted that this does not guarantee 100% that there is no abnormality. Also, in NIPT results, false positives, false negatives, and not reportable cases appear in 0.01–7% of the total number of tests. Factors for these cases include the following: (1) the fetal cell-free DNA in maternal plasma is derived from placental villi, e.g., placental mosaic (CPM), vanishing twin, etc.; (2) 87% of cell-free DNA in maternal plasma is maternally derived and therefore shows maternal tumors, maternal chromosomal disease, copy number variation (CNV), etc.; (3) low fetal DNA rate, e.g., maternal obesity, etc.; (4) test errors, changes in the whole genome may be due to maternal tumors, obesity, or the effects of heparin use. On the other hand, changes in specific genomic regions could be due to small chromosomal deletions in the infant, maternal CNV, CPM, obesity, or maternal tumors. In addition, it has been reported that a vanishing twin, CPM, chromosome duplication, heparin use, autoimmune disease, or maternal tumor involvement can be presumed [11].

18.2.4 Present and Future of NIPT

Recently, the targets of NIPT have been expanded, with some countries beginning analysis for subchromosomal deletions and duplications by NIPT. Currently, the prenatal diagnosis of large subchromosomal deletions and duplications in clinical practice still relies on invasive testing, such as fetal cell analysis through chorionic villus sampling (CVS) and amniocentesis using karyotyping. Large or small subchromosomal deletions and duplications are associated with genetic disorders; these are derived from genomic structural changes, such as copy number variants, resulting from abnormal gene dosage with a significant impact on phenotype.

Furthermore, with the development of whole-genome sequencing technology, smaller pathogenic genomic rearrangements that were unable to be detected by conventional karyotyping are now able to be detected. However, the detection rate and PPV are far from satisfactory, the application of the NIPT by whole-genome sequencing for subchromosomal deletions, duplications, and genetic diseases as a clinical test is still under discussion.

18.3 NIPT and Genetic Counseling

18.3.1 Genetic Counseling for Perinatal Care

It is said that the principles of bioethics in modern medicine are beneficence, autonomy, and nonmaleficence. Ethical discussions on NIPT have been conducted in various countries, but from the viewpoint of bioethics, adequate information is first provided through appropriate genetic counseling (good deeds) and under a proper informed choice. The decision-making of the pregnant woman (autonomy) must be ensured [12]. Genetic counseling was defined as "a kind of genetic social work without eugenics" by Sheldon Reed in 1947, and the emergence of new sophisticated genetic diagnostic techniques and alterations in human behavior has resulted in an increasing awareness of the importance of autonomy in healthcare along with changes in understanding, public health policies, ethical consciousness, and counseling theory [13].

With the advent of amniocentesis (1966), modern genetic counseling for prenatal testing began, and in order to make autonomous decision-making in a nondirective atmosphere, the attention is first paid to genetic counseling in perinatal care.

Traditional invasive prenatal diagnostic methods, such as amniocentesis or chorionic villus sampling, involve a small but definite risk of pregnancy loss; [14, 15] thus, it is mandatory to obtain informed consent before these procedures are performed. In contrast, NIPT for fetal aneuploidy from cell-free DNA in maternal plasma involves no risk of pregnancy loss from the test itself and no medical disadvantages that offset the advantages of the test. However, due to its convenience, there is a great concern that the test may be offered without sufficient explanation and informed consent before testing. It is therefore questionable whether sufficient explanation will be given prior to the test to ensure that the individual woman's autonomy and ethical rights are respected. Moreover, there is a concern that the test's high precision could be overvalued, which could lead to an increased number of cases that are misdiagnosed based on NIPT results.

18.3.2 The Goal of Genetic Counseling for NIPT

Some studies have shown that pregnant women have high expectations regarding NIPT [12]. The goal of genetic counseling for pregnant women who undergo NIPT is to provide them with adequate information about NIPT on aspects such as the accuracy of the test, the procedure, limitations, target diseases, and options depending on the result to facilitate an informed and autonomous decision on whether or not they should proceed with testing. Clinicians also need to ensure that pregnant women are adequately counseled to make autonomous and informed decisions regarding NIPT and to ensure that they understand the results and limitations of the test. Yotsumoto et al. reported that genetic counseling prior to NIPT enhances a pregnant women's understanding of the test and has the possibility to effectively facilitate informed decision-making after adequate consideration. A more careful and thorough approach is considered to be necessary for women who receive a positive test result [16]. Based on the existing genetic counseling model of prenatal testing, various statements and guidelines have been published regarding the clinical use of NIPT. These recommendations uniformly require pretest counseling by a genetic counselor or another skilled individual and stipulate that genetic counseling should be available to any pregnant woman who receives a positive result.

18.3.3 Genetic Counseling for Positive Result

Women with positive NIPT results have various difficulties regarding genetic counseling in relation to the test. It is required that the patient is provided with a sufficient explanation before the NIPT test and genetic counseling if the result is positive [10]. A "positive" or "aneuploidy detected" result does not confirm that the fetus definitively has a chromosomal condition. An abnormal result (positive result) indicates an increased risk for a specified condition. However, it is not diagnostic, and patients should be offered confirmatory testing through a diagnostic procedure, such as amniocentesis or CVS. This not only may indicate an affected fetus but can also represent a false positive result in an unaffected pregnancy, confined placental mosaicism, placental and fetal mosaicism, a vanishing twin, an unrecognized maternal condition, or another unknown biological occurrence.

The anxiety of the test taken after being informed of the positive test result can be high, and dissatisfaction regarding the uncertainty of the test's precision is also evident, especially since the test results and the positive predictive value are explained to the women with positive test results. Even with a sufficient advanced explanation, there is a great impact on women who receive a positive test result, and a significant long-term emotional burden is caused by their uncertainty as they wait for a definitive diagnosis [15]. The required time for genetic counseling was shown to be longer among these women; however, since it is considered that women with positive test results may make decisions in a state of reluctance and confusion, a more careful approach is considered to be necessary.

Confirmatory testing via CVS or amniocentesis should be offered to all women with an abnormal NIPT result. Patients selecting to have CVS for confirmation should be counseled regarding the limitations of this technology since CPM (confined placental mosaicism) may explain the abnormal NIPT result and may also be detected by CVS, especially when aneuploidy FISH (Fluorescence in situ hybridization) is ordered. Trophoblast cells are the primary source of cell-free DNA in maternal blood and are also the cells analyzed for aneuploidy FISH testing. CPM may cause an abnormal NIPT result and abnormal CVS FISH and/or karyotype result. Cells analyzed by amniocentesis are not typically affected by CPM since they are primarily derived from the fetal skin and genitourinary tract.

If it is difficult to perform a diagnostic test, management of the pregnancy should be dictated by ultrasound findings and maternal indications. Additional ultrasounds and fetal echocardiogram screening may be considered when NIPT results are abnormal. Postnatal evaluation by physical exam and/or karyotyping is also indicated after delivery.

When a pregnant woman goes into a diagnostic test, it can take an extended method of time to receive a result. It is predicted that the psychological burden on pregnant women during that time will increase. It is essential that the patient discusses with the partner whether to continue the pregnancy or not thoroughly before the final diagnosis of the fetus will be made.

18.4 Conclusion

NIPT genetic counseling requires a variety of precautions. The content is complex and diverse given the information provided, and so a thorough understanding and knowledge are required. The content of genetic counseling includes the expectation of pregnant women regarding the subject of the test, the principle of the test, the accuracy and the limitations of the test, the interpretation of the results, the correct knowledge and understanding of chromosomal diseases, and various problems that can arise from undergoing the test. It is important to discuss all of these factors with the counselor.

Despite the simplicity of the test itself and the difficulties in its content, the results that NIPT produces are as heavy as other prenatal tests. It cannot be explained simply as it is a noninvasive and simple test. It should not be dictated by the personal values or ethics of the genetic counselor. It is the pregnant woman that is the main subject of the entire prenatal examination, and shared decision-making, which further evolved from informed decision-making, is required in order to be able to make autonomous decisions in close proximity to the swinging decision-making process.

The emergence of a new technology, NIPT, poses new challenges for us. It is too short-circuited to use this new technology as it is convenient. New technologies will appear one after another, and the number of diseases to be diagnosed is expected to increase dramatically. At that point, we must start a discussion about our choice.

The wide variety of screening test options, each offering varying levels of information and accuracy, has resulted in the need for complex counseling by the health care provider and complex decision-making by the patient.

It is important that obstetrician-gynecologists and other obstetric care providers be prepared to discuss not only the risk of aneuploidy but also the benefits, risks, and limitations of the available screening tests. Screening for aneuploidy should be an informed patient choice, with an underlying foundation of shared decision-making that fits the patient's clinical circumstances, values, interests, and goals [10].

References

1. Lo YM, Corbetta N, Chamberlain PF, Rai V, Sargent IL, Redman CW, et al. Presence of fetal DNA in maternal plasma and serum. Lancet. 1997;350(9076):485–7.
2. Gil MM, Revello R, Poon LC, Akolekar R, Nicolaides KH. Clinical implementation of routine screening for fetal trisomies in the UK NHS: cell-free DNA test contingent on results from first-trimester combined test. Ultrasound Obstet Gynecol. 2016;47(1):45–52.
3. Kagan KO, Sonek J, Wagner P, Hoopmann M. Principles of first trimester screening in the age of non-invasive prenatal diagnosis: screening for chromosomal abnormalities. Arch Gynecol Obstet. 2017;296(4):645–51.
4. Galeva S, Konstantinidou L, Gil MM, Akolekar R, Nicolaides KH. Routine first-trimester screening for fetal trisomies in twin pregnancy: cell-free DNA test contingent on results from combined test. Ultrasound Obstet Gynecol. 2019;53(2):208–13.
5. Norton ME. What is new in prenatal aneuploidy screening?: Best articles from the past year. Obstet Gynecol. 2015;126(1):211–2.
6. Samura O, Sekizawa A, Suzumori N, Sasaki A, Wada S, Hamanoue H, et al. Current status of non-invasive prenatal testing in Japan. J Obstet Gynaecol Res. 2017;43(8):1245–55.
7. Petersen AK, Cheung SW, Smith JL, Bi W, Ward PA, Peacock S, et al. Positive predictive value estimates for cell-free noninvasive prenatal screening from data of a large referral genetic diagnostic laboratory. Am J Obstet Gynecol. 2017;217(6):691 e1–6.
8. Hu H, Wang L, Wu J, Zhou P, Fu J, Sun J, et al. Noninvasive prenatal testing for chromosome aneuploidies and subchromosomal microdeletions/microduplications in a cohort of 8141 single pregnancies. Hum Genomics. 2019;13(1):14.
9. Wellesley D, Dolk H, Boyd PA, Greenlees R, Haeusler M, Nelen V, et al. Rare chromosome abnormalities, prevalence and prenatal diagnosis rates from population-based congenital anomaly registers in Europe. Eur J Hum Genet. 2012;20(5):521–6.
10. Committee on Practice Bulletins-Obstetrics CoG, the Society for Maternal-Fetal M. Practice Bulletin No. 163: Screening for fetal aneuploidy. Obstet Gynecol. 2016;127(5):e123–37.

11. Suzumori N, Sekizawa A, Takeda E, Samura O, Sasaki A, Akaishi R, et al. Classification of factors involved in nonreportable results of noninvasive prenatal testing (NIPT) and prediction of success rate of second NIPT. Prenat Diagn. 2019;39(2):100–6.
12. Yotsumoto J, Sekizawa A, Koide K, Purwosunu Y, Ichizuka K, Matsuoka R, et al. Attitudes toward non-invasive prenatal diagnosis among pregnant women and health professionals in Japan. Prenat Diagn. 2012;32(7):674–9.
13. Reed SC. A short history of genetic counseling. Soc Biol. 1974;21(4):332–9.
14. Tabor A, Alfirevic Z. Update on procedure-related risks for prenatal diagnosis techniques. Fetal Diagn Ther. 2010;27(1):1–7.
15. Akolekar R, Beta J, Picciarelli G, Ogilvie C, D'Antonio F. Procedure-related risk of miscarriage following amniocentesis and chorionic villus sampling: a systematic review and meta-analysis. Ultrasound Obstet Gynecol. 2015;45(1):16–26.
16. Weinans MJ, Huijssoon AM, Tymstra T, Gerrits MC, Beekhuis JR, Mantingh A. How women deal with the results of serum screening for Down syndrome in the second trimester of pregnancy. Prenat Diagn. 2000;20(9):705–8.

Chapter 19
Trisomy and Genetic Counseling

Nobuhiro Suzumori

Abstract Genetic counseling for the prenatal diagnosis of fetal trisomy is important for all pregnant women, especially in view of the increasing prevalence of women with an advanced maternal age. Noninvasive prenatal testing (NIPT) is now performed worldwide and provides highly accurate results for the detection of fetal chromosomal abnormalities at any maternal age. Genetic counseling for fetal trisomy includes a health service context, after considering clinical, ethical, social, legal, and economic issues. In this section, we present prenatal diagnostic testing for fetal trisomy, genetic counseling following a prenatal diagnosis of trisomy, and decision-making after a prenatal diagnosis of trisomy.

Keywords Advanced maternal age · Down syndrome · Decision-making · Genetic counseling · Trisomy

19.1 Advanced Maternal Age and Fetal Trisomy

Recently, the prevalence of women with an advanced maternal age, which is a risk factor for fetal trisomy, has been increasing in developed countries. Any evidence of a greater recurrence risk of a trisomic spontaneous miscarriage after a first trisomic spontaneous miscarriage has generally been found to be weak [1] or nonsignificant [2] after data correction for differences in maternal age [3, 4]. Robinson et al. reported that the etiology of trisomy is mostly a result of meiotic errors related to increased maternal age, regardless of whether the couple has experienced one or more aneuploid spontaneous miscarriages [5].

N. Suzumori (✉)
Department of Obstetrics and Gynecology, Nagoya City University Graduate School of Medical Sciences, Nagoya, Japan
e-mail: og.n.suz@med.nagoya-cu.ac.jp

H. Masuzaki (ed.), *Fetal Morph Functional Diagnosis*, Comprehensive Gynecology and Obstetrics, https://doi.org/10.1007/978-981-15-8171-7_19

The effects of maternal age on fetal trisomy 21 occur via oogenesis, causing a predisposition to the nondisjunction of chromosome 21 predominantly during the first meiotic division [6]. Older pregnant women have an increased risk of pregnancy with fetal trisomies 13, 16, 18, X, and 47,XXY, as well as trisomy 21. Risk factors for fetal trisomies in addition to maternal age have been widely reported. A reduced total follicular number in the ovaries has been linked to an increased risk of fetal trisomy [7, 8]. Environmental factors, for instance, caffeine intake, have also been suggested to modify the risk of trisomy 21 [9]. Paternal age commonly does not enter into the equation, at least with respect to autosomal aneuploidies [10]. However, Martin et al. reported that mutations in *MSH2*, a mismatch repair gene, were associated with a significant increase in chromosomally abnormal sperms [11].

Genetic counseling for the prenatal diagnosis of fetal trisomy is beneficial and effective for all pregnant women, especially in view of the increasing prevalence of women with an advanced maternal age. Noninvasive prenatal testing (NIPT) is now performed worldwide and is highly accurate for the detection of fetal chromosomal abnormalities at any maternal age [12, 13]. Figure 19.1 shows important data for genetic counseling about fetal chromosome abnormalities. Although numerous studies have focused on the development and quality of laboratory techniques for prenatal diagnosis, these techniques must be placed into a health service context after considering clinical, ethical, social, legal, and economic issues.

Allowing individuals to choose the prenatal diagnosis of fetal trisomies can tailor medical care to meet the needs of individuals, thereby reducing anxiety and stress [15, 16]. However, post-traumatic stress, depression, and anxiety are common after prenatal diagnosis for congenital heart defects. The establishment of interdisciplinary treatment settings where access to psychological support is facilitated may be

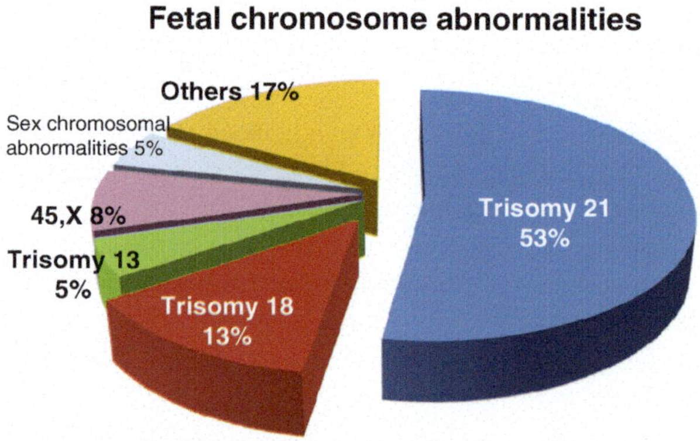

Fig. 19.1 Chromosome abnormalities, prevalence, and prenatal diagnosis rates from population-based congenital anomaly registers [14]. (Note: There were approximately 2.4 million births in the registry areas, representing 9% of the total births in 11 countries, during the 7-year study period, of which 10,323 were diagnosed as having a chromosome abnormality within the first year of life. The overall prevalence of an unbalanced chromosome abnormality was 43.8/10,000 births, ranging from 25.6 in Antwerp to 75.1 in Paris)

beneficial. While such activities increase patient autonomy and reassurance, this expansion of fetal chromosomal information may also increase patient anxiety or generate unjust outcomes with regard to fetal selection and elective abortions.

19.2 Prenatal Diagnostic Testing for Fetal Trisomy

The analysis of cell-free DNA in maternal blood for the purpose of NIPT has been shown to be very accurate for the detection of the main fetal trisomies 21, 18, and 13 [13, 17]. Although NIPT has been reported to be very accurate for detection, a small percentage of women have false-positive, false-negative, or nonreportable results [18]. If the results of NIPT using maternal blood testing are positive or repeatedly unreportable, further invasive testing by amniocentesis or chorionic villus sampling (CVS) is needed to confirm the fetal findings [13, 18].

Indications for amniocentesis and CVS include an advanced maternal age, maternal serum screening results, ultrasonographic findings for fetal anomalies, and chromosomal aberrations in a previous pregnancy [19]. In contrast, traditional fetal aneuploidy screening tests, based on ultrasonography and maternal biochemistry, have a detection rate of 50–95% and a 5% false-positive rate [20]. Fetal abnormal findings detected using ultrasound are also important for parents with fetal trisomy prior to genetic counseling and decision-making, since the ultrasound data may include a predictive assessment of neonatal outcome. In terms of a precise prenatal diagnosis of fetal NT thickness, cytogenetic karyotyping and microarray analyses by amniocentesis or chorionic villus sampling are recommended over cell-free fetal DNA testing results [12].

When an abnormal karyotype is identified by prenatal diagnosis, parents are faced with decision options that include termination versus continuation of the pregnancy [21–23]. Couples with a recent diagnosis tend to be eager to search the internet for information about chromosomal abnormalities, and they may find inaccurate or biased information. We should inform the parents of the precise fetal findings and conditions during genetic counseling for each trisomy case. Decisions concerning prenatal testing and the termination of pregnancy in cases of affected fetuses are complex and may be influenced by a variety of factors, such as the country's health system and abortion laws as well as the social and cultural backgrounds [24–26].

19.3 Genetic Counseling Following a Prenatal Diagnosis of Trisomy

Chromosome abnormalities, prevalences, and prenatal diagnosis rates from population-based congenital anomaly registers are shown in Fig. 19.1 [14]. The frequency of trisomy increases exponentially with maternal age, as has been widely reported, although

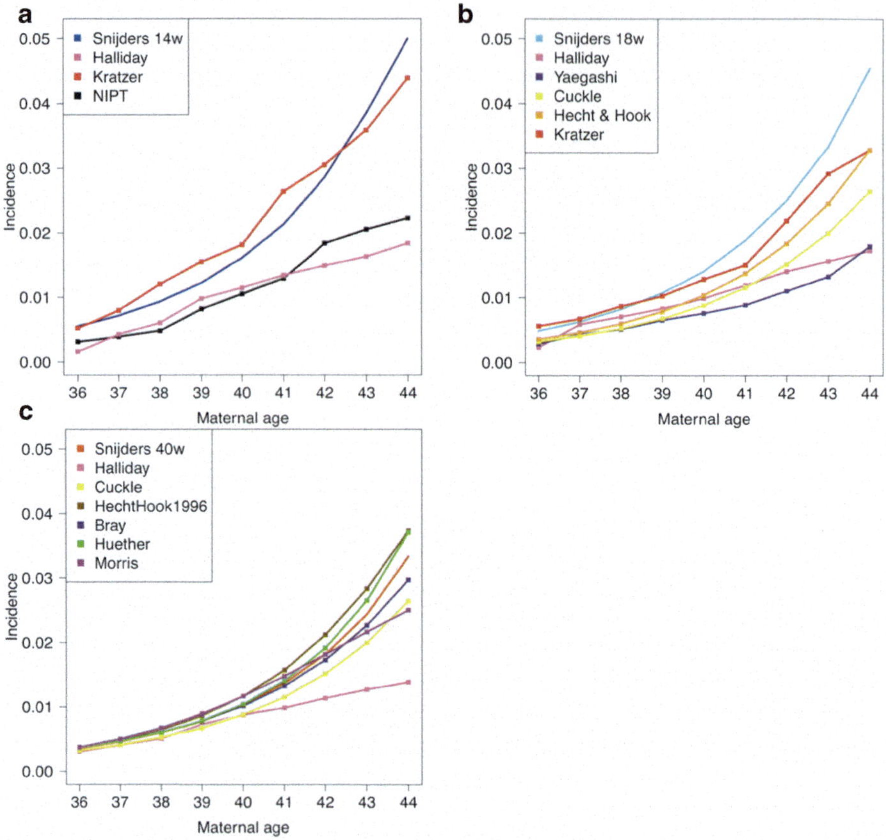

Fig. 19.2 Maternal age-specific risk of trisomy 21 based on the clinical performance of NIPT during the chorionic villus sampling period (10–14 weeks of gestation) (**a**), the amniocentesis period (15–20 weeks of gestation) (**b**), and the live-birth period (term) (**c**)

recent data on the maternal age-specific risk of trisomy 21 were much lower than those reported by Snijders et al. (Fig. 19.2a–c; [27, 28]). Although the maternal age-specific risk of trisomy reported by Kratzer was similar to that reported by Snijders et al., Halliday confirmed the results of the recent study [29]. When comparing studies based on the amniocentesis period (Fig. 19.2b) and term (Fig. 19.2c), large variations among studies can be seen, especially for mothers older than 41 years, while the maternal age-specific risks reported by Snijders were much higher [30].

19.3.1 Trisomy 21 (Down Syndrome)

Trisomy 21 is associated with intellectual disability, a characteristic facial appearance, and hypotonia during infancy [31–33]. Genetic counseling for prenatally diagnosed cases of trisomy 21 should address the medical, developmental, and psychological manifestations of the condition. All affected individuals experience cognitive delays, but the intellectual disability is usually mild to moderate. Down syndrome babies can have a variety of birth defects. Almost half of affected children are born with a heart defect. Neonates with trisomy 21 have an increased risk of developing several medical conditions including gastroesophageal reflux and celiac disease. About 15% of trisomy 21 cases have hypothyroidism.

Down syndrome babies may have an increased risk of hearing and vision problems. Approximately 5–10% of children with Down syndrome develop leukemia. Delayed development and behavioral problems are often confirmed in the children. The children's speech and language develop later and more slowly, and they can be more difficult to understand. Some people with Down syndrome also have developmental conditions such as autism spectrum disorders, which affect communication and social interactions. People with trisomy 21 often experience a gradual decline in cognition as they age, usually starting around the age of 50–60 years.

The risk of pregnancy loss is greater than 30% during the second half of pregnancy [34]. In addition, there may be an increased risk of aneuploidies in future conceptions [34].

19.3.2 Trisomy 18 (Edwards' Syndrome) and Trisomy 13 (Patau Syndrome)

Trisomy 18 and trisomy 13 are chromosomal conditions associated with abnormalities in many parts of the body. Genetic counseling for clients with prenatally diagnosed cases of trisomy 18 and trisomy 13 should address the medical and developmental manifestations, including intrauterine growth restriction, intrauterine fetal demise, and a low birth weight. Affected neonates with trisomy 18 may have heart defects and abnormalities of other organs that develop before birth. Other features of trisomy 18 include a small, abnormally shaped head; a small jaw and mouth; and clenched fists with overlapping fingers [35]. Trisomy 13 is also associated with severe intellectual disability and physical abnormalities in many parts of the body. Neonates with trisomy 13 often have heart defects, brain or spinal cord abnormalities, microphthalmia, extra fingers or toes, a cleft lip with or without a cleft palate, and hypotonia [36–38]. Due to the presence of several life-threatening medical problems, most infants with trisomy 13 or 18 die within their first days or weeks of life. Only 5–10% of children with these conditions live past their first year [35].

19.3.3 Trisomy X (47,XXX)

Trisomy X is a sex chromosome anomaly with a variable phenotype caused by the presence of an extra X chromosome, occurring in 1 in 1000 female births [39]. Intrauterine fetal demise is rare, and genetic counseling for prenatally diagnosed cases of trisomy X is essential for parents. There is a significant variability in development delays, learning disability, and psychological characteristics in trisomy X. However, couples should be informed of the high frequency of trisomy X and the fact that most girls are undiagnosed; some couples have found it helpful to talk with other parents of trisomy X children (KS&A: Knowledge, Support & Action. http://www.genetic.org; Clements H: Triplo-X Support Group. http://www.triplo-x.org).

19.3.4 Klinefelter Syndrome (47,XXY)

Klinefelter syndrome is a sex chromosome anomaly causing small testes and infertility, although testicular sperm extraction and in vitro fertilization have enabled some men to become fathers [6]. Androgen deficiency can be managed through replacement therapy with testosterone. Gynecomastia, learning difficulties, and persistent reading and spelling problems may be present [40]. As for psychosocial adaptation, several studies have indicated that Klinefelter syndrome cases are shy, immature, restrained, and reserved [6].

19.3.5 XYY

XYY males have an increased stature and normal sexual activity; their motor proficiency may be impaired. Klinefelter syndrome and XYY have overlapping cognitive profiles characterized by deficits in executive function and language-related skills and psychosocial adaptation, including a low frustration tolerance, aggressive behavior during the teenage years, and antisocial behavior [6, 41].

19.4 Decision-Making Following a Prenatal Diagnosis of Trisomy

After a prenatal genetic diagnosis, termination of pregnancy was chosen in 86% of autosomal trisomy cases and 60% of sex chromosome aneuploidy cases [6]. The rates of termination increased progressively from XXX (40%) to XYY (57%), 45,X (65%), and XXY (70%), in parallel with the perceived severity of the phenotype [6]. On the other hand, Gruchy et al. reported that the termination rates in France fell between 1976 and 2012 from 41% to 12% for trisomy X and from 26% to 7% for XYY [42]. Neurodevelopmental concerns in males with sex chromosome aneuploidy (Klinefelter syndrome, XYY, and XXYY) include symptoms seen in autism spectrum disorder, such as language impairments and social difficulties [39].

After genetic counseling with both a geneticist and a genetic counselor in our Unit, the rates of pregnancy termination for aneuploidies were 81.7% [43]. Among the prenatal diagnoses of Down syndrome, pregnancy was terminated in 93.3% of cases in Japan. In both trisomy 13 and trisomy 18, pregnancy was terminated in almost all the cases. Among cases with sex chromosome aneuploidy, pregnancy was terminated in 46.7% cases, and pregnancy was terminated in 20% of cases with Klinefelter syndrome.

When diagnosed with a chromosome aneuploidy in which a severe prognosis is expected, most couples in Japan decide to terminate the pregnancy. The termination rate (93.3%) for Japanese cases of autosomal trisomy [43] was higher than those of previously published reports [22, 26, 44]. The rate of termination in cases of sex chromosome aneuploidy (46.7%) supports previous data showing a higher rate of termination because of autosomal trisomy than for sex chromosome aneuploidy, which has a relatively low-risk prognosis [26, 45]. Long-term follow-up studies have demonstrated that the postnatal development of cases with sex chromosome aneuploidies is mostly normal [46, 47].

Women who wish to undergo invasive prenatal testing and amniocentesis might tend to decide to terminate their pregnancy if the results show chromosome aneuploidy, regardless of sufficient genetic counseling. An advanced maternal age at diagnosis was associated with the decision to continue an affected pregnancy in one report [26], but other studies have been divisive [48, 49]. Our previous study showed a likely trend for women aged 35 years and older to terminate pregnancies in cases of sex chromosome aneuploidy [43].

Individual choice for prenatal diagnosis meets the needs of individuals, thereby reducing anxiety and stress. However, post-traumatic stress, depression, and anxiety are common after a prenatal diagnosis for congenital heart disease [50]. Women undergoing prenatal diagnostic procedures experience more psychological distress, which may be currently underestimated [51]. Appropriate knowledge of the risk of trisomy 21 and consideration of NIPT by couples and their parents may be important for decreasing maternal nonspecific psychological distress [15]. The establishment of interdisciplinary treatment settings where access to psychological support is facilitated may be beneficial [51].

Nonmedical factors play a role in parental decisions concerning prenatal screening and termination of pregnancy in affected pregnancies [47]. Several reports suggest that these factors include the societal acceptance of the resulting handicap, parental perceptions, environmental familiarity, the orientation of medical facilities, and the attitude of the society in question [10, 52, 53]. The societal acceptance of the resulting handicap should also be discussed, as some people have not received education regarding handicaps during their own childhoods. Tertiary medical centers are recommended to employ professionals who have completed a master's program in medical genetics and have appropriate counseling skills.

References

1. Morton NE, Chiu D, Holland C, Jacobs PA, Pettay D. Chromosome anomalies as predictors of recurrence risk for spontaneous abortion. Am J Med Genet. 1987;28(2):353–60.
2. Warburton D, Kline J, Stein Z, Hutzler M, Chin A, Hassold T. Does the karyotype of a spontaneous abortion predict the karyotype of a subsequent abortion? Evidence from 273 women with two karyotyped spontaneous abortions. Am J Hum Genet. 1987;41(3):465–83.
3. Cuckle HS, Wald NJ, Thompson SG. Estimating a woman's risk of having a pregnancy associated with Down's syndrome using her age and serum alpha-fetoprotein level. Br J Obstet Gynaecol. 1987;94(5):387–402.
4. Hecht CA, Hook EB. Rates of Down syndrome at livebirth by one-year maternal age intervals in studies with apparent close to complete ascertainment in populations of European origin: a proposed revised rate schedule for use in genetic and prenatal screening. Am J Med Genet. 1996;62(4):376–85.
5. Robinson WP, McFadden DE, Stephenson MD. The origin of abnormalities in recurrent aneuploidy/polyploidy. Am J Hum Genet. 2001;69(6):1245–54.
6. Gardner RJM, Amor DJ. Chromosome abnormalities and genetic counseling. 5th ed. Oxford: Oxford University Press; 2018.
7. Freeman SB, Yang Q, Allran K, Taft LF, Sherman SL. Women with a reduced ovarian complement may have an increased risk for a child with Down syndrome. Am J Hum Genet. 2000;66(5):1680–3.
8. Kline J, Kinney A, Levin B, Warburton D. Trisomic pregnancy and earlier age at menopause. Am J Hum Genet. 2000;67(2):395–404.
9. Torfs CP, Christianson RE. Effect of maternal smoking and coffee consumption on the risk of having a recognized Down syndrome pregnancy. Am J Epidemiol. 2000;152(12):1185–91.
10. Dzurova D, Pikhart H. Down syndrome, paternal age and education: comparison of California and the Czech Republic. BMC Public Health. 2005;5:69.
11. Martin RH, Green J, Ko E, Barclay L, Rademaker AW. Analysis of aneuploidy frequencies in sperm from patients with hereditary nonpolyposis colon cancer and an hMSH2 mutation. Am J Hum Genet. 2000;66(3):1149–52.
12. Bianchi DW, Platt LD, Goldberg JD, Abuhamad AZ, Sehnert AJ, Rava RP. Genome-wide fetal aneuploidy detection by maternal plasma DNA sequencing. Maternal blood is source to accurately diagnose fetal aneuploidy (MELISSA) Study Group. Obstet Gynecol. 2012;119:890–901.
13. Bianchi DW, Chiu RWK. Sequencing of circulating cell-free DNA during pregnancy. N Engl J Med. 2018;379:464–73.
14. Wellesley D, Dolk H, Boyd PA, Greenlees R, Haeusler M, Nelen V, Garne E, Khoshnood B, Doray B, Rissmann A, Mullaney C, Calzolari E, Bakker M, Salvador J, Addor MC, Draper E, Rankin J, Tucker D. Rare chromosome abnormalities, prevalence and prenatal diagnosis rates from population-based congenital anomaly registers in Europe. Eur J Hum Genet. 2012;20(5):521–6.
15. Suzumori N, Ebara T, Kumagai K, Goto S, Yamada Y, Kamijima M, Sugiura-Ogasawara M. Non-specific psychological distress in women undergoing noninvasive prenatal testing because of advanced maternal age. Prenat Diagn. 2014;34:1055–60.
16. Takeda E, Suzumori N, Kumagai K, Oseto K, Ebara T, Yotsumoto J, Numabe H, Sugiura-Ogasawara M. Background of couples undergoing non-invasive prenatal testing (NIPT) in Japan. J Obstet Gynecol Res. 2016;42:1222–8.
17. Suzumori N, Ebara T, Yamada T, Samura O, Yotsumoto J, Nishiyama M, Miura K, Sawai H, Murotsuki J, Kitagawa M, Kamei Y, Masuzaki H, Hirahara F, Saldivar J-S, Dharajiya N, Sago H, Sekizawa A, Japan NIPT consortium. Fetal cell-free DNA fraction in maternal plasma is affected by fetal trisomy. J Hum Genet. 2016;61:647–52.

18. Suzumori N, Sekizawa A, Takeda E, Samura O, Sasaki A, Akaishi R, et al. Classification of factors involved in nonreportable results of noninvasive prenatal testing (NIPT) and prediction of success rate of second NIPT. Prenat Diagn. 2019;39:100–6.
19. American College of Obstetricians and Gynecologists (ACOG). Prenatal diagnosis of fetal chromosomal abnormalities (ACOG practice bulletin; no 27). Obstet Gynecol. 2002;97(Suppl):1–12.
20. Nicolaides KH. Nuchal translucency and other first-trimester sonographic markers of chromosomal abnormalities. Am J Obstet Gynecol. 2004;191(1):45–67.
21. Akdeniz N, Kale A, Erdemoglu M, Yalinkaya A, Yayla M. Retrospective analysis of the 126 cases terminated in pregnancy by the ethical committee decision. Perinat J. 2005;13:80–5.
22. Balkan M, Kalkanli S, Akbas H, Yalinkaya A, Alp MN, Budak T. Parental decisions regarding a prenatally detected fetal chromosome abnormality and the impact of genetic counseling: an analysis of 38 cases with aneuploidy in Southeast Turkey. J Genet Counsel. 2010;19:241–6.
23. Eldahdah LT, Ormond KE, Nassar AH, Khalil T, Zahed LF. Outcome of chromosomally abnormal pregnancies in Lebanon: obstetricians' roles during and after prenatal diagnosis. Prenat Diagn. 2007;27:525–34.
24. Britt DW, Risinger ST, Miller V, Mans MK, Krivchenia EL, Evans M. Determinants of parental decisions after the prenatal diagnosis of Down syndrome: bringing in context. Am J Med Genet. 2000;93:410–6.
25. Schechtman KB, Gray DL, Baty JD, Rothman SM. Decision-making for termination of pregnancies with fetal anomalies: analysis of 53,000 pregnancies. Obstet Gynecol. 2002;99:216–22.
26. Shaffer BL, Caughey AB, Norton ME. Variation in the decision to terminate pregnancy in the setting of fetal aneuploidy. Prenat Diagn. 2006;26:667–71.
27. Snijders RJ, Sebire NJ, Nicolaides KH. Maternal age and gestational age-specific risk for chromosomal defects. Fetal Diagn Ther. 1995;10(6):356–67.
28. Yamada T, Sekizawa A, Fujii Y, Hirose T, Samura O, Suzumori N, Miura K, Sawai H, Hirahara F, Sago H. Maternal age-specific risk for trisomy 21 based on the clinical performance of NIPT and empirically derived NIPT age-specific positive and negative predictive values in Japan. J Hum Genet. 2018;63:1035–40.
29. Halliday JL, Watson LF, Lumley J, Danks DM, Sheffield LJ. New estimates of Down syndrome risks at chorionic villus sampling, amniocentesis, and livebirth in women of advanced maternal age from a uniquely defined population. Prenat Diagn. 1995;15(5):455–65.
30. Kratzer PG, Golbus MS, Schonberg SA, Heilbron DC, Taylor RN. Cytogenetic evidence for enhanced selective miscarriage of trisomy 21 pregnancies with advancing maternal age. Am J Med Genet. 1992;44(5):657–63.
31. Antonarakis SE, Lyle R, Dermitzakis ET, Reymond A, Deutsch S. Chromosome 21 and down syndrome: from genomics to pathophysiology. Nat Rev Genet. 2004;5(10):725–38.
32. Capone G, Goyal P, Ares W, Lannigan E. Neurobehavioral disorders in children, adolescents, and young adults with Down syndrome. Am J Med Genet C Semin Med Genet. 2006;142C(3):158–72.
33. Roizen NJ, Patterson D. Down's syndrome. Lancet. 2003;361(9365):1281–9.
34. Benn PA, Hsu LYF. Prenatal diagnosis of chromosomal abnormalities through amniocentesis. In: Milunsky A, editor. Genetic disorders of the fetus. 5th ed. Baltimore: The Johns Hopkins University Press; 2004. p. 217–8, 226–227.
35. Wapner R, Thom E, Simpson JL, Pergament E, Silver R, Filkins K, et al. First trimester maternal serum biochemistry and fetal nuchal translucency screening (BUN) study group. First-trimester screening for trisomies 21 and 18. N Engl J Med. 2003;349(15):1405–13.
36. Chen M, Yeh GP, Shih JC, Wang BT. Trisomy 13 mosaicism: study of serial cytogenetic changes in a case from early pregnancy to infancy. Prenat Diagn. 2004;24(2):137–43.
37. Crider KS, Olney RS, Cragan JD. Trisomies 13 and 18: population prevalences, characteristics, and prenatal diagnosis, metropolitan Atlanta, 1994-2003. Am J Med Genet A. 2008;146A(7):820–6.

38. Di Giacomo MC, Susca FC, Resta N, Bukvic N, Vimercati A, Guanti G. Trisomy 13 mosaicism in a phenotypically normal child: description of cytogenetic and clinical findings from early pregnancy beyond 2 years of age. Am J Med Genet A. 2007;143A(5):518–20.
39. Tartaglia NR, Wilson R, Miller JS, Rafalko J, Cordeiro L, Davis S, Hessl D, Ross J. Autism spectrum disorder in males with sex chromosome aneuploidy: XXY/Klinefelter Syndrome, XYY, and XXYY. J Dev Behav Pediatr. 2017;38(3):197–207.
40. Leggett V, Jacobs P, Nation K, Scerif G, Bishop DV. Neurocognitive outcomes of individuals with a sex chromosome trisomy: XXX, XYY, or XXY: a systematic review. Dev Med Child Neurol. 2010;52(2):119–29.
41. Ratcliffe S. Long-term outcome in children of sex chromosome abnormalities. Arch Dis Child. 1999;80(2):192–5.
42. Gruchy N, Blondeel E, Le Meur N, Joly-Hélas G, Chambon P, Till M, Herbaux M, Vigouroux-Castera A, Coussement A, Lespinasse J, Amblard F, Jimenez Pocquet M, Lebel-Roy C, Carré-Pigeon F, Flori E, Mugneret F, Jaillard S, Yardin C, Harbuz R, Collonge-Rame MA, Vago P, Valduga M, Leporrier N, Vialard F. Pregnancy outcomes in prenatally diagnosed 47, XXX and 47, XYY syndromes: a 30-year French, retrospective, multicentre study. Prenat Diagn. 2016;36(6):523–9.
43. Suzumori N, Kumagai K, Goto S, Nakamura A, Sugiura-Ogasawara M. Parental decisions following prenatal diagnosis of chromosomal abnormalities: implications for genetic counseling practice in Japan. J Genet Counsel. 2015;24:117–21.
44. Mansfield C, Hopfer S, Marteau TM. Termination rates after prenatal diagnosis of Down syndrome, Spina Bifida, Anencephaly, and Turner and Klinefelter syndromes: a systematic literature review. Prenat Diagn. 1999;19:808–12.
45. Mezei G, Papp C, Toth-Pal E, Beke A, Papp Z. Factors influencing parental decision making prenatal diagnosis of sex chromosome aneuploidy. Obstet Gynecol. 2004;104:94–101.
46. Brun J, Gangbo F, Wen ZQ, Galant K, Taine L, Maugey-Laulom B, et al. Prenatal diagnosis and management of sex chromosome aneuploidy: a report on 98 cases. Prenat Diagn. 2004;24:213–8.
47. Quadrelli R, Quadrelli A, Mechoso B, Laufer M, Jaumandreu C, Vaglio A. Prenatal decisions to abort or continue a pregnancy following prenatal diagnosis of chromosome abnormalities in a setting where termination of pregnancy is not legally available. Prenat Diagn. 2007;27:228–32.
48. Drugan A, Greb A, Johnson MP, Mrivchenia EL, Uhlmann WR, Moghissi KS, et al. Determinants of parental decisions to abort for chromosome abnormalities. Prenat Diagn. 1990;10:483–90.
49. Forrester MB, Merz RD. Pregnancy outcomes and prenatal diagnosis of sex chromosome abnormalities in Hawaii, 1986-1999. Am J Med Genet. 2003;119A:305–10.
50. Rychik J, Donaghue DD, Levy S, et al. Maternal psychological stress after prenatal diagnosis of congenital heart disease. J Pediatr. 2013;162:302–7.
51. Allison SJ, Stafford J, Anumba DO. The effect of stress and anxiety associated with maternal prenatal diagnosis on feto-maternal attachment. BMC Womens Health. 2011;11:33.
52. Shojai R, Boubli L, d'Ercole C. Prognosis work-up in prenatal medicine: the example of Down's syndrome. Gynecol Obstet Fertil. 2005;33:514–9.
53. Zahed L, Nabulsi M, Tamim H. Attitudes towards prenatal diagnosis and termination of pregnancy among health professionals in Lebanon. Prenat Diagn. 2002;22:880–6.

Chapter 20
Sex Chromosome Abnormalities and Genetic Counseling

Hidehiko Miyake

Abstract Sex chromosome abnormalities that are represented as Turner syndrome, Kleinfelder syndrome, XXX female, and XYY male are common conditions in newborn. While Turner syndrome is more likely to have complications that require early medical intervention, the phenotype of other sex chromosomal aneuploidies is mild. In the prenatal testing context, future parents are interested in autosomal trisomy, but not sex chromosomal aneuploidy. Therefore, when parents were informed of the sex chromosome abnormality incidentally, in genetic counseling about sex chromosome abnormality, physician/genetic counselor ought to provide not only medical matters, but also psychosocial issues. In the genetic counseling, explanations by multiple way might be useful.

Keywords Turner syndrome · Kleinfelder syndrome · XXX female · XYY male

20.1 Introduction

Sex chromosome abnormalities are common conditions in newborn. Turner syndrome, Kleinfelder syndrome, XXX female, and XYY male are representative sex chromosomal aneuploidy. A person with one of the aforementioned syndromes is likely to display a near-normal appearance with several developmental problems. This feature is associated with difficulties in genetic counseling. To provide information about sex chromosome abnormalities, it is necessary to understand the biological characteristics of the sex chromosomes. This section describes the characteristics of sex chromosomes and discusses genetic counseling for the sex chromosomal abnormalities.

H. Miyake (✉)
Tokyo, Japan
e-mail: miyake.hidehiko@ocha.ac.jp

H. Masuzaki (ed.), *Fetal Morph Functional Diagnosis*, Comprehensive Gynecology and Obstetrics, https://doi.org/10.1007/978-981-15-8171-7_20

20.2 Characteristics of Sex Chromosomes

In humans, the common chromosome composition is 46,XX (female) and 46,XY (male), respectively. According to data from the *Ensembl Genome Browser* on *GRCh38* [1], the human X chromosome consists of approximately 156 million base pairs and contains 852 coding genes, 665 noncoding genes, and 891 pseudogenes. On the contrary, the Y chromosome consists of approximately 57 million base pairs and contains 66 coding genes, 107 noncoding genes, and 394 pseudogenes. On the X chromosome, genes required to maintain biological activity are present. In contrast, the Y chromosome, excluding homologous region on the X and Y chromosome, contains genes for androgenization (e.g., *SRY*) and spermatogenesis (e.g., *DAZ1*, *SPGFY2*). Thus, there is a substantial difference between the X chromosome and the Y chromosome in both chromosome number and function. However, both chromosomes have homologous structures. This homologous structure is called a pseudoautosomal region (PAR), and homologous recombination occurs during meiosis I to form a chiasma. The 2.6 MB region on the terminal of the short arm is called PAR-1, and the 320 kb region on the terminal of the long arm side is called PAR-2 (Fig. 20.1) [2]. In addition, the Y chromosome has a large heterochromatic region at Yq12, and this part varies greatly between individuals.

From the viewpoint of allelic composition, alleles on the X chromosome are homozygous in females. However, in males, almost all loci on the X and Y

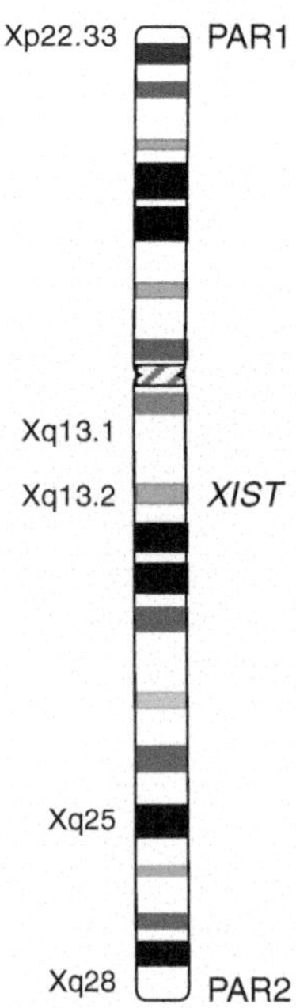

	X chromosome	Y chromosome
Length (bps)	156,040,895	57,227,415
Coding gene	852 (14 readthrough)	66
Non coding gene	665 (4 readthrough)	107 (3 readthrough)
Peudogenes	891	394
Short Variants	27,033,410	487,868

Data form GRCh38.p13

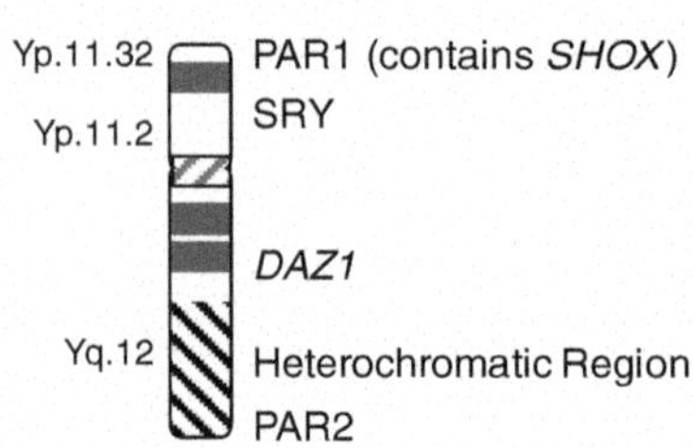

Fig. 20.1 Idiogram of the X and Y chromosomes (850 band level). *PAR* pseudoautosomal region, *SRY* sex-determining region Y

chromosomes are hemizygous, except for PAR. This imbalance in gene amount is adjusted by X chromosome inactivation. X-inactivation center (XIC) located in the Xq13 region regulates gene expression as well as contains several factors associated with inactivation [2]. Among these factors, the *XIST* (X-inactive specific transcript) gene localized at Xp13.2 is the primary inactivating factor. Providing that noncoding RNA molecules from the *XIST* gene epigenetically inactivate in a cis-regulation manner, genes on the same X chromosome are not translated into proteins. The inactivated X chromosome has a heterochromatin structure and can be observed under a microscope as a Barr body. It is important to note that inactivated genes are present on the X chromosome. Inactivation is mainly on the long arm of the X chromosome, and genes on the telomere side of the short arm are not generally inactivated.

In female cells with 46,XX karyotype, one X chromosome originating from either the father or the mother is inactivated and the other X chromosome is activated. This inactivation occurs during the early development stage. Which of the two chromosomes are inactivated is random, and its epigenetic status is stably inherited to daughter cells. Since the distribution of epigenetic status follows a Gaussian distribution, most women have biallelic expression of the X chromosome (Fig 20.2a). Therefore, almost all women with 46,XX are in a somatic mosaic state of X chromosome expression. In case of biased inactivation, bias may be involved in the onset of X-linked recessive disease in a carrier woman.

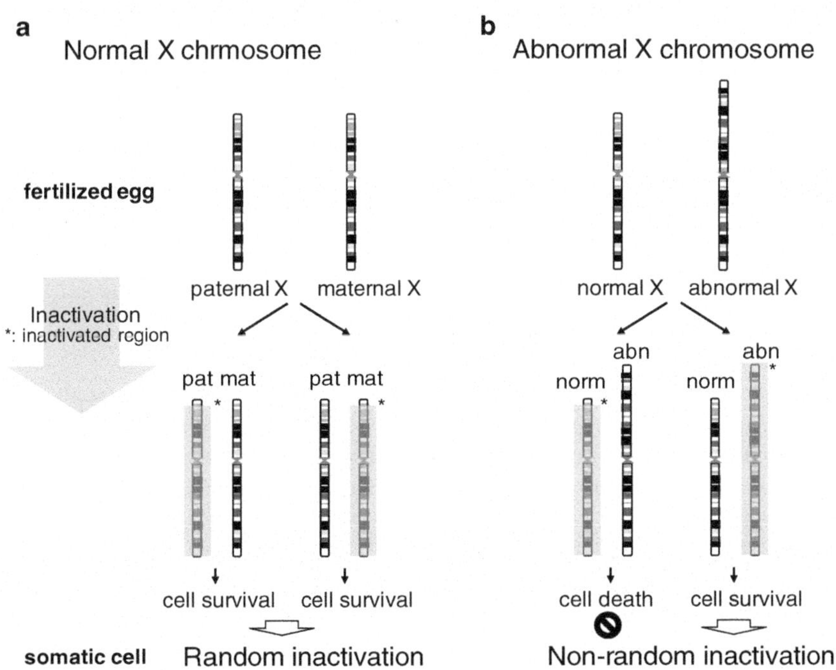

Fig. 20.2 Theoretical cell selection in X chromosome inactivation

When there are three or more X chromosomes, all but one X chromosome is inactivated. Due to these biological properties, it is considered that the sex chromosome aneuploidy does not substantially affect the phenotype. If a patient has a structural chromosome aberration on the X chromosome, inactivation of X may occur selectively. This selection occurs when cells with a chromosomal organization that can survive in the presence of inactivation survive when the chromosomal organization adversely affects cell survival due to inactivation (Fig. 20.2b).

20.3 Turner Syndrome and Variants

Turner syndrome is caused by X chromosome monosomy. The general frequency is 1 in 2500 women born. Clinical symptoms include short stature, gonadal dysfunction, and characteristic physical features [3]. Hemizygous of the *SHOX* (short stature homeobox-containing) gene located at Xp22.33 is thought to be the cause of short stature. Growth hormone therapy is recommended for girls with Turner syndrome who have short stature. Representative external findings include the pterygium and valgus elbow and edema of the extremities in neonates. Birth weight tends to be relatively low. Congenital malformations include aortic stenosis, mitral valve prolapse, and bicuspid aortic valve. In addition, malformations of the kidneys and renal vasculature, such as the horseshoe kidney, are observed. Because ear and hearing problem including otitis media is a common problem among girls and women with Turner syndrome, early otological examinations and audiological evaluations are important [4]. Diseases such as diabetes, osteoporosis, and thyroid dysfunction also pose a risk for those in adulthood.

Gonadal dysfunction causes a lack of secondary sexual characteristics and infertility. Low estrogenic status also leads to the risk of osteoporosis. For women with Turner syndrome, deliberate estrogen and progesterone replacement therapy is recommended. Including the case of the mosaic type, there are cases of spontaneous conception with spontaneous ovulation. If a patient without spontaneous ovulation desires pregnancy, egg donation might be considered. To prepare for the conception of Turner women, it is essential to evaluate medical complications, especially cardiac function.

Turner syndrome is associated with an increased risk of difficulties with visual-spatial reasoning, visual-spatial memory, attention, executive functioning, motor, and math skills [5]. Additionally, increased rates of social difficulties, anxiety, and depression were observed. Typically, the linguistic IQ shows a higher value than the behavioral IQ does [6].

During the fetal period, nuchal translucency (NT) and cystic hygroma are often confirmed by ultrasound, and it is thought that this involves lymphatic malformation. Sabire et al. showed that a fetus with Turner syndrome has a high rate of miscarriage during pregnancy, with the fetal NT above the 95th percentile in 87.9% of the 33 cases with 45,X [7]. In their consideration, assuming that all intrauterine deaths were from those with increased NT, screening for trisomy 21 by maternal age and fetal NT would have identified only 20% of potential livebirths in the 45,X group. Accordingly, a meticulous follow-up is required after fetal diagnosis. Tokita et al. investigated the effect of prenatal diagnosis on the postnatal outcome in cases with 45,X/46,XX. In the report, prenatal patients were more likely to have normal growth and normal secondary sexual development, as well as less likely to manifest distinctive Turner syndrome features such as nuchal webbing and edema and had a significantly fewer renal defects [8].

The common karyotype is 45,X (not described as 45,XO), accounting for 40–50% of patients with Turner syndrome [3]. Approximately 75% of patients with Turner syndrome with 45,X have a maternal X chromosome. Women with mosaic [45,X/46,XX] with a normal karyotype and a mosaic with triple X cells [45,X/47,XXX] are phenotypically mild. Since the characteristics of Turner syndrome are caused by the functional lack of genetic material on the short arm of the X chromosome, short arm deletion [46,XXp-], isochromosome [46,X,i(Xq) or 46,idic(Xp)], and ring chromosome [46,X,r(X)] also have a phenotype of Turner syndrome. The isochromosome is present in 10% of Turner syndrome cases and cannot be phenotypically distinguished from females with a 45,X karyotype. However, there are reports that autoimmune diseases are frequently seen in these women. Turner syndrome, due to ring chromosome, was often found in the mosaic karyotype 45,X/46,X,r(X). The ring chromosome lacks the telomeric region of both the short and long arms, and the size of the deletion is variable. Turner syndrome due to ring chromosomes is known to have little lymphedema and pterygium and is characterized by developmental delays [9]. It is also known that among the cases of Turner syndrome due to ring chromosomes, Kabuki syndrome is caused by mutations at the *MLL2* gene present at 12q13.12 and the *KDM6A* gene located at Xp11.3.

In women with a normal phenotype, mosaic karyotype 45,X/46,XY is occasionally found. This type of mosaic is due to the lack of the X chromosome as a result of aging [10]. This condition is called low-level X chromosome mosaicism, which is not Turner syndrome.

Advanced maternal age did not affect the incidence of Turner syndrome [11]. After the birth of a child or the loss of a pregnancy with 45,X, the risk of recurrence is very low [12]. If female offspring with Turner syndrome has a structural X chromosome rearrangement, the maternal karyotype is indicated. In women who carry any structural chromosome rearrangements, the recurrence risk increases if the parents have any chromosomal abnormality [12].

Few women with Turner syndrome are able to have a natural conception. In a French study, among 480 women with Turner syndrome, 27 women (5.6%) had a total of 52 spontaneous pregnancies with 30 full-term deliveries in 18 women [13]. In this report, 19 of the 27 pregnant women had a mosaic karyotype, and two cases were monosomy. Women with Turner syndrome have been reported to have a 30% risk of chromosomal and congenital abnormalities if they become naturally pregnant [14]. In a previous study by Bernard et al., karyotyping of offspring was performed in 0/13 boys and 11/17 newborn girls, and 2 of these 11 female newborns were diagnosed with TS, with ring X mosaicism and X-Y translocation mosaicism.

Mixed gonadal dysgenesis 45,X/46,XY

Mixed gonadal dysplasia, which is a typical karyotype of 45,X/46,XY, may also exhibit a phenotype similar to that of Turner syndrome. Mixed gonadal dysplasia is a condition in which testicular components and streak gonads coexist in one body and is a pathological condition associated with abnormal differentiation of the internal and external genital. The phenotypes are wide range and vary from normal females or males to those with ambiguous external genitalia. For the case with ambiguous external genitalia, surgical management is indicated. Given that this condition has a high risk of gonadoblastoma, follow-up is necessary. Similarly, if Turner syndrome exists in which a marker chromosome exists, it is important to confirm whether the marker chromosome contains the Y chromosome component [3].

X chromosome long arm deletion

Deletion of the long arm of the X chromosome can also cause Turner syndrome. In patients with a deletion proximal to Xq25, Turner syndrome commonly results [15]. Geerkens et al. reviewed that in women with Xq13 to Xq25 breakpoints had both a short stature and average stature [16]. Deletion close to the proximal region causes inactivation of the short arm region, resulting in a Turner syndrome phenotype. However, large Xq deletions are not indicative for survival.

20.4 Klinefelter Syndrome

Klinefelter syndrome (KS) is caused by an excess of the X chromosome in the male karyotype. The incidence is 1/600–800 in men. A Danish National Registry study revealed that only 25% of Klinefelter syndrome cases were diagnosed postnatally, and less than 10% of these cases were diagnosed before puberty [17]. Accordingly, most men with Klinefelter syndrome might go undiagnosed in their lifetime. Klinefelter syndrome is characterized by male gonadal dysfunction and tall stature. Tall stature of Klinefelter syndrome causes three copies of the *SHOX* gene. Other physical features include long limbs, gynecomastia, small testes, and small penis. For gynecomastia, surgical intervention is considered. Moreover, since the risk of male breast cancer increases, periodic surveillance is recommended. It has been demonstrated that Klinefelter syndrome is one of the most frequent causes of infertility, affecting 11% of azoospermia and 3.1% of all infertile men, and 90% of Klinefelter syndrome are azoospermic [18]. For infertile patients with Klinefelter syndrome, testicular sperm extraction (TESE) and intracytoplasmic sperm injection (ICSI) might be considered as treatment options. Using TESE, the retrieval rates of spermatozoa for adolescents younger than 16 years of age are much lower (0–20%) compared with those for adolescents and young adults between 16 and 30 years of age (40–70%) [19]. There is a risk of chromosomal aberrations in children when using ICSI. Study that investigated sperm chromosome segregation of a 34-years-old man with non-mosaic Klinefelter syndrome showed that 94.9% of the sperm were normal haploid, but higher rate of 24,XX and 24,XY spermatozoa (4.7%) in the patient was seen (0.3 and 0.7% in controls), and the frequency of sperm with disomy 21 was 6.2% that was higher than 0.4% in controls [20]. Prenatal diagnosis should be offered to expectant fathers with Klinefelter syndrome, under balanced information [12].

The intelligence of a person with Klinefelter syndrome is almost normal, but tends to be slightly lower when compared between siblings [21]. It is known that verbal IQ decreases, and in some cases, learning disabilities are found. Children with Klinefelter syndrome need to follow their neural development, including language development, if necessary, referral to additional educational support is recommended. The other complications associated with Klinefelter syndrome are abdominal adiposity, metabolic syndrome, type 2 diabetes, cryptorchidism, mitral valve prolapse, bone fractures, and other neurological and mental disorders [22].

In general, the fetal phenotype is extremely mild and difficult to distinguish from normal. Klinefelter syndrome is generally diagnosed by incidentally investigating male infertility or prenatal testing. No sonographic findings are characteristic of a fetus with Klinefelter syndrome. Sabire et al. reported that the fetal NT was above the 95th centile in 40% of the 20 cases with 47,XXX, 47,XYY, or 47,XXX. Assuming that all intrauterine deaths are from those with increased NT, screening for trisomy 21 by maternal age and fetal NT would have identified 9% of those with 47,XXY, 47,XYY, or 47,XXX [7].

The common karyotype of Klinefelter syndrome is [47,XXY], and a mosaic type [46,XY/47,XXY] is recognized in about 7% of cases. Other variants include 48,XXXY and 49,XXXXY, whose frequencies are 1/20,000 and 1/85,000, respectively [23]. Regarding the origin of additional X chromosome of men with Klinefelter syndrome, 53% of the nondisjunction is attributable to paternal meiosis I errors, 34% to maternal meiosis I errors, 9% to maternal meiosis II errors, and 3% to a post-zygotic mitotic error [24] (Fig. 20.3). The risk of recurrence is theoretically expected to be higher than the general frequency due to parental chromosome nondisjunction, but clear evidence is not available.

20.5 XXX Female

Women with one extra X chromosome are termed triple X syndrome/XXX females. Two of the three X chromosomes are inactivated, except for a specific region. The birth frequency was 1/1000 to 1/1200 of women. It is substantially under-ascertained and the majority of 47,XX women are unaware of their karyotype [12]. The appearance of XXX females is almost normal, and high height is recognized as a characteristic. This height is due to the dose effect of the *SHOX* gene. Intellectual abilities of XXX female group are slightly lower than those of the general population, but the ability varies among individuals. Learning and developmental disabilities in XXX females are not specific characteristics of the condition. If girls with XXX experience learning and developmental disabilities, providing additional general support is recommended.

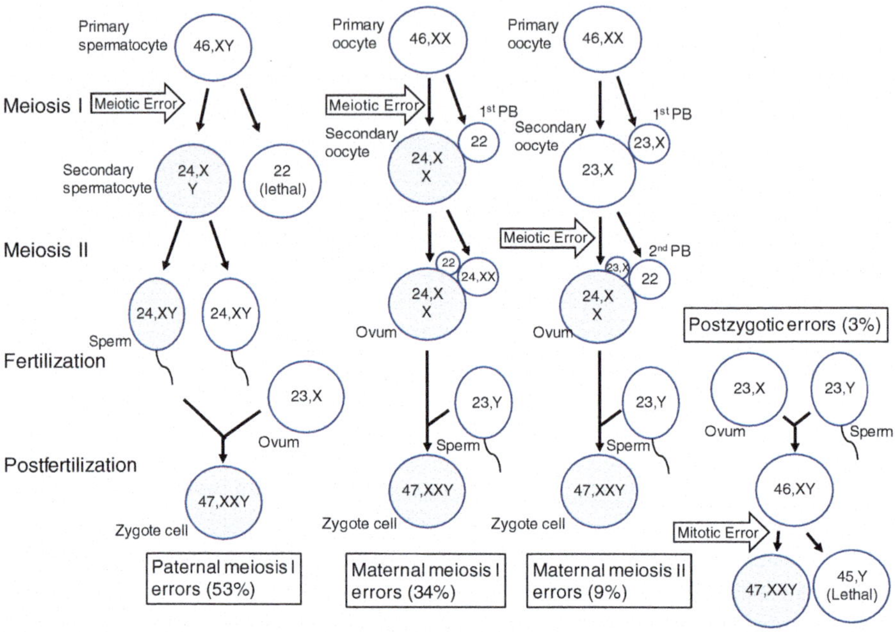

Fig. 20.3 Multiple origin of Klinefelter syndrome in gametogenesis and postfertilization. *PB* polar body. The cell directly caused to Klinefelter syndrome is shaded gray

Sexual maturity and fertility are normal in XXX women. Oocytes formed are mostly [23, X] [25] and the risk of transmission from XXX women to their offspring <1% [12]. XXX female patients have premature ovarian failure risk. The ages of onset of premature ovarian failure (POF) ranged from 19 to 40 years [26]. One study reported that the POF risk was around 3% [27].

NT may increase during the fetal stage. Moreover, XXX females have a risk of genitourinary structural anomalies. When supernumerary X chromosome is confirmed, ultrasonographic examination is recommended.

The most common karyotype is 47,XXX, and there is also a mosaic with 45,X, and 46,XX cells, which are derived from post-zygotic error. 47,XXX conceptions result from maternal nondisjunction at meiosis I. The birth frequency slightly increases with the aging of the mother. XXX female is generally diagnosed incidentally. The risk of recurrence of the next offspring increases slightly in theory, but most of those might have a normal karyotype.

20.6 XYY Male

XYY males have 1 for every 1000 male births. Excessive Y chromosome is not associated with advanced paternal age. Intellectual abilities are reported to be slightly lower than siblings, but most of them are in the normal range [21]. There is also a risk of reduced language skills and learning disabilities. Males with XYY karyotype have no signs of malformation, but high stature is noted. During the prenatal period, this condition is discovered unintentionally, as an incidental finding. When the XYY karyotype was found from the investigation of the boys with learning and behavioral disabilities, this finding may be of clinical significance [12]. Parents of XYY males do not have a high risk of recurrent offspring. XXY males have normal fertility, and sperm karyotypes are also normal haploid. In fact, in sons of XYY male, the risk of having an XYY karyotype does not increase.

20.7 Genetic Counseling for Sex Chromosome Abnormalities

In the prenatal testing context, future parents were interested in autosomal trisomy, but not sex chromosomal aneuploidy. Therefore, when parents were informed of the sex chromosome abnormality incidentally, they faced difficulty in understanding medical information and psychosocial issues. Among sex chromosome abnormalities, Turner syndrome is likely to require early medical intervention. However, while all sex chromosome abnormalities are associated with development risks for mild delay in motor skills and speech/language skills and the risk for learning disabilities, it is not possible to determine which child will exhibit any or all of these concerns [28]. In one study, autism spectrum disorder rates were 10% in XXY/KS, 38% in XYY, and 52% in XXYY using ADOS-2/DSM-5 and were not statistically different compared to DSM-IV criteria [29]. Counseling before a prenatal diagnosis procedure should always include the possibility of the presence of a sex chromosome abnormality and a brief discussion of the prognosis [28].

In genetic counseling-associated disclosure of the prenatal result of sex chromosome abnormality, physician/genetic counselor ought to provide an overview of the conditions, including clinical symptoms, medical intervention, public support, and social resources. For cases with Turner syndrome, parents need to understand the opportunity for fetal loss. When genetic counselors talk about developmental conditions, the counselor should present that the conditions occur in either normal karyotype or sex chromosome abnormality. Furthermore, the phenotype and intervention were not different between normal karyotype and sex chromosome abnormalities. Because intellectual phenotype is a continuous trait (Fig. 20.4) [30], issues of IQ not

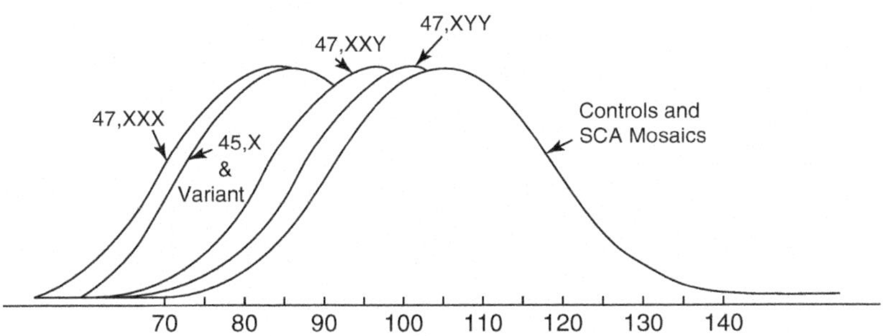

Fig. 20.4 Estimated full scale IQ distributions for SCA and control children [30]

only about average, but also the distribution, should be explained. Parents who decide to carry a pregnancy to term after receiving a diagnosis of a sex chromosome abnormalities need to be counseled in strategies of accepting genetic diversity, prepared for seeking early intervention for a child who may show problems associated with these syndromes (physical, reproductive, and behavioral), and encouraged to keep in touch with a center of expertise and with specialists who are aware of the specific needs of these children and their families [21].

For declarations for persons with sex chromosome abnormalities, disclosure of the karyotype on a 'need to know' basis is advised generally, so that the child is not treated differently or regarded differently by others. Telling a child about their karyotype should be a gradual process extending over many years, with parents being supported by health professionals [12]. In the genetic counseling, explanations by multiple approach might be useful. It is recommended to use verbal approach with a visual/graphical approach, such as genetic counseling aid materials.

References

1. Ensembl. http://asia.ensembl.org/index.html
2. Gardner RJM, Amor DJ. Sex chromosome translocations. Gardner and Sutherland's Chromosome abnormalities and genetic counseling. 5th ed. New York: Oxford University Press; 2018a. p. 113–41.
3. Gravholt CH, Andersen NH, Conway GS, Dekkers OM, Geffner ME, Klein KO, Lin AE, Mauras N, Quigley CA, Rubin K, Sandberg DE, Sas TCJ, Silberbach M, Söderström-Anttila V, Stochholm K, van Alfen-van der Velden JA, Woelfle J, Backeljauw PF, International Turner Syndrome Consensus Group. Clinical practice guidelines for the care of girls and women with Turner syndrome: proceedings from the 2016 Cincinnati International Turner Syndrome Meeting. Eur J Endocrinol. 2017 Sep;177(3):G1–G70.
4. Stenberg AE, Nylén O, Windh M, Hultcrantz M. Otological problems in children with Turner's syndrome. Hear Res. 1998 Oct;124(1-2):85–90.
5. Hutaff-Lee C, Bennett E, Howell S, Tartaglia N. Clinical developmental, neuropsychological, and social-emotional features of Turner syndrome. Am J Med Genet C Semin Med Genet. 2019 Mar;181(1):126–34.
6. Davenport ML. Approach to the patient with Turner syndrome. J Clin Endocrinol Metab. 2010 Apr;95(4):1487–95.
7. Sebire NJ, Snijders RJ, Brown R, Southall T, Nicolaides KH. Detection of sex chromosome abnormalities by nuchal translucency screening at 10-14 weeks. Prenat Diagn. 1998 Jun;18(6):581–4.
8. Tokita MJ, Sybert VP. Postnatal outcomes of prenatally diagnosed 45,X/46,XX. Am J Med Genet A. 2016 May.;170A;(5):1196–201.
9. Dennis N, Coppin B, Turner C, Skuse D, Jacobs P. A clinical, cytogenetic and molecular study of 47 females with r(X) chromosomes. Ann Hum Genet. 2000 Jul;64(Pt 4):277-293.
10. Russell LM, Strike P, Browne CE, Jacobs PA. X chromosome loss and ageing. Cytogenet Genome Res. 2007;116:181–5.
11. Allen EG, Freeman SB, Druschel C, Hobbs CA, O'Leary LA, Romitti PA, Royle MH, Torfs CP, Sherman SL. Maternal age and risk for trisomy 21 assessed by the origin of chromosome nondisjunction: a report from the Atlanta and National Down Syndrome Projects. Hum Genet. 2009 Feb;125(1):41–52.

12. Firth HV, Hurst JA. Chromosomes. Oxford desk reference: clinical genetics & genomics. 2nd ed. Oxford: Oxford University Press; 2017. p. 623–701.
13. Bernard V, Donadille B, Zenaty D, Courtillot C, Salenave S, Brac de la Perrière A, Albarel F, Fèvre A, Kerlan V, Brue T, Delemer B, Borson-Chazot F, Carel JC, Chanson P, Léger J, Touraine P, Christin-Maitre S, CMERC Center for Rare Disease. Spontaneous fertility and pregnancy outcomes amongst 480 women with Turner syndrome. Hum Reprod. 2016 Apr;31(4):782–8.
14. Saenger P. Turner's syndrome. N Engl J Med. 1996 Dec 5;335(23):1749–54.
15. Maraschio P, Tupler R, Barbierato L, Dainotti E, Larizza D, Bernardi F, Hoeller H, Garau A, Tiepolo L. An analysis of Xq deletions. Hum Genet. 1996 Mar;97(3):375–81.
16. Geerkens C, Just W, Vogel W. Deletions of Xq and growth deficit: a review. Am J Med Genet. 1994 Apr 1;50(2):105–13.
17. Viuff MH, Stochholm K, Uldbjerg N, Nielsen BB, Danish Fetal Medicine Study Group, Gravholt CH. Only a minority of sex chromosome abnormalities are detected by a national prenatal screening program for Down syndrome. Hum Reprod. 2015 Oct;30(10):2419–26.
18. Lanfranco F, Kamischke A, Zitzmann M, Nieschlag E. Klinefelter's syndrome. Lancet. 2004;364(9430):273–83.
19. Franik S, Hoeijmakers Y, D'Hauwers K, Braat DD, Nelen WL, Smeets D, Claahsen-van der Grinten HL, Ramos L, Fleischer K. Klinefelter syndrome and fertility: sperm preservation should not be offered to children with Klinefelter syndrome. Hum Reprod. 2016 Sep;31(9):1952–9.
20. Hennebicq S, Pelletier R, Bergues U, Rousseaux S. Risk of trisomy 21 in offspring of patients with Klinefelter's syndrome. Lancet. 2001 Jun 30;357(9274):2104–5.
21. Lalatta F, Tint GS. Counseling parents before prenatal diagnosis: do we need to say more about the sex chromosome aneuploidies? Am J Med Genet A. 2013 Nov.;161A;(11):2873–9.
22. Groth KA, Skakkebæk A, Høst C, Gravholt CH, Bojesen A. Clinical review: Klinefelter syndrome–a clinical update. J Clin Endocrinol Metab. 2013 Jan;98(1):20–30.
23. Kleczkowska A, Fryns JP, Van den Berghe H. X-chromosome polysomy in the male. The Leuven experience 1966-1987. Hum Genet. 1988 Sep;80(1):16–22.
24. Jacobs PA, Hassold TJ, Whittington E, Butler G, Collyer S, Keston M, Lee M. Klinefelter's syndrome: an analysis of the origin of the additional sex chromosome using molecular probes. Ann Hum Genet. 1988 May;52(2):93–109.
25. Gardner RJM, Amor DJ. Sex chromosome aneuploidy and structural rearrangement. Gardner and Sutherland's Chromosome abnormalities and genetic counseling. 5th ed. New York: Oxford University Press; 2018b. p. 337–58.
26. Tartaglia NR, Howell S, Sutherland A, Wilson R, Wilson L. A review of trisomy X (47,XXX). Orphanet J Rare Dis. 2010 May 11;5:8.
27. Goswami R, Goswami D, Kabra M, Gupta N, Dubey S, Dadhwal V. Prevalence of the triple X syndrome in phenotypically normal women with premature ovarian failure and its association with autoimmune thyroid disorders. Fertil Steril. 2003 Oct;80(4):1052–4.
28. Linden MG, Bender BG, Robinson A. Genetic counseling for sex chromosome abnormalities. Am J Med Genet. 2002 Jun 1;110(1):3–10.
29. Tartaglia NR, Wilson R, Miller JS, Rafalko J, Cordeiro L, Davis S, Hessl D, Ross J. Autism spectrum disorder in males with sex chromosome aneuploidy: XXY/Klinefelter Syndrome, XYY, and XXYY. J Dev Behav Pediatr. 2017 Apr;38(3):197–207.
30. Bender BG, Puck MH, Salbenblatt JA, Robinson A. Cognitive development of children with sex chromosome abnormalities. In: Holmes CS, editor. Psychoneuroendocrinology. New York: Springer; 1990. p. 138–63.

Chapter 21
Genetic Counseling: Chromosomal Structural Rearrangements

Haruka Hamanoue

Abstract Structural rearrangements are classified into balanced and unbalanced types. Balanced structural rearrangements mainly result from translocations (e.g., reciprocal translocation, Robertsonian translocation, and inversion), and unbalanced structural rearrangements result from deletion, duplication, insertion, ring chromosomes, and small supernumerary marker chromosomes, in addition to derivative chromosomes associated with translocations and inversion. Chromosomal variants are structural rearrangements that do not affect phenotypes or reproduction, and it is important not to confuse other structural rearrangements. Besides, it is desirable to provide medical information to help the parents understand the situation, essential points in the future of their reproductive health, and to propose psychological and social support as needed.

Keywords Chromosomal structural rearrangements · Translocation · Inversion
Small supernumerary marker chromosome · Derivative chromosome
Chromosomal variant

21.1 What Are the Chromosomal Structural Rearrangements Identified During the Fetal Period?

Chromosomal abnormalities are broadly classified into numerical aberration and structural rearrangements. Most often, chromosomal abnormalities cause development to stop at any stage of pregnancy, starting from the early stage after fertilization. Depending on the degree of impairment, they lead to miscarriage or stillbirth. Chromosomal abnormalities are more varied in the fetuses and occur more frequently than in post-birth children. Since clinical information and analysis for

H. Hamanoue (✉)
Department of Clinical Genetics, Yokohama City University Hospital, Yokohama, Japan
e-mail: haruka@mb.ejnet.ne.jp

H. Masuzaki (ed.), *Fetal Morph Functional Diagnosis*, Comprehensive Gynecology and Obstetrics, https://doi.org/10.1007/978-981-15-8171-7_21

chromosomal abnormalities in fetuses are limited, it should be noted that evaluation, judgment, and natural prognosis are likely to be unclear.

Structural rearrangements are classified into balanced and unbalanced types. Balanced structural rearrangements mainly result from translocations (e.g., reciprocal translocation, Robertsonian translocation, and inversion), and unbalanced structural rearrangements result from deletion, duplication, insertion, ring chromosomes, and small supernumerary marker chromosomes, in addition to derivative chromosomes associated with translocations and inversion (Fig. 21.1). Chromosomal variants are structural rearrangements that do not affect phenotypes or reproduction, and it is important not to confuse other structural rearrangements.

21.2 Balanced Structural Rearrangements

Balanced structural rearrangements refer to a state in which structural changes occur among two or more chromosomes or within one chromosome, but there is no imbalance in the quantity of genome (chromosomes or genes). Patients are often asymptomatic and identified as carriers, but balanced structural rearrangements can become unbalanced in the next generation. Balanced structural rearrangements are detected in about 5% of the amniotic fluid tests. In contrast, de novo balanced structural rearrangements are found in 0.06–0.09% of the amniotic fluid tests, of which 6.1% of the children have abnormalities (5.6% for reciprocal translocation, 3.9% for Robertsonian translocation, and 9.7% for inversion) [2].

21.2.1 Reciprocal Translocation

Reciprocal translocation is where at least two chromosomes break and rejoin with different chromosomes. This is the most frequent among the chromosomal structural rearrangements (1 in 400 in the general population (0.25%), or 1 in 200 pairs). In people who have repeat miscarriages or stillbirths, detection rate of balanced translocations is higher (1.25% in males, 2.38% in females).

Most of the balanced translocations do not affect phenotypes. When a parent has the same balanced reciprocal translocation, the fetus is unlikely to have pathogenic phenotypes. However, when both parents have normal chromosomes (de novo), the probability that their fetus might have pathogenic phenotypes is 6.1%. This may be due to subtle deletions or complex chromosomal rearrangements near the translocation breakpoints. The degree of the clinical effect cannot be predicted. The frequency of this congenital anomaly is notably high in the general population (3–5%).

In general, the possibility of a child being born with an unbalanced translocation from carrier parent is as follows: if the father is a carrier, the rate is approximately 5%, and if the mother is a carrier, it is approximately 10%. However, the probability varies (<1% to 20%, sometimes 50%) depending on breakpoints, the translocated

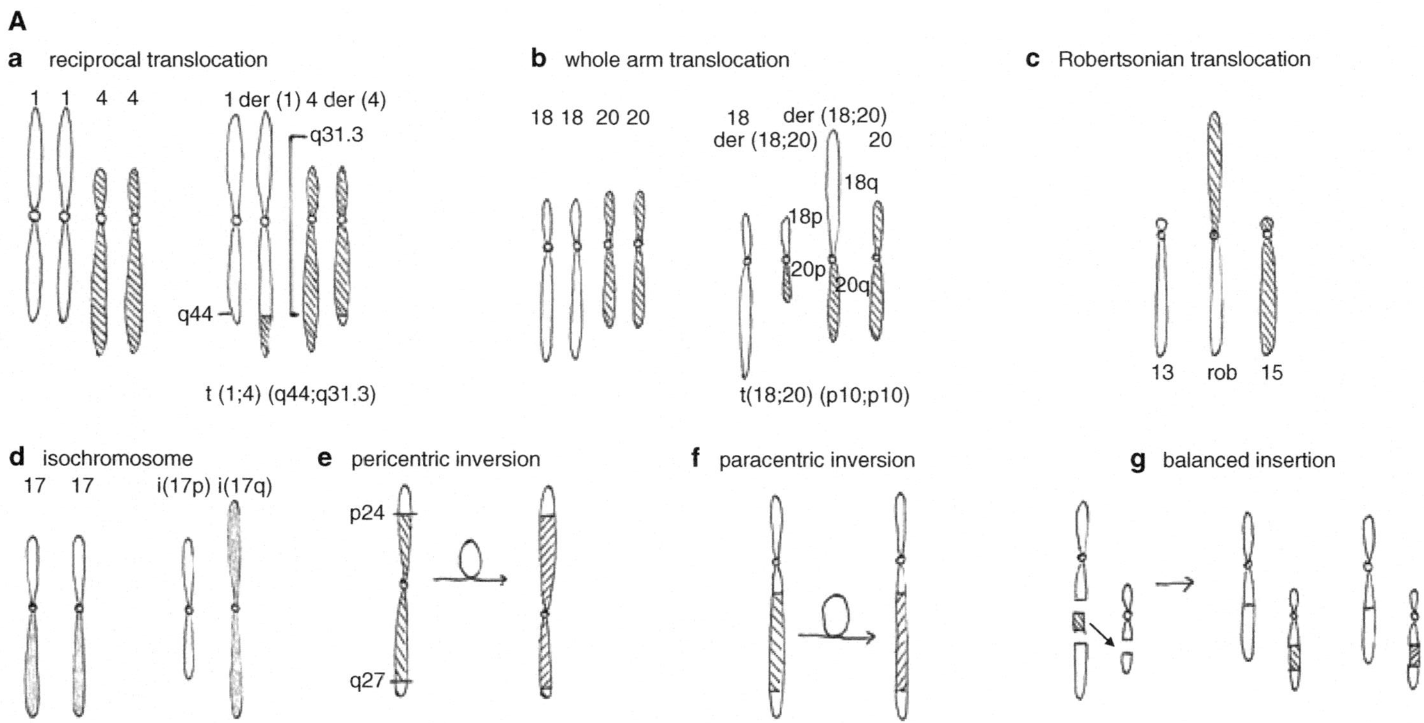

Fig. 21.1 A: Balanced. B: Unbalanced. C: Complex chromosomal rearrangements. D: Translocations among X-Y-autosomal chromosomes. E: Chromosomal variants [1]

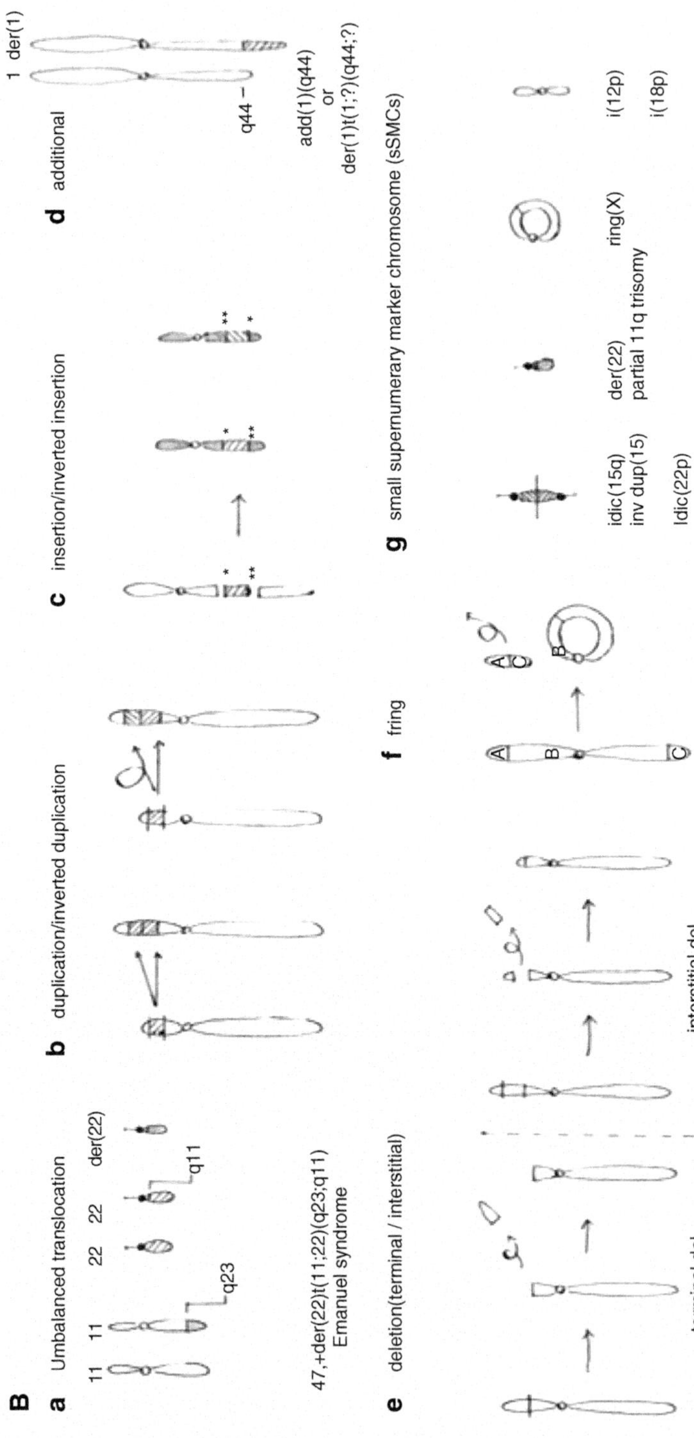

Fig. 21.1 (continued)

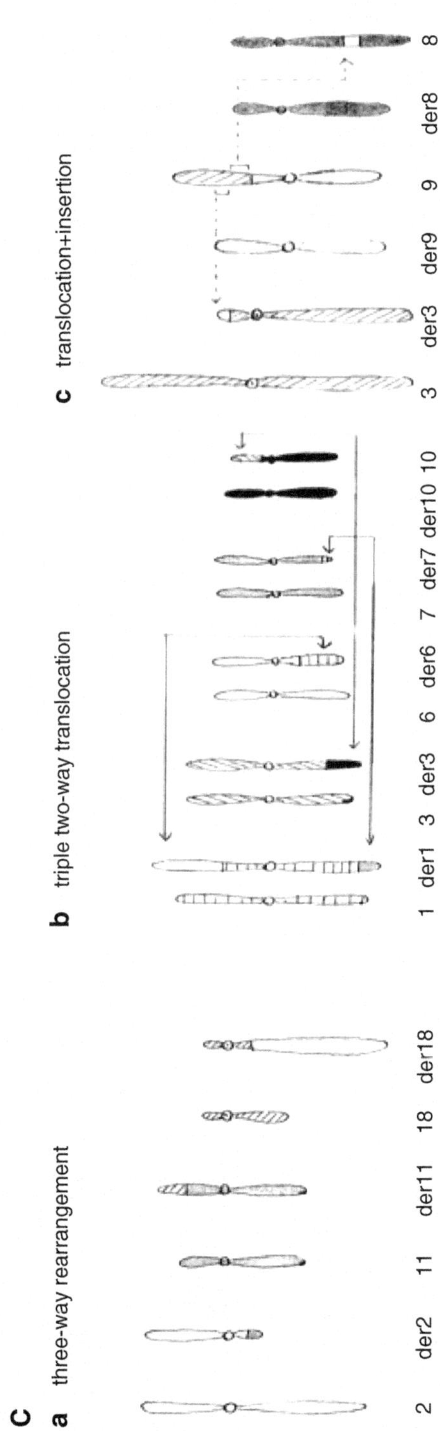

Fig. 21.1 (continued)

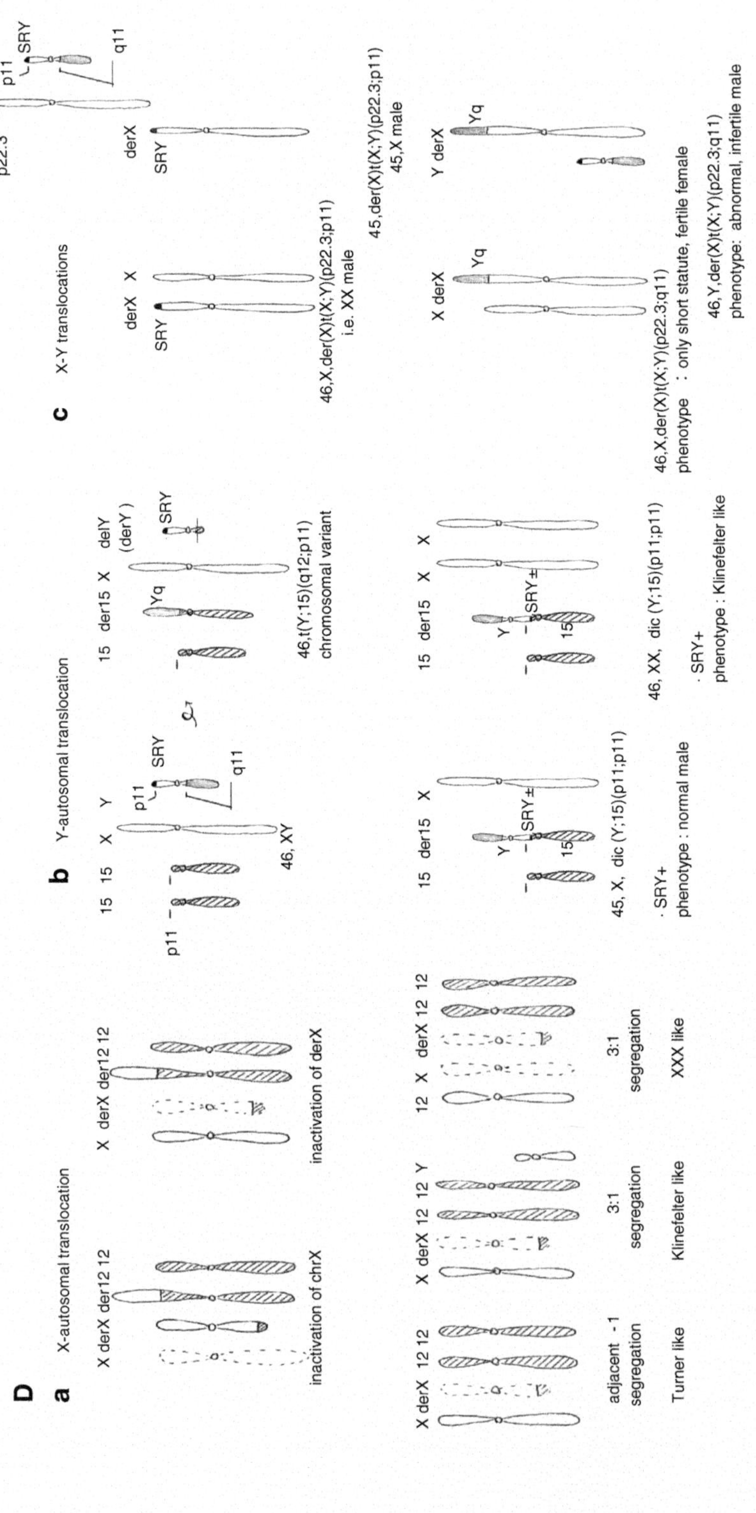

Fig. 21.1 (continued)

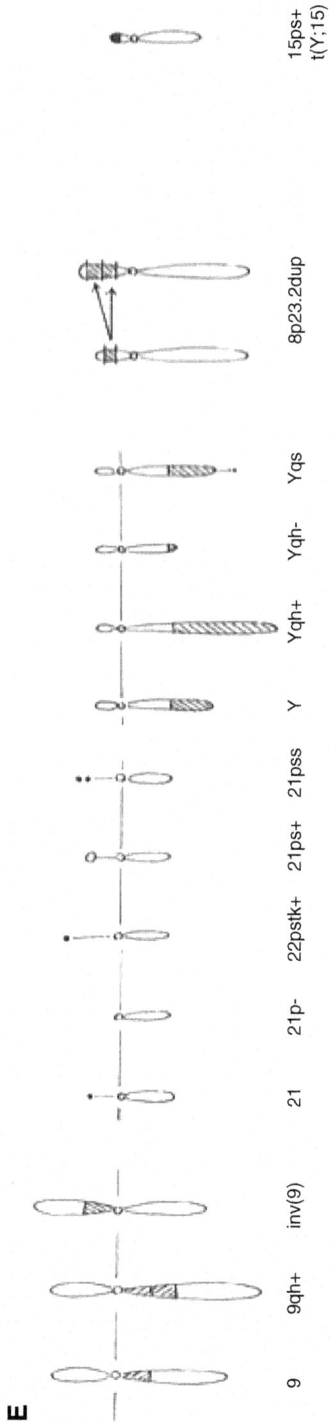

Fig. 21.1 (continued)

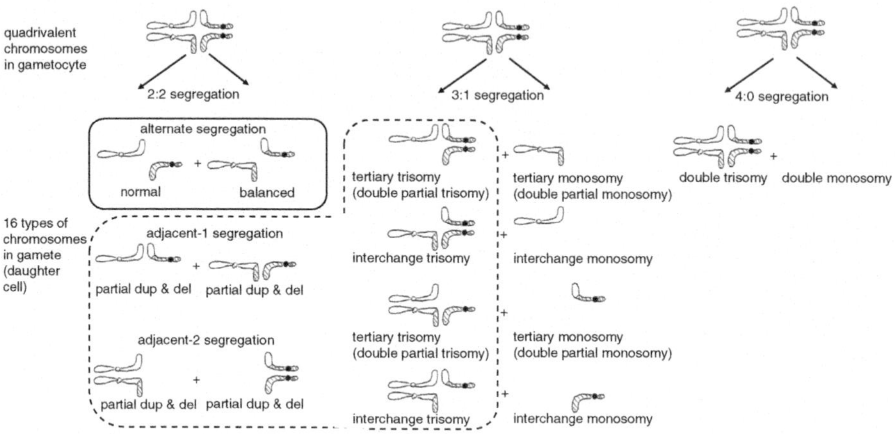

Fig. 21.2 Gametogenesis in reciprocal translocation (quadrivalent in gametocyte at meiosis I and 16 possible chromosomal combinations) [1]

region, origin (paternal or maternal), and the trigger to detect. The probability of having a child with an unbalanced translocation is difficult to accurately assess, but the ratio of balanced translocation to normal karyotype is almost 1:1 in the healthy children.

Figure 21.2 shows the chromosome synapsis related to the translocation and gametogenesis process. The presence of a translocation may result in the formation of quadrivalent chromosomes in the first meiosis to theoretically produce 16 kinds of gametes. Of these, only a part of gamete types has possibility to be born: 71% for adjacent-1 segregation, 22% for tertiary trisomy or monosomy due to 3:1 segregation, 2.5% for interchange trisomy, and 4% for adjacent-2 type [3]. The 3:1 segregation is reported to increase when the mother is a carrier [4]. Zygotes with different unbalanced translocations are generated from a translocation carrier of the same family, but zygotes with unbalanced translocations leading to birth are usually identical (others will be eliminated).

The likelihood of the birth of a child with an unbalanced translocation from a parent with a balanced reciprocal translocation is calculated in various tools. The smaller the translocation region is, the more likely that the baby is born with an unbalanced translocation. This is because the possibility of survival is low unless the fragment causing monosomy is small. In adjacent-1 segregation, the birth is possible only when the excess/shortage piece is small. Adjacent-2 segregation is rare, and survival is possible only when breakpoints are near the centromeres of chromosomes 13, 14, 15, 21, and 22 or on the long arm of chromosome 9. In the 3:1 segregation, the total number of chromosomes is 47, resulting in partial trisomy of two chromosomes or trisomy with one derivative chromosome.

Generally, i) when sick baby has been already alive, ii) when the mother is a translocation carrier, and iii) when the translocation segment is small, they having the chromosome findings may easily survive more. In the case of i), the probability is said to be as high as 19% [5], but this is just an estimation. With regard to iii), we judge it from the percentage of haploid autosome length (%HAL). In the many

Table 21.1 The percentage of haploid autosome length for each chromosome

Chromosome	Percentage of HAL	Chromosome	Percentage of HAL
1	9.24	12	4.66
2	8.02	13	3.74
3	6.83	14	3.56
4	6.3	15	3.46
5	6.08	16	3.36
6	5.9	17	3.46
7	5.36	18	2.93
8	4.93	19	2.67
9	4.8	20	2.56
10	4.59	21	1.9
11	4.61	22	2.04

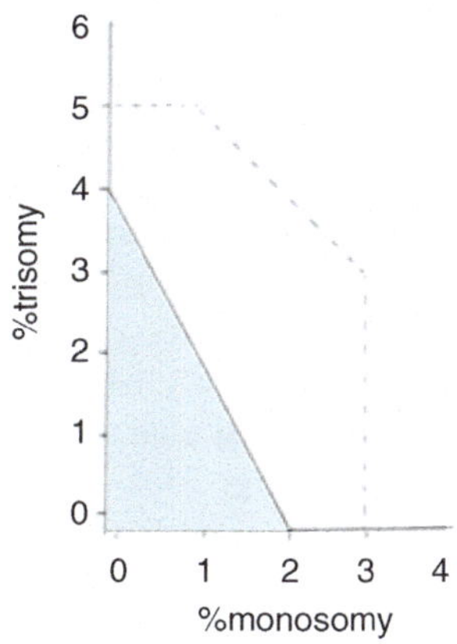

Fig. 21.3 %HAL

survivor cases, %HAL of deletion is 2% or less (partial monosomy) or %HAL of duplication is 4% or less (partial trisomy). It indicates that the cases entering the triangle formed by X-axis (%HAL of the deletion), Y-axis (%HAL of the duplication), and a straight line (allied with 2% of the X-axis and 4% of the Y-axis) are probably survived. (Table 21.1, Fig. 21.3).

In balanced translocations, it is not possible to accurately predict about sterility, repetition miscarriage, stillbirth, or birth defects. However, the information is important to a judgment about a prenatal test and interruption of the pregnancy.

21.2.2 *Whole Arm Translocation*

Whole arm translocation occurs when two chromosomes break near the centromeres and are reciprocally translocated. This can be considered as a type of reciprocal translocation, but it can also be considered as a reciprocal translocation involving large translocation segments, such as t(18;20) (p10;p10). Usually, unbalanced zygotes do not lead to birth, and carrier couples are infertile. In the case of whole arm translocations between homologous chromosomes, such as t(7;7) (p10;p10), all generated zygotes become unbalanced and do not result in live births.

21.2.3 Robertsonian Translocation/Isochromosomes

In the case of Robertsonian translocation, the breaks take place near the centromeres of two acrocentric chromosomes (Groups D and G), and the long arms rejoin with each other. If two long arms of homologous chromosomes (acrocentric chromosome) are rejoined, it is called isochromosome. The short arms are lost, but this does not usually affect the phenotype. Robertsonian translocation is considered to be a balanced structural abnormality, and a person with this translocation is called a translocation carrier. Since two chromosomes are bound, the total number of chromosomes is 45. It is cytogenetically expressed such as der (13;14) or rob (14;21).

Robertsonian translocations are observed only in 0.1% of the general population, but they are observed in 3.4% of men with oligo/azoospermia and 0.7% of the parents in cases of recurrent miscarriage [6]. The classification of translocation chromosomes is shown in Table 21.2 [7, 8]. The reported frequency of each translocation chromosome varies greatly, so it remains unclear. Clinically, these translocations may cause trisomy 13, trisomy 21, UPD (14), and UPD (15).

In a Robertsonian translocation, trivalent chromosomes are formed during gametogenesis (Fig. 21.4). When an unbalanced chromosome is seen in a fetus, the

Table 21.2 The reported frequency of each Robertsonian translocation chromosome

Chromosomes	Reviews (n = 1266)	Amniotic fluid test
t(13;13)	3%	2%
t(14;14)	0.5%	–
t(15;15)	2%	–
t(13;14)	33%	74%
t(13;15)	2%	2%
t(14;15)	2%	5%
t(13;21)	2%	1%
t(13;22)	1%	2%
t(14;21)	30%	8%
t(14;22)	1%	2%
t(15;21)	3%	0.5%
t(15;22)	0.5%	1%
t(21;21)	17%	3%
t(22;22)	1%	–
t(21;22)	2%	0.5%

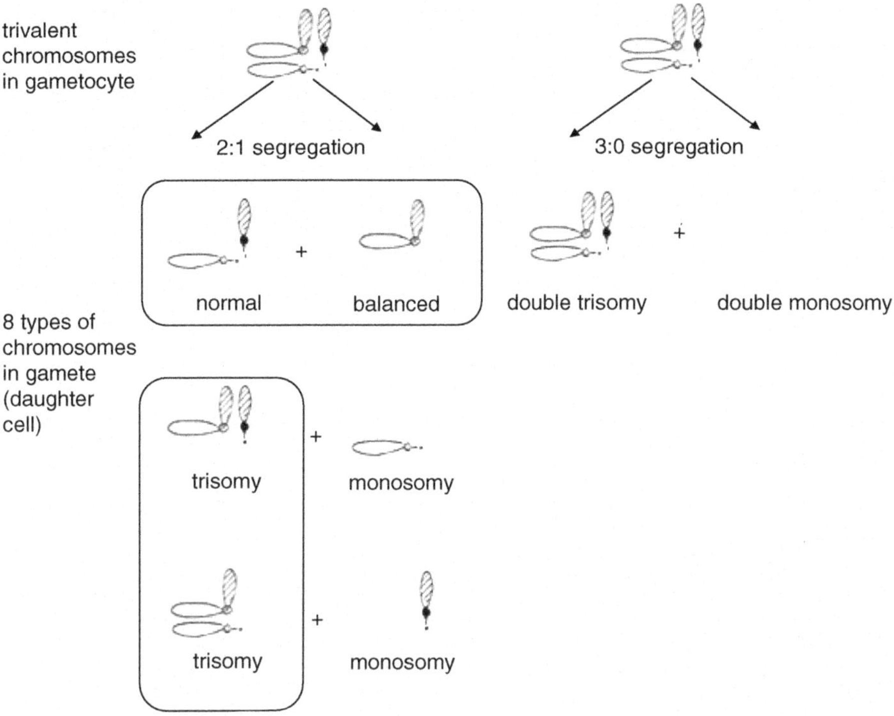

Fig. 21.4 Gametogenesis in Robertsonian translocation (trivalent in gametocyte at meiosis I and 8 possible chromosomal combinations) [1]

mother is often a translocation carrier. The amniotic fluid test of parents who are translocation carriers also reveals that the probability of the unbalanced type is higher when mothers are the carriers. This is because the formation of unbalanced spermatozoa is disturbed and they are disadvantageous to the fertilization.

For the most commonly seen chromosomal translocation 14q21q, the probability of having a child with Down syndrome is reported to be 14% if the mother is a translocation carrier and 4.3% if the father is a translocation carrier. For balanced zygotes, balanced translocations are more common than normal karyotypes. This phenomenon is called the meiotic drive, but its etiology is not clear [9].

Balanced Robertsonian translocations of rob(14;15), iso(14;14), or iso(15;15) may involve pathogenic phenotypes even if the case is inherited from carrier's parent. This is because in many cases, uniparental disomy (UPD) occurs (Fig. 21.5).

21.2.4 Inversion

On the same chromosome, if breaks occur at two sections, and the middle part that is cleaved is rotated 180° along its long axis and rejoins, this results in an inversion. When the inverted part contains the centromere, it is called a pericentric inversion,

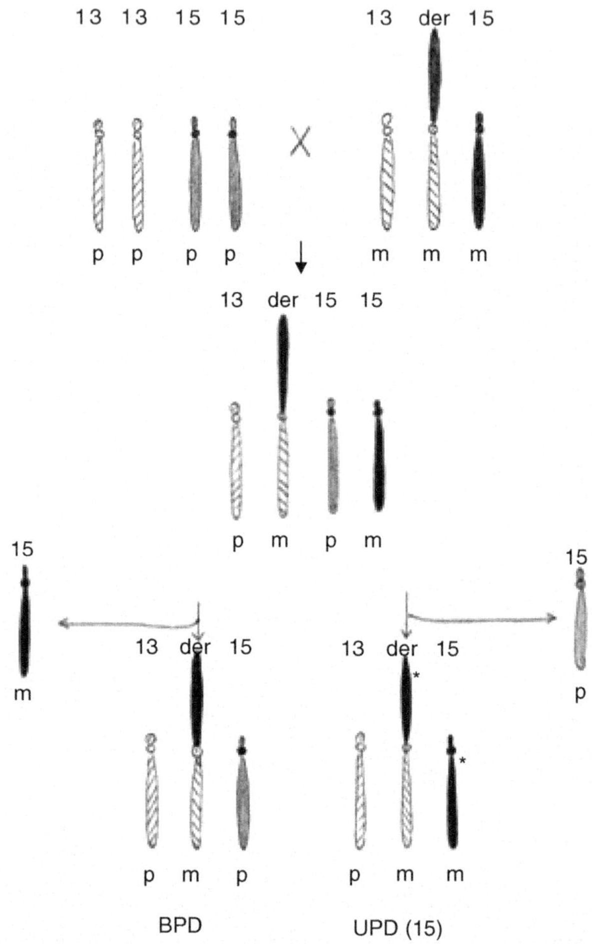

Fig. 21.5 Uniparental disomy 15 from a rob(13q15q) parent, due to "trisomy rescue"

and when it does not, it is called a paracentric inversion. When a de novo inversion is noted in a fetus, the probability of pathogenic phenotypes in the fetus is reported to be 9.4%.

In the pericentric inversion, four chromatids of the homologous chromosomes in meiosis form loops and establish pairing (Fig. 21.6). Of these, the two lateral chromatids do not cross over and become a normal gamete or a gamete with a balanced inversion. However, when an odd number of recombinations between the two inner-side chromatids results in chromosomes with duplications or deletions, these are called unbalanced recombinants. Since recombination in the first meiosis is generally more common in women than in men, it is more likely to cause an unbalanced translocation during egg formation. Daniel et al. reported that the probability of having children with unbalanced translocations when mothers have an inversion is 3.3%. In addition, crossover and unbalanced inversions are likely to occur (6.9%) in pericentric inversions because the inverted region is large [10], while they are considered unlikely to occur in paracentric inversions.

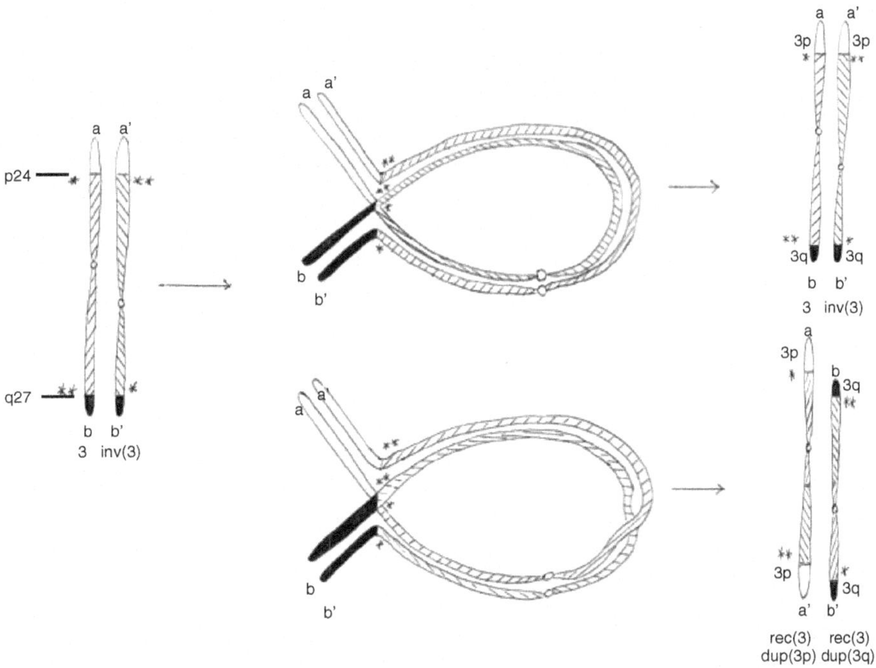

Fig. 21.6 Gametogenesis in pericentric inversion (inversion loop in meosis) [1]

Whether a recombinant can be born depends on the segment size of duplication and deletion by recombination. This is similar to the case in unbalanced translocations. In general, in children born with recombinants caused by pericentric inversion, the duplication segment is larger than the deletion segment. In contrast, a pericentric inversion near the centromere is a chromosomal variant, and there is no possibility that a child would have the unbalanced type translocation.

Paracentric inversion is often hereditary, and the clinical feature is normal, but there are the pathogenic phenotypes in 6–7% of de novo cases. In particular, a paracentric inversion on the long arm of the X chromosome can cause amenorrhea. It is also known that a minor parental inversion can induce an SRY-positive X chromosome (Xp/Yp translocation), microdeletion syndrome (unbalanced translocation), and inv dup or indel in the next generation. In addition, we should be careful with the abnormal case looking like a paracentric inversion, but is an unbalanced structural abnormality called intrachromosomal insertion, where there is a deletion on the same site, and another segment is inserted.

In a paracentric inversion, loops are formed in the first meiosis, similar to the pericentric inversion, but when recombination occurs among them, they become either dicentric (two centromeres) or acentric (no centromeres), and thus cell division is not possible in either case and development will stop. In other words, unbalanced recombinants are rarely produced by parents with a paracentric inversion. However, in rare cases, unbalanced recombinants occur via U-loop recombination when the recombination occurs within the loops and the chromosomes rejoin in the form of a U-shape (Fig. 21.7).

Fig. 21.7 Gametogenesis in paracentric inversion (mechanism of U-loop exchange) [1]

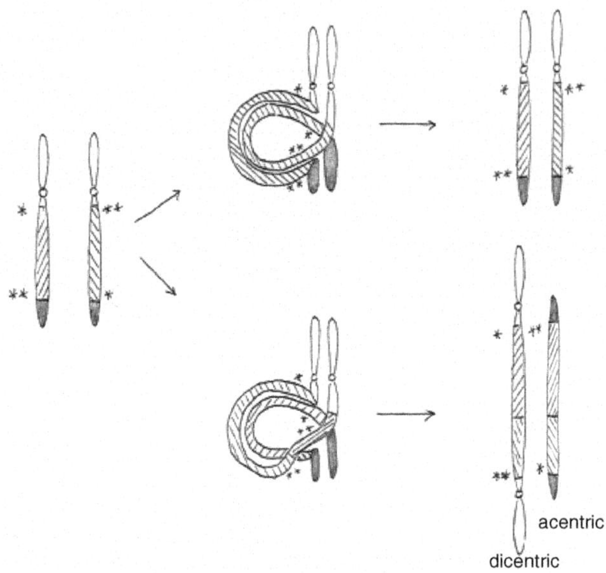

21.2.5 Balanced Insertion

Balanced insertion is a state where an interstitial deletion occurs in one of the two chromosomes, and the deleted region is inserted into the other chromosome. Inheriting only the derivative chromosome that contains the insertion region results in partial trisomy, and inheriting the derivative chromosome that contains the interstitial deletion results in partial monosomy. In a fertilized egg of parents with a balanced insertion, a normal, balanced insertion carrier, partial trisomy, and partial monosomy are seen at a ratio of 1:1:1:1, and some unbalanced insertions are eliminated during the fetal development. Therefore, the percentage of children born with an unbalanced insertion is reported to be 36% when mothers are balanced insertion carriers and 26% when fathers are carriers.

21.3 Unbalanced Structural Rearrangements

Unbalanced structural rearrangements, such as microdeletion syndrome and contiguous genes syndrome, are identified by the region of duplication and deletion, and the natural history may be explained (Table 21.3), but in many cases, it is difficult to estimate the accurate clinical symptoms.

In structural rearrangements detected by prenatal testing, the degree of unbalance is often small. On the other hand, chromosome analysis of them (such as couples of infertility or recurrent miscarriage, males with oligo/azoospermia, etc.) more

Table 21.3 List of main micro deletion syndromes

	Micro deletion syndrome
del1p36.3	
del2q37	Albright-like Syndrome
del4p	Wolf Hirschhorn Syndrome
del5p	cri du chat Syndrome
del7q11.23	Williams Syndrome
del8p24	Langer-Giedion Syndrome
del11p13	WAGR (Wilms tumor, aniridia, genital defects, retardation) Syndrome
del13q14	Retinoblastoma plus other features
del15q11.2	Prader-Willi/Angelman Syndrome
del16p13.3	Rubinstein-Taybi Syndrome
del17p13.3	Miller-Dirker Syndrome/Charcot-Marie-Tooth Syndrome/Hereditary pressure sensitive neuropathy
del17p11.2	Smith-Magenis Syndrome
del18p	
del18q	
del20p12	Alagille Syndrome
del22q11	di-George Syndrome
del22q13	McDermid Syndrome

often identifies balanced structural rearrangements that will be eliminated due to a large-scale unbalance in zygotes.

In many cases, an unbalanced structural abnormality observed in a fetus does not affect the phenotype, if a similar structural abnormality is identified in either parent. However, asymptomatic parents (or parents with a mild phenotype) may have the same chromosomal findings, which may lead to some symptoms in the baby. De novo unbalanced structural rearrangements are detected in 0.04–0.09% by the amniotic fluid test, and abnormalities are observed in about 60% of the children. It is also reported that structural rearrangements are observed in about 5% of spermatozoa of normal healthy men.

21.3.1 Small Supernumerary Marker Chromosomes (sSMCs)

The frequency of small marker chromosomes (sSMCs), the origin of which is challenging to identify, is 0.04–0.28% [11]. Prenatal tests detect sSMCs at a frequency of 0.075%, but they are found more often in patients with developmental disabilities or infertility. sSMCs are classified into either parentally derived sSMCs or de novo sSMCs, and more than half of all cases are de novo. Also, there are many cases of mosaicism observed in the normal karyotype cells. Parentally derived sSMCs generally result in no abnormality in the child unless both parents have abnormal phenotypes. However, de novo sSMCs may result in abnormalities in the child (pathogenic phenotypes are not observed in 70% of de novo sSMCs). It was reported

Table 21.4 Major small marker chromosomes (sSMCs)

	Frequency of all sSMCs	Phenotype	(%)
idic(15)	30.5%	Prader-Willi syndrome or Angelman syndrome (almost SNRPN positive)	5
i(12p)	10.6%	Pallister-Killian syndrome	100
i(18p)	6.0%	Tetrasomy18p syndrome	100
idic(22q11.2)	7.1%	Cat eye syndrome	30
der(22)t(11;22)(q23;q11)	10.1%	Emanuel Syndrome	100
inv dup/ring(15q, 3q, 8p, 13q, Yq) etc.			

that some phenotypes are exhibited in 26% among de novo sSMCs confirmed by prenatal diagnosis.

As the origin of sSMCs, acrocentric chromosome-derived sSMCs, especially idic(15)-derived sSMCs are observed at a high rate (Table 21.4). In some cases, 3:1 segregation is caused by a balanced reciprocal translocation in parents [e.g., der (22)]. To identify the origins of sSMCs, FISH (fluorescence in situ hybridization), SKY (spectral karyotyping), or microarray methods are very useful. The rate of abnormalities is low in sSMCs containing satellites that are stained using C-banding. When the duplicated size is large or when it is derived from the imprinted chromosome (chr15 and 14) or the PWS/AS region (15q11.2-q14), the rate of abnormalities is increased.

21.3.2 Additional Chromosomes and Unbalanced Translocations

These are states where a part of a specific chromosome is missing and a fragment of unknown origin is attached to it. There is a possibility of observing a derivative chromosome in cases with an unbalanced reciprocal translocation, and parental chromosomal analysis identifies a balanced reciprocal translocation in a parent with a probability of 38% (the child's karyotype is corrected more accurately referring to that karyotype). If a parent has a balanced reciprocal translocation, recurrence may possibly occur in their next child. In contrast, if both parents have normal karyotypes, the result is de novo translocation. The probability of the next child having the same unbalanced translocation can be considered to be zero. For the identification of additional fragments, SKY is effective if they are 10 Mb or more, but for smaller fragments, chromosome FISH using a subtelomeric probe should be considered. In recent years, copy number analysis by microarray has become common.

Supernumerary derivative chromosome 22 syndrome [+ der (22)], resulting in Emanuel syndrome, is an unbalanced translocation caused by 3:1 segregation in the first meiosis of a t(11;22) balanced reciprocal translocation carrier. The 11q23 and

22q11 regions have structures that can easily translocate and exchange with each other. In a t(11;22) translocation carrier, spontaneous abortion is common (23–37%), and about 1.8–5.6% of children are born with Emanuel syndrome (t(11; 22) balanced reciprocal translocation carriers account for about 50%) [12, 13]. In Emanuel syndrome, de novo cases are rare, and it has been revealed that in 95% of the cases mothers carry the translocation and fathers account for 5%.

21.3.3 Unbalanced Robertsonian Translocations

Unbalanced Robertsonian translocation mostly causes trisomy, such as t(13;14), t(14;21), and t(21;21). Usually, a search for parental origin is required in both parents. In translocation trisomy 21(rob (14; 21), + 21), the ratio of cases where a parent has rob(14;21) translocation to cases where he/she has a normal karyotype (and the child has a de novo karyotype) is 3:4. Since t(21;21) translocation carriers only produce trisomy 21 zygotes or monosomy 21 zygotes, all of their children are born with Down syndrome.

This translocation type accounts for 4% of children with Down syndrome. In the parental analysis, t(21;21) translocation carriers are detected very rarely (3 of 112 cases with t(21;21) translocation trisomy). The frequency of the parental origin identified in unbalanced Robertsonian translocation is not high (most cases are de novo).

21.3.4 Deletion, Duplication, Insertion, Inverted Insertion

Structural rearrangements involving deletions and duplications identified with chromosome analysis are not common. (The detection limit of G-banding is 10–3 Mb.) They have, so far, been conventionally diagnosed as microdeletion syndrome or contiguous gene syndrome using a prenatal test only when either parent has the same disease (including low level mosaicism), and the deletion area is relatively large, or when a disease is suspected based on fetal findings (that syndromes are shown in Table 21.3). Therefore, these are rare cases in routine obstetric practice. In recent years, however, de novo microdeletion syndromes are sometimes detected by microarray analysis and genome wide analyses (including noninvasive prenatal genetic testing (NIPT)) for prenatal-screening. In deletion regions, it may result in nullisomy (zero copy), monosomy (one copy), or functional null with imprinting, which may cause the loss of function or haploinsufficiency. Similarly, in duplication regions (e.g., three copies), it causes overexpression of the gene or a gain-of-function. It is partially understood that deletions and duplications are caused by nearby homologous or repetitive sequences. Therefore, some sites are more likely to develop structural rearrangements (deletions and duplications).

Deletions include terminal and interstitial deletions, and their mechanisms are different. Mostly, they are difficult to distinguish. When a deletion region is detected, we should be careful whether the deletion region involves insertion, duplication, or inverted duplication.

Terminal deletion lacks a p- or q-terminal, but contains a reacquired telomere. In many cases, it is de novo and mostly derived from spermatozoa. The risk of recurrence in the next child is considered to be very low, and parental chromosomal analysis may not be performed. However, in rare cases, a terminal deletion may be caused by reciprocal translocation, half-cryptic translocation, duplication, or inversion of parental chromosomes.

Most of the interstitial deletions are de novo, but they can be also egg-derived or sperm-derived. In the several regions, it is easy to rearrange associated with homologous and repetitive sequences around deletion. There are rare cases where interstitial deletion may be derived from a balanced insertion of the parent.

Similarly, if there is a derivative chromosome with an insertion region, whether it is a simple insertion (or an insertion with interstitial deletion), a duplication, an inverted duplication, or an inversion needs to be distinguished. Many insertions are inherited and mothers are often balanced insertion carriers. Chromosomal analysis of both parents may be useful.

21.3.5 Ring Chromosomes

Ring chromosomes in fetuses are detected using conventional G-banding of the amniotic fluid. If they are difficult to distinguish, they can be confirmed by subtelomeric FISH, as two signals cannot be detected on the same chromosome. The origin of ring chromosomes may be easily identified by the band pattern, and sometimes the SKY method is required.

The ends of the short and long arms are cut, and each end rejoins to form a ring chromosome. Thus, it involves partial monosomy of the p- and q-terminals. Some phenotypes due to the partial monosomy are observed, but it is also known that, depending on the instability of the ring chromosomes, they are likely to induce the mosaic loss or dicentrics in each cell division (dynamic mosaicism), resulting in more cell-death each time. This causes growth retardation, disorder of central nervous systems (e.g., convulsion), and anomalies, with large ring chromosomes (general ring syndrome). The ring chromosomes of 22 and 21 are often stable, and the phenotypes are normal when their breakpoints are at the terminals.

Breaking and rejoining within the telomere region is not often accompanied by genomic loss, so they have no symptoms or mild phenotypes (as mentioned above, cells with ring chromosomes are lost with cell division, which may result in short stature).

Approximately 50% of the small supernumerary marker chromosomes (sSMCs) are ring chromosomes. It brings the partial trisomy of the ring chromosome and makes abnormal findings. One of the common ring chromosomes is the mosaic ring chromosome 20. This chromosome causes intractable epilepsy, growth retardation, often with behavioral abnormalities, immature personality, and minor anomaly.

It has been reported that 5–6% of cases with mosaic ring chromosomes are inherited [14], and many of them are derived from mothers. The recurrence risk in the next generation is said to be 40% for non-mosaic ring chromosome cases. If a ring chromosome is identified in a fetus, a parental chromosomal analysis should be suggested.

21.3.6 Uniparental Disomy

In the eukaryote, embryo from haploid cells or diploid cells derived from only one parent does not develop (parthenogenesis does not occur). Chromosomes are usually inherited as haploid chromosomes, each from the mother and father, to become diploid pairs of chromosomes. In other words, one chromosome of a pair of autosomal chromosomes is derived from the mother and the other from the father. However, there is a case where a particular chromosome or region is derived from one parent, and this may occasionally cause abnormalities in embryo or fetal development (UPD: Uniparental disomy). It is known that there are genes that exhibit different expression patterns depending on parental origins (imprinting genes). In many cases, the state of DNA methylation in the gene expression regulatory region differs depending on the origins. The UPD region may cover the whole chromosome or a part of a chromosome. In addition, there are cases where the same alleles of either parent are carried as diploid alleles (isodisomy), and cases where the homologous alleles of either parent are carried as diploid alleles (heterodisomy). In the latter case, detection by single nucleotide polymorphism (SNP) typing is insufficient, and other methods such as methylation analysis may be required. In many cases, uniparental disomy is not detected unless that region is imprinted.

UPD regions that have phenotypic impacts have been identified to some chromosomes (chr6, 7, 9, 11, 14, 15). The mechanism of occurrence is often trisomy rescue (mostly heterodisomy) or monosomy rescue (usually isodisomy). These are relatively common when a parent has a translocation containing a chromosome involved in imprinting. Methods such as SNP microarray are useful for diagnosis because UPD cannot be identified by routine G-banding. Recently, there is a possibility that it may be incidentally identified by NIPT using the SNP method.

21.4 Mosaicism

Mosaicisms found in amniotic fluid chromosome analysis include true mosaicism and pseudo mosaicism. When the same chromosomal abnormality is observed in multiple cells in multiple cultures, it is diagnosed as true mosaicism. Although the frequency of chromosome mosaicism is 0.1–0.3% in the general population, chromosomal mosaicisms that cannot be detected by G-banding are observed in several tens percent of embryos. Among them, mosaic aneuploidy is common, and mosaic marker chromosomes and mosaic structural rearrangements are relatively uncommon. According to the observation in 166 cases with mosaic aneuploidy, pathogenic phenotypes in children were detected in 12 cases (8.3%), and most of them were confined placental mosaicism (CPM). Mosaic cases affecting the phenotypes of children are likely to be eliminated. The same can be considered for mosaic structural rearrangements. Among them, Pallister-Killian syndrome is a representative disease of mosaic structural rearrangements that are identified during the fetal period. This is an i(12p) mosaicism and is considered as mosaic partial tetrasomy of 12q.

21.4.1 Complex Chromosomal Rearrangements (CCRs)

Even if we judged a normal karyotype or a balanced reciprocal translocation in G-staining, it may have become the unbalanced type having several breakpoints. These are said as complex chromosomal rearrangements (CCRs), and they involve some phenotypes. Although the majority of CCRs are de novo, balanced CCRs are sometimes identified in parents. The pattern of gamete segregation in a balanced CCR is very complex due to the involvement of at least six relevant homologous chromosomes, and unbalanced zygotes being generated, many of which are eliminated in the early phase of development.

The phenomenon that many double-stranded DNA breaks (DSBs) occur due to a dense accumulation of one chromosome or multiple chromosomes, with their cut ends joined randomly, is called chromothripsis. This is often seen in cancer cells, but it also causes congenital anomaly. DSBs are known to occur during somatic cell division in fathers before spermatogenesis. Working the repair process in the replication, copy number variations (duplication and/or deletion) are easy to occur.

Among the fetuses that are balanced CCR carriers, 50% result in spontaneous abortion and 20% are born with pathogenic phenotypes [15]. If there is a child with a phenotype, the next child is more likely to be born with a phenotype as well. Mothers with a history of recurrent miscarriage are more likely to experience a miscarriage during the next pregnancy.

CCRs have been identified by methods such as SKY (M-FISH), but in recent years, more detailed structural rearrangements can be confirmed by fiber FISH or a next-generation long-read sequencer.

21.5 Others

Sometimes, it is difficult to distinguish whether it is balanced or not. Please see below (e.g., X/Y chromosome-autosomal chromosome translocations).

21.5.1 X-Autosomal Translocation

X chromosomes are complex due to the effect of inactivation. Usually, women (XX) have a mechanism where one of the two X chromosomes becomes inactivated at 2 weeks after fertilization to maintain a quantitative balance of X chromosomes with those of men (XY). The X chromosome to be inactivated is determined randomly for each cell, and its inactivated state is maintained in daughter cells even if the cell repeats mitosis. In the inactivated X chromosome, genes except for XIST in the X13.2 region, PAR1 (2.6 Mb of the end of the X short-arm), and PAR2 (320 kb of the end of the X long arm) become inactivated. However, homologous genes on scattered Y chromosomes escape inactivation. It has also been reported that 65% of genes on the inactivated X chromosome become entirely inactivated.

Men with balanced X-autosomal translocations are phenotypically normal but sterile. In women with balanced X-autosomal translocations, if an X chromosome without translocation is selectively inactivated, the balance of gene dosage is maintained, and the phenotype is normal, but these women are likely to be infertile. Moreover, if they are pregnant, they have a possibility of giving birth to children with pathogenic phenotypes. Those who have a pathogenic variant of an X-linked hereditary disease are heterozygous carriers, and at the same time, they develop the disease. However, if the X chromosome with a translocation is inactivated, genes on the autosomal chromosomes with translocations will not be expressed, resulting in different phenotypes. Based on the above, approximately 25% of women with a balanced X-autosomal translocation are considered to exhibit pathogenic phenotypes. In the unbalanced X-autosomal translocation, the X chromosome with the translocation is inactivated, and a phenotype is always observed.

If a balanced X-autosomal translocation is detected using an amniotic fluid test, even if mothers carry the same balanced translocation, 25% of them are considered to exhibit pathogenic phenotypes [16]. If they are de novo carriers, they are more likely to exhibit pathogenic phenotypes.

The following method is used to detect the inactivated state: When an X chromosome treated with BrdU is lightly stained by Giemsa, it is determined as the inactivated X chromosome; and when it is densely stained, it is determined as the activated X chromosome. Alternatively, gene expression levels may be determined by reverse-transcription polymerase chain reaction (RT-PCR), or methylation analysis may be considered.

21.5.2 Y-Autosomal Translocation

There are cases where the long arm of the Y chromosome is translocated on the short-arm of an acrocentric chromosome, accounting for 70% of Y-autosomal translocations. This type is most commonly seen in chromosome 15. It is considered to be one of the chromosomal variants and does not affect phenotypes/reproduction. It is confirmed by Q- or C-banding techniques when it appears to be a giant satellite.

Other balanced Y-autosomal translocations are phenotypically normal, but result in infertility. They occur as de novo translocations because they are not inherited.

21.5.3 X-Y Translocations

21.5.3.1 Xp-Yq Translocation: t(X;Y)(p22.3;q11)

X-Y translocation occurs when the long arm of the Y chromosome is translocated to the end of the short-arm of the X chromosome, which can be identified by Q- or C-banding.

Men with X-Y translocations (46,Y,der(X)t(X;Y)(p22.3;q11)) develop symptoms such as chondrodysplasia punctata, mental retardation, ichthyosis congenita, Kallmann's syndrome, and X-linked albinism depending on the degree of deletion on the translocated X chromosome. These men will develop azoospermia because the X and Y chromosomes cannot be paired in meiosis.

In women with an X-Y translocation (46,X,der(X)t(X;Y)(p22.3;q11)), the translocated Y long arm region does not affect the phenotype (Normally, the translocated X is selectively inactivated), but the deletion of the *SHOX* gene in the PAR1 region at the end of the X short-arm results in short stature (Leri-Weill syndrome). A random inactivation results in microphthalmia with linear skin defects. Although Leri-Weill syndrome offers normal intelligence and fertility, a male child of a mother with this syndrome often exhibits symptoms associated with the deletion of the X short-arm, with an X-Y translocation.

21.5.3.2 Xp-Yp Translocation: t(X;Y)(p22.3;p11)

This is the case where the Y short-arm, including SRY, is translocated to the end of the X short-arm due to unequal crossing-over. It is a derivative X chromosome made by X-Y unequal crossing-over during the spermatogenesis in the father.

If a man has another X short-arm chromosome, he becomes a 46,XX male (46,X,der(X)t(X;Y)(p22.3;p11)). In some cases, the Y short-arm that is translocated to the X short-arm cannot be detected by G-banding, but it can be identified by SRY-FISH. An SRY-positive XX male has normal intelligence, and his height is close to that of women. The testes are small and devoid of the Y long arm region (Yq 11.23) that is involved in spermatogenesis, making him infertile. The translocation is de novo, and X-Y unequal crossing-over is presumed to have occurred during the spermatogenesis process in his father.

If the maternal X chromosome is not inherited, he will become a 45,X male (45,der(X)t(X;Y)(p22.3;p11)). This will result in short stature due to the deletion of the SHOX gene on the short-arm of the X chromosome. He is infertile because he does not have the Y long arm region (Yq 11.23) that is involved in spermatogenesis.

21.5.3.3 Xq-Yq Translocation: t(X;Y)(q28;q11.21)

Xq-Yq translocation is when the Y long arm is translocated to the end of the X long arm. A 46,X male (der(Y)t(X;Y)(q28;q11.21)) with the Xq-Yq translocation presents with severe intellectual disabilities and pathogenic phenotypes.

Women with the Xq-Yq translocation (46,X,der(X)t(X;Y)(q28;q11.21)) rarely present with pathogenic phenotypes due to the selective inactivation of the translocated X, but the association with premature ovarian failure has been reported [17].

21.6 Chromosomal Variants

Chromosomal variants are a type of structural change, relatively detected by an amniotic fluid test. They are dominant traits that do not affect the phenotype/reproduction of a carrier and roughly classified as shown in Table 21.5. Many of them are considered heterochromatin, but some are euchromatin. The C-banding (by which the centromere is stained), Q-banding (by which the heterochromatins on the long arm of the Y chromosome are stained), and Ag-NOR staining (by which the stalk

Table 21.5 Normal chromosomal variants

Heterochromatin
1. Paracentromeric region
(a) Size: 1qh+, 9qh+, 16qh+
(b) Pericentric inversion: inv(9), inv(1)(p13q21), inv(1)(p13q12)
(c) Supernumerary heterochromatin of short arm: 3ph, 10ph, 16ph, 18ph
2. Acrocentric chromosomes (chr13-15, 21, 22)
(a) Deletion of all short arm: 21p-
(b) Double, triple satellites: 21pss, 21pstkstk
(c) Giant satellites: 21ps+
(d) Y;15 translocation: t(Yq15p)
3. chrY: Yqh+, Yqh−, inv(Y)
4. Nucleolus organizer region(NOR)and/or satellites
(a) Translocation: 1ps, 2qs, 4qs, 10qs, 12ps, 17ps, 22qs, Yqs
(b) Insertion : 6q15, 7p13, 8q11, 12p11
Euchromatin
1. Insertion to heterochromatin: 9q12
2. Pericentric inversion with euchromatin: inv(2)(p11.2q13), inv(19)(p11.2q21.2)
Fragile region (a part of all)

region of an acrocentric chromosome [NOR: nucleolus organizing region] is stained) may also be used to identify the details and regions of variants.

Even if normal variants are found in a fetus, it is useless to perform a karyotyping of the parents. Since most of them are inherited in an autosomal dominant manner, the analysis will prove which of the parents has the same variant, but this has no relation to the phenotype of the child.

When there are minute deletions or duplications, a rigor distinction between a chromosomal structural abnormality and a chromosomal variant is sometimes challenging (e.g., 8p23.2 duplication*). It is necessary to confirm whether there are chromosome findings in parents or minor phenotype abnormalities in family members.

The most representative chromosomal variant is inv(9) (p12q13), which occurs in 1–2.5% of the general population. It is known that there are ethnic differences, and this variant is more common in the Japanese population than in the Caucasian population. The usual G-banding technique can detect the total inv(9), in which all the C-band-positive blocks are inverted, but there are many ranges of inversion, and in fact, there may be a lot of undetectable inv(9)s. This variant is not associated with phenotypes/reproduction. If an inv(9) is found, both parents have the same inv(9) (Not de novo). In some cases, they have homozygous inv(9), but they still present with no clinical findings. In contrast, there are rare cases of an inversion involving a region wider than p12q13 [18]. In this case, upon first meiosis, a recombinant zygote in the inversion segment may acquire an unbalanced type translocation, and it is not treated as a chromosomal variant.

The 8p23.2 duplication is a chromosomal variant detected by a high-resolution G-banding technique. According to Harada et al., this duplication is relatively common. This region is where various duplications and deletions occur, and it is necessary to carefully distinguish between a chromosomal variant and a variant affecting the phenotype.

21.7 Chromosome Abnormalities and Selection

It has been reported that chromosomal abnormalities are found in 45% of embryos during the cleavage stage after fertilization. They are also found in 0.83% of babies, and balanced structural rearrangements are the most common (0.43%). Many of chromosomal disorders are not inherited to the next generation, but balanced structural rearrangements are exceptions. It is considered that de novo structural rearrangements occur in the population at some probabilities, and the balance is maintained. It is also possible to think that chromosome variations are necessary for evolution and adaptation in human beings, rather than an accident that occurs in a specific individual.

21.8 Key Points in Genetic Counseling for Chromosomal Structural Rearrangements in Fetus

If a chromosomal structural abnormality is identified in a fetus, the ability to determine whether it is a chromosomal variant, balanced/unbalanced variant, or a de novo variant is required first. Importantly, chromosomal variants and findings that are unlikely to affect phenotypes should not be confused with unbalanced chromosomal structural rearrangements. As mentioned above, advanced differential staining for structural rearrangements, parental analysis, and the confirmation of the presence or absence of similar cases within the family and stillbirth are useful. However, we experience a lot of cases where we cannot show a clear information in clinical situation.

When an unbalanced structural abnormality is identified by chromosomal analysis in a fetus, the couple must determine whether or not the pregnancy should be continued based on the unclear and limited information of the child's natural history, perinatal prognosis, the acceptance of disease or disorder, and social support system. The distress is very hard when the possibility of the child's disability is explained, while the time left for making an autonomous decision is short, as abortion in the second trimester of pregnancy is permitted only up to less than 22 weeks gestation under the Japanese Maternal Protection Act.

It is important to try to provide accurate and comprehensible information as much as possible, to show an empathetic understanding of the couple facing a difficult situation and to support their decision making entirely.

Chromosomal analysis is considered if the discovery of a structural abnormality in a fetus results in the discovery that the parent is a balanced translocation carrier and the previous child has a normal phenotype. In general, the probability that the previous child is the carrier of the same balanced translocation as the parent is always greater than 50%. This phenomenon is called meiotic drive. The reason is unknown.

Besides, it is desirable to provide medical information, to help the parents understand the situation, essential points in the future of their reproductive health, and to propose psychological and social support as needed. These activities should be performed continuously, not only during pregnancy but also after pregnancy.

References

1. Gardner RJM, Sutherland GR. Chromosome abnormalities and genetic counseling. 4th ed. (Oxford Monographs on Medical Genetics); 2011.
2. Warburton D. De novo balanced chromosome rearrangements and extra marker chromosomes identified at prenatal diagnosis: clinical significance and distribution of breakpoints. Am J Hum Genet. 1991;49:995–1013.

3. Cohen O, Cans C, Mermet MA, Demogeot J, Jalbert P. Viability thresholds for partial trisomies and monosomies. A study of 1,159 viable unbalanced reciprocal translocations. Hum Genet. 1994;93:188–94.
4. Daniel A, Hook EB, Wulf G. Risks of unbalanced progeny at amniocentesis to carriers of chromosome rearrangements: data from United States and Canadian laboratories. Am J Med Genet. 1989;31:14–53.
5. Youings S, Ellis K, Ennis S, Barber J, Jacobs P. A study of reciprocal translocations and inversions detected by light microscopy with special to origin, segregation, and recurrent abnormalities. Am J Med Genet A. 2004;126A:46–60.
6. Tharapel AT, Tharapel SA, Bannerman RM. Recurrent pregnancy losses and parental chromosome abnormalities: a review. Br J Obstet Gynaecol. 1985;92(9):899–914.
7. Hook EB, Cross PK. Rates of mutant structural chromosome rearrangements in human fetuses: data from prenatal cytogenetic studies and associations with maternal age and parental mutagen exposure. Am J Hum Genet. 1983;35:96–109.
8. Therman E, Susman B, Denniston C. The nonrandom participation of human acrocentric chromosomes in Robertsonian translocations. Ann Hum Genet. 1989;53:49–65.
9. Therman E, Trunca C, Kuhn EM, Sarto GE. Dicentric chromosomes and the inactivation of the centromere. Hum Genet. 1986;72(3):191–5.
10. Sherman SL, lselius L, Gallano P, et al. Segregation analysis of balanced pericentric inversion in pedigree data. Clin Genet. 1986;30:87–94.
11. Lierr T, Weise A. Frequency of small supernumerary marker chromosome in prenatal, newborn, developmentally retarded and infertility diagnostics. Int J Mol Med. 2007;19:719–31.
12. Fraccaro M, Lindsten J, Ford CE, Iselius L. The 11q;22q translocation: a European collaborative analysis of 43 cases. Hum Genet. 1980;56:21–51.
13. Zackai EH, Emanuel BS. Site-specific reciprocal translocation, t(11;22) (q23;q11), in several unrelated families with 3:1 meiotic disjunction. Am J Med Genet. 1980;7:507–21.
14. Kosztolányi G, Mehes K, Hook EB. Inherited ring chromosomes: an analysis of published cases. Hum Genet. 1991;87:320–4.
15. Madan K, Nieuwint AW, van Bever Y. Recombination in a balanced complex translocation of a mother leading to a balanced reciprocal translocation in a child. Review of 60 cases of balanced complex translocations. Hum Genet. 1997;99:806–15.
16. Schmidt M, Du Sart D. Functional disomies of the X chromosome influence the cell selection and hence the X-inactivation pattern in females with balanced X-autosome translocations: a review of 122 cases. Am J Med Genet. 1992;42:161–9.
17. Cheng DH, Tan YQ, Di YF, Li LY, Lu GX. Crypt Y chromosome fragment resulting from an X;Y translocation in a patient with premature ovarian failure. Fertil Steril. 2009;92(2):828.e3–6.
18. Groupe de Cytogéinéticiens Français. Pericentric inversions in man. A French collaborative study. Ann Genet. 1986;29:129–68.

Chapter 22
Gene Disorders and Genetic Counseling

Shoko Miura and Kiyonori Miura

Abstract Because prenatal diagnosis has ethical issues, it is important for pregnant women and their partners to understand the clinical significance of genetic tests before and after prenatal diagnosis. Therefore, genetic counseling should be performed for prenatal diagnosis of gene disorders. To date, human genome project develops a high-throughput genome analysis in addition to the conventional genetic diagnostic analysis including G-banding, FISH analysis, PCR test, etc. For example, the whole genome/exosome sequencing and the genome wide association study enable us to find the causative mutations/polymorphisms for a lot of gene disorders as a high-throughput genome analysis. In this section, the critical information for the genetic counseling of gene disorders is provided.

Keywords Gene disorders · Genetic counseling · Prenatal diagnosis · Mendelian disorders · Nonmendelian disorders

22.1 Introduction

Recently, molecular genetic diagnostic testing can be used for prenatal diagnosis. However, as prenatal diagnosis has ethical issues, it is important for pregnant women and their partners to understand the clinical significance of genetic tests for prenatal diagnosis before and after prenatal diagnosis. Therefore, genetic counseling should be performed for prenatal diagnosis of gene disorders [1].

Double strands of DNA had been found in 1953. To get the entire human genome sequences, the Human Genome Project was started in 1990, and then, the complete human genome sequences were clarified in 2003 [2]. This project gave us a detailed

S. Miura · K. Miura (✉)
Department of Obstetrics and Gynecology, Nagasaki University Graduate School of Biomedical Sciences, Nagasaki, Japan
e-mail: shokom@nagasaki-u.ac.jp; kiyonori@nagasaki-u.ac.jp

H. Masuzaki (ed.), *Fetal Morph Functional Diagnosis*, Comprehensive Gynecology and Obstetrics, https://doi.org/10.1007/978-981-15-8171-7_22

map of the genes and human genome variations including polymorphism. Also, sequence information by the human genome project develops a novel molecular diagnostic testing, e.g., microarray technology and whole genome sequencing [3, 4]. These high-throughput genome analyses including the whole genome/exosome sequencing and the genome wide association study (GWAS) enable us to find the mutations, which are causative for both mendelian and nonmendelian diseases, fastly and easily [5]. As genetic tests become an option of prenatal diagnosis in genetic disorders, it is essential that obstetrician and other medical staff should understand the fundamental principles of molecular testing [6].

In this section, in cases of prenatal diagnosis for gene disorders, the critical information for genetic counseling is provided.

22.2 Human Genome, Genes, Alleles, and Polymorphism

Human genome includes approximately 20,000–30,000 genes. Approximately 1.5% of the human genome is composed of exons, which are transcribed into messenger RNA (mRNA) [6]. However, other regions of the genomes also have the essential information for human including DNA polymorphism, small RNA sequences, etc. To date, various mutations and polymorphisms in human genome are causative for human genetic diseases, which include both mendelian and nonmendelian diseases. Also, gene expression is controlled by other DNA modifications including DNA methylation and histone modification. This molecular regulation of DNA methylation and histone modification is known as epigenetics, and the disruption of this mechanism causes "imprinting disorders" in human.

"Alleles" are normal variants within the human population, which are related to the blood types, the ear wax types (dry or wet), etc. [7]. Human has two alleles, and each allele is transmitted from each parent. Also, human genome has small differences of DNA sequences, which are called "polymorphism". Polymorphism is the variations of more than one allele at the same locus, and these are seen in the same population. Single nucleotide polymorphism (SNP) and copy number variation (CNV) are found as polymorphism in human genome, most of which are benign variants [8]. However, some polymorphisms change the gene function and then cause human diseases. Especially, when allele frequency of polymorphisms is less than 1 in 100, those are defined as "mutation".

22.3 Mendelian Disorders

In general, mendelian disorders are caused by a mutation of single gene. The phenotype of many single-gene disorders depends on the kind of gene mutation and/or environmental factors.

22.3.1 Autosomal Dominant Inheritance

Autosomal dominant disorders occur in only individual having one allele of pathogenic variants (Fig. 22.1) [9, 10]. When the affected parent has the gene mutation of autosomal dominant disorder, inheritance risk of causative gene mutation to each offspring is 50%. The chance that an offspring will not inherit the mutated gene is also 50%.

However, the individual, who has the gene mutation, does not always express the affected phenotype. The affected phenotype of an individual with a dominant gene mutation is determined by penetrance, which indicates whether or not the mutant gene is expressed. When an affected phenotype is seen in all individuals having the dominant gene mutation, its inheritance is called "complete penetrance". On the other hand, an affected phenotype is seen in some individuals having the dominant gene mutation, and its inheritance is called "incomplete penetrance". When affected phenotype is expressed in 50% of individuals having the gene mutation, it is called "50% penetrance". Penetrance is one of the important information to decide if its disorder adapts for prenatal diagnoses or not.

22.3.2 Autosomal Recessive Inheritance

Autosomal recessive disorders occur in only individual having both alleles of pathogenic variants (Fig. 22.2). When each affected parent has the gene mutation of autosomal recessive disorder, the risk of affected phenotype, which is caused by two allele inheritance of causative gene mutation to each offspring, is 25%. The chance

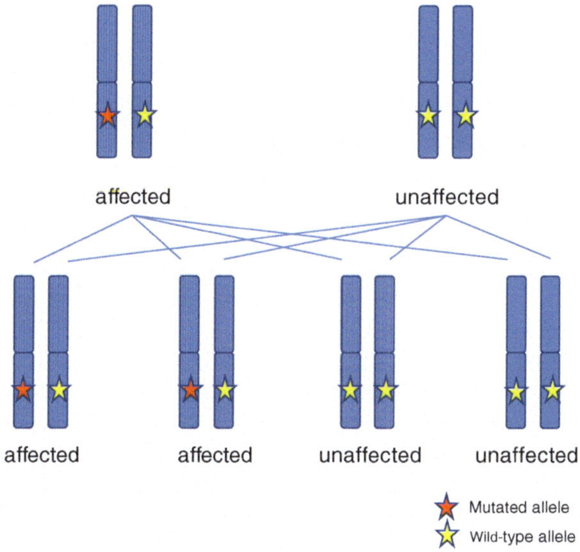

Fig. 22.1 Autosomal dominant inheritance

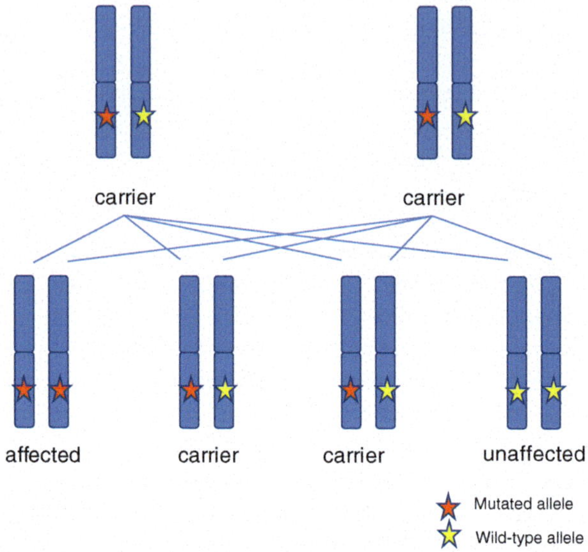

Fig. 22.2 Autosomal recessive inheritance

that an offspring will not inherit the mutated gene is also 25%. Individuals who have only one allele of mutated gene are called "carriers", and its risk is 50% (Fig. 22.2). In cases of autosomal recessive disorders, carriers will not have affected offspring unless their partners are mutated gene carriers or are affected. Also, an individual who has two different mutated alleles for the same disorder is called a "compound heterozygote".

22.3.3 X-Linked Inheritance

X-linked recessive disorders are caused by one allele of mutated gene on the X-chromosome (Fig. 22.3) [11]. Male offspring has only one copy of the X chromosome, and female one has two copies of X chromosome. The affected phenotype is seen in only men. Women who have an X-linked recessive gene generally are unaffected, and they are called "carriers". In general, as for each human cell, one of the two X chromosomes is active and the other allele is inactive, randomly. However, in female individual having only mutated allele of X chromosome, when mutated allele remains active in most cells, females with X-linked recessive disorders can express the affected phenotype. This phenomenon is known as "skewed X-inactivation". When pregnant woman is a carrier of X-linked recessive disorder, she has a 50% risk of passing on the gene with each pregnancy. In the case of male offspring, affected phenotype occurs in 50% and normal one in 50%. In the case of female offspring, the risk of affected phenotype is nothing, and each female offspring has a 50% chance of carrier and a 50% chance of unaffected.

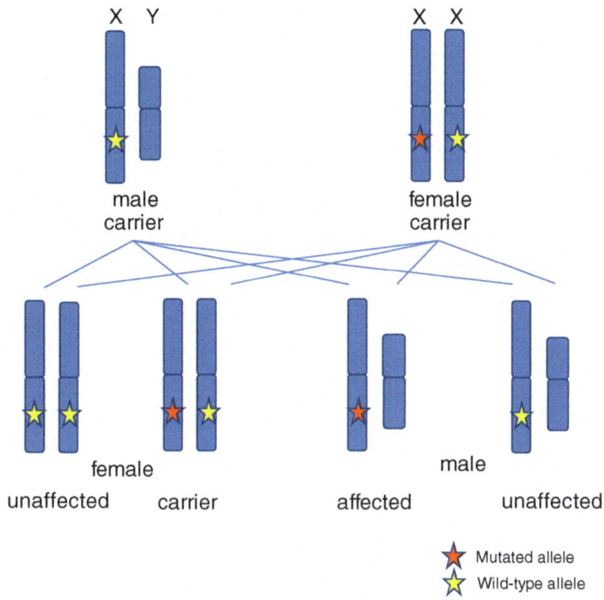

Fig. 22.3 X-linked recessive inheritance

In general, X-linked dominant disorders are seen in females, because male offspring having mutated allele of X-linked dominant disorders seems to be lethal phenotypes. Therefore, when male-to-male transmission is found in the same family, the possibility of X-linked inheritance can be denied.

22.4 Nonmendelian Disorders

Inherited pattern of imprinting diseases and mitochondrial disorders is known as nonmendelian disorders. Genetic inheritance except for mendelian diseases is described below.

22.4.1 Triplet Repeat Diseases

Myotonic dystrophy, which expresses the symptoms of muscle dysfunction, is caused by expansion of the number of triplet repeats (a CTG repeat) in myotonic dystrophy protein kinase (DMPK) gene. Although inheritance pattern of myotonic dystrophy is autosomal dominant, the expression of affected phenotype depends on the length of triplet repeats. Individuals with between 5 and 37 repeats are considered to have normal phenotypes, while individuals with 50 repeats or more express an affected phenotype. Therefore, 50 or more triplet repeats in DMPK gene are classified as "mutation" allele. Individuals with repeats between 38 and 49 are considered to have a "premutation", who are at risk of having their offspring with further expanded repeats causing an affected phenotype. The offspring from individuals with p number of triplet repeats seems to inherit the expanded triplet repeat alleles of DMPK gene, which are longer than their parents. Therefore, the offspring from individuals with premutations or mutations of DMPK gene are likely to express an earlier onset and more severity of phenotypes, and this phenomenon known as "anticipation".

22.4.2 *Imprinting Diseases*

In general, gene expresses from maternal and paternal alleles equally. However, some human genes show a parent-specific expression pattern (gene expressing from only maternal or paternal specific allele), which phenomenon is known as "genomic imprinting" [12, 13].

Angelman syndrome and Prader–Willi syndrome are known as imprinting diseases. Interestingly, both imprinting diseases are caused by the same chromosomal deletion at 15q11–13. Angelman syndrome originates from the deletion of maternally derived chromosome 15 segment [14], while Prader–Willi syndrome originates from the deletion of paternally derived chromosome 15 segments. If an individual has two normal chromosome 15, uniparental disomy (UPD) and disruption of DNA methylation are also found as cause of genomic imprinting diseases.

Generally, one pair of chromosome in human genome is inherited from mother and father. However, "rescue" of "trisomic" or "monosomic" pregnancy can cause a "loss of one of the three chromosomes" or a "duplication of one chromosome". In the case of "trisomy rescue", when two chromosomes transmitted by the same parent are retained in the cell by chance, uniparental heterodisomy that two different homologous chromosomes are transmitted from one parent is formed (Fig. 22.4). On the other hand, in the case of "monosomy rescue", because one chromosome is transmitted by the same parent, uniparental isodisomy that the same homologous chromosomes are transmitted from one parent is formed. UPD is defined as the situation that both chromosome pairs are inherited from the same parent. Therefore, UPD including "imprinting genes" results in "imprinting disease" (Fig. 22.4).

22.4.3 *Mitochondrial Inheritance*

The mitochondria act as essential components of aerobic respiration. Therefore, mitochondrial diseases commonly affect the organs (or tissues) with high energy requirement (the central nervous system, heart, muscles, etc.). The inheritance of mitochondrial DNA (mtDNA) defects is more complex, because a mutation occurs in the mtDNA causing "mitochondrial heteroplasmy", which is the situation having

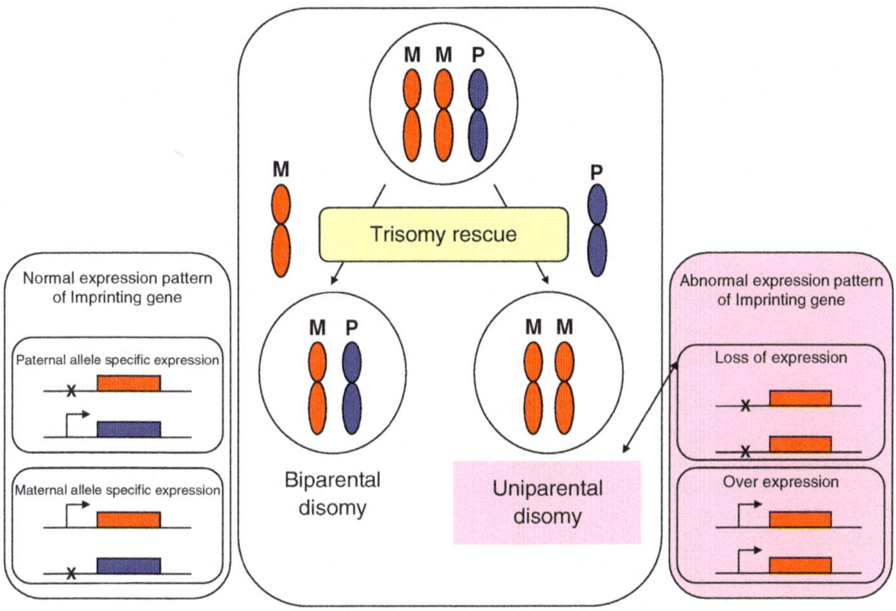

Fig. 22.4 Imprinting disorders and uniparental disomy

normal and abnormal mitochondria in single cell. Pregnant woman with a heteroplasmic mtDNA mutation can transmit a variable amount of mutated mtDNA to each of her offspring. Therefore, regarding mitochondrial disease, clinical variation among siblings is seen as the same.

22.4.4 Germline Mosaicism and Chimerism

"Mosaic" is defined as the situation that individual (or tissue) is originated from one fertilized egg, and "Chimera" is defined as the situation that individual (or tissue) is from two or more distinct fertilized eggs [15, 16].

Sometimes, individuals with normal phenotype have mosaicism, where organs or tissues consist of cells with two or more different DNA sequences (normal and mutated alleles). When a mitotic error occurs in zygotic cells, mosaicism is confined to the gonadal organs; this situation is called "germline mosaicism".

22.5 Conclusion

Molecular genetic testing for gene disorders becomes to be applicable in the field of prenatal diagnosis. Therefore, it is essential that obstetrician and other medical staff should pay attention regarding the advances in genetic testing and the ethical issues of prenatal diagnosis [16]. In addition, it is necessary for pregnant woman and her partner to understand the clinical significance of genetic testing, and therefore, genetic counseling should be performed before and after gene testing for prenatal diagnosis.

References

1. Minakami H, Maeda T, Fujii T, Hamada H, Iitsuka Y, Itakura A, Itoh H, Iwashita T, Kanagawa T, Kanai M, Kasuga Y, Kawabata M, Kobayashi K, Kotani T, Kudo Y, Makino Y, Matsubara S, Matsuda H, Miura K, Murakoshi T, Murotsuki J, Ohkuchi A, Ohno Y, Ohshiba Y, Satoh S, Sekizawa A, Sugiura M, Suzuki S, Takahashi T, Tsukahara Y, Unno N, Yoshikawa H. Guidelines for obstetrical practice in Japan: Japan Society of Obstetrics and Gynecology (JSOG) and Japan Association of Obstetricians and Gynecologists (JAOG) 2014 edition. J Obstet Gynaecol Res. 2014;40:1469–99.
2. Witokowski J. Long view of the Human Genome Project. Nature. 2010;466:921–2.
3. Miura S, Miura K, Masuzaki H, Miyake N, Yoshiura KI, Sosonkina N, Harada N, Shimokawa O, Nakayama D, Yoshimura S, Matsumoto N, Niikawa N, Ishimaru T. Microarray comparative genomic hybridization (CGH)-based prenatal diagnosis for chromosome abnormalities using cell-free fetal DNA in amniotic fluid. J Hum Genet. 2006;51:412–7.
4. Miura S, Miura K, Yamamoto T, Yamanaka M, Saito K, Hirabuki T, Kurosawa K, Harada N, Ishizaki Yamasaki Y, Matsumoto N, Hirahara F, Yoshiura K, Masuzaki H, Niikawa N. Origin and mechanisms of formation of fetus-in-fetu: two cases with genotype and methylation analyses. Am J Med Genet. 2006;140A:1737–43.
5. Miura K, Mishima H, Kinoshita A, Hayashida C, Abe S, Tokunaga K, Masuzaki H, Yoshiura KI. Genome-wide association study of HPV associated cervical cancer in Japanese women. J Med Virol. 2014;86:1153–8.
6. Vora NL, Ralston SJ. Modern genetics in obstetrics and gynecology. Obstet Gynecol. 2018;132:e143–68.
7. Miura K, Yoshiura KI, Miura S, Shimada T, Yamasaki K, Yoshida A, Nakayama D, Shibata Y, Niikawa N, Masuzaki H. A strong association between human earwax-type and apocrine colostrum secretion from the mammary gland. Hum Genet. 2007;121:631–3.
8. Abe S, Miura K, Kinoshita A, Mishima H, Miura S, Yamasaki K, Hasegawa Y, Higashijima A, Jo O, Sasaki K, Yoshida A, Yoshiura KI, Masuzaki H. Copy number variation of the antimicrobial-gene, *defensin beta 4*, is associated with susceptibility to cervical cancer. J Hum Genet. 2013;58:250–3.
9. Miura K, Acierno JS Jr, Seminara SB. Characterization of the human nasal embryonic LHRH factor gene, *NELF,* and a mutation screening among 65 patients with idiopathic hypogonadotropic hypogonadism (IHH). J Hum Genet. 2004;49:265–8.
10. Miura K, Miura S, Yoshiura K, Seminara S, Hamaguchi D, Niikawa N, Masuzaki H. A case of Kallmann syndrome carrying a missense mutation in alternatively spliced exon 8A encoding the immunoglobulin-like domain IIIb of FGFR1. Hum Reprod. 2010;25:1076–80.
11. Miura K, Higashijima A, Shimada T, Miura S, Yamasaki K, Abe S, Jo O, Kinoshita A, Yoshida A, Yoshimura S, Niikawa N, Yoshiura K, Masuzaki H. Clinical application of fetal sex determination using cell-free fetal DNA in pregnant carriers of X-linked genetic disorders. J Hum Genet. 2011;56:296–9.
12. Miura K, Miyoshi O, Yun K, Inazawa J, Miyamoto T, Hayashi H, Masuzaki H, Yoshimura S, Niikawa N, Jinno Y, Ishimaru T. Repeat-directed isolation of a novel gene preferentially expressed from the maternal allele in human placenta. J Hum Genet. 1999;44:1–9.

13. Miura K, Obama M, Yun K, Masuzaki H, Ikeda Y, Yoshimura S, Akashi T, Niikawa N, Ishimaru T, Jinno Y. Methylation imprinting of H19 and SNRPN genes in human benign ovarian teratomas. Am J Hum Genet. 1999;65:1359–67.
14. Miura K, Kishino T, Li E, Webber H, Dikkes P, Holmes GL, Wagstaff J. Neurobehavioral and electroencephalographic abnormalities in ube3a maternal-deficient mice. Neurobiol Dis. 2002;9:149–59.
15. Miura K, Yoshiura KI, Miura S, Kondoh T, Harada N, Yamasaki K, Fujimoto Y, Yamasaki Y, Tanigawa T, Kitajima Y, Shimada T, Yoshida A, Nakayama D, Tagawa M, Yoshimura S, Wagstaff J, Jinno Y, Ishimaru T, Niikawa N, Masuzaki H. Clinical outcome of infants with confined placental mosaicism and intrauterine growth restriction of unknown cause. Am J Med Genet. 2006;140A:1827–33.
16. Miura K, Niikawa N. Do monochorionic dizygotic twins increase after pregnancy by assisted reproductive technology? J Hum Genet. 2005;50:1–6.

Part VI
Technical

Chapter 23
G-Banding: Fetal Chromosome Analysis by Using Chromosome Banding Techniques

Naoki Harada

Abstract Clinical application of Next Generation Sequencing (NGS) technology is progressing. In the field of cytogenetics, NGS is used for noninvasive prenatal testing (NIPT) and preimplantation genetic testing for aneuploidy (PGT-A). Also, chromosomal microarray (CMA) testing is routinely performed in postnatal as chromosome testing for the patients with developmental delay, and in prenatal, it is widely used as testing for multiple fetal anomalies. Although prenatal screening for fetal aneuploidies by NIPT using cell-free DNA is gradually becoming more common, the standard for prenatal diagnostic testing is karyotype analysis by G-banding at this moment. This chapter outlines the necessary process of fetal chromosome analysis by G-banding, the features of other banding techniques, and points to consider in the interpretation issues regarding frequently encountered aneuploidy mosaic and structural variations such as chromosomal heteromorphisms.

Keywords Prenatal diagnosis · G-banding · Aneuploidy · Mosaicism
Heteromorphism

The number of human chromosomes was determined in 1956, and the success of the culture of peripheral blood mononuclear cells with the addition of PHA was achieved in 1960, followed by the success of the culture of amniotic fluid cells in 1966 and placental villus cells in 1974. Chromosome analysis was established as clinical testing in the mid-1970s. Since then, various technological innovations occurred in the cytogenetics and cytogenomics field, and clinical applications have promoted in order. Among the various cytogenomic technologies, karyotyping by chromosome banding, fluorescence in situ hybridization (FISH), multiplex ligation-dependent probe amplification (MLPA), the chromosomal microarray (CMA), and the noninvasive prenatal testing (NIPT) are categorized as cytogenetic testing.

N. Harada (✉)
Department of Fundamental Cell Technology, Center for iPS Cell Research and Application (CiRA), Kyoto University, Kyoto, Japan
e-mail: nharada@cira.kyoto-u.ac.jp

H. Masuzaki (ed.), *Fetal Morph Functional Diagnosis*, Comprehensive Gynecology and Obstetrics, https://doi.org/10.1007/978-981-15-8171-7_23

In the prenatal diagnosis, the gold standard for the diagnosis of fetal chromosome abnormalities is karyotype analysis of G-banded cells, which were harvested after the cultivation of amniotic fluid, chorionic villus, and fetal umbilical cord blood cells.

CMA is used as the first choice only when multiple fetal morphological abnormalities are detected by ultrasound [1]. In the cytogenetic analysis, we need to choose a test method according to the size of the variant to be detected. Most prenatal diagnostic tests focus on chromosomal aneuploidies, and so cytogenetic testing by G-banding is an appropriate choice at this time.

23.1 The Procedure of the Chromosome Analysis by G-banding

The chromosome analysis is usually started by appropriately culturing each of the aseptically collected materials. Please refer to other documents for the sampling of amniotic fluid, chorionic villi, umbilical cord blood, and precautions for that primary culture [2–4].

In the cell culture of umbilical cord puncture blood, phytohemagglutinin (PHA) is added in the same way as germline cytogenetic testing using peripheral blood lymphocytes to induce cell division, so that mitotic cell harvesting becomes possible in the short term of 48 or 72 h.

The cell culture for the chromosome analysis of amniotic fluid cells and chorionic villus cells is classified into an in situ method (directly harvesting the grown cell colonies) and a flask method (trypsinizing the grown cells and collecting them as free cells). In prenatal diagnosis, it is necessary to perform karyotyping by in situ cell culture and harvesting, which excels in discriminating between true mosaics and pseudo mosaics, except when performing molecular genetic diagnosis using DNA or biochemical genetic diagnosis via cell culture.

When amniotic fluid cells and chorionic villus cells are cultured by the in situ method, usually, it takes about 10 days until they are proliferated enough to harvest. The general procedure for testing amniotic fluid cells and chorionic villus cells is as follows.

Cell harvest:

1. To accumulate mitotic cells at the metaphase stage, a microtubule formation inhibitor, colcemid, is added and treated for several hours before harvest.
2. The culture medium in the container is put in the coverslips where the cells that have proliferated are removed by suction, and a hypotonic solution (75 mM KCl) is added to expose the cells, followed by treatment for 20 min.
3. Inject Carnoy's fixative (3:1 mixture of alcohol and acetic acid). While slowly injecting the fixative, the mixture of the hypotonic solution and Carnoy's solu-

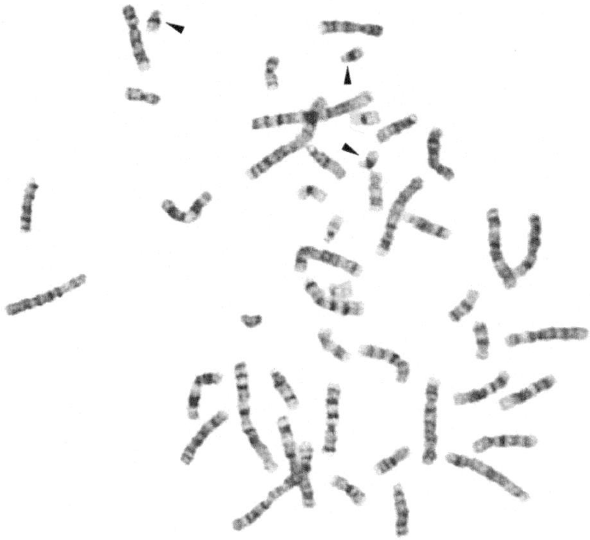

Fig. 23.1 A G-banded metaphase spread of the trisomy 21 cell. Band resolution is about 500 bands/haploid set. Arrowheads indicate chromosome 21

tion is removed by suction, and the concentration of Carnoy's solution is increased stepwise for fixation.

4. After completely replacing the hypotonic solution with Carnoy's solution, remove the coverslip with forceps, carefully absorb excess Carnoy's droplets with filter paper, and slowly air dry to make chromosome preparation (press onto glass surface with surface tension).
5. Perform solid Giemsa staining and G-banding (Fig. 23.1).

Chromosome analysis:

Regarding images of a metaphase spread taken under an image analysis system or a microscope are analyzed by following procedures.

1. Count the chromosome number of a minimum of 15 cells from at least 15 colonies, distributed as equally as possible between at least two or more independently established cultures.
2. Analyze five cells, each from a different colony, preferably from two independently established cultures.
3. Karyotype 2 cells, these cells can be from the analyzed five cells. If more than one abnormal cell line is found, karyotype is at least one cell representative of each cell line.

When using fresh chorionic villus cells, mitotic cells can be harvested by short-term culture (direct method), but it is difficult to obtain a morphologically well-metaphase. Therefore, in principle, the results of karyotyping must be obtained by long-term cultured cells [5].

23.2 Chromosome Banding

The chromosome banding is a general term for a method of performing various processes to making a chromosome preparation, displaying striped patterns (bands and sub-bands) on the chromosome. The primary method of chromosome banding is the G-banding, which is simple to operate and provides a clear staining image. The chromosomes are grouped by relative size and shape (depending on the position of constriction of kinetochore region), and band patterns identify homologous chromosomes and then are compared with each of the homologous chromosomes.

The number of appearing bands determines the resolution, and the required resolution depends on the reason for the referral of the testing. The principle of the G-banding depends on the resistance to the digestion of nonhistone proteins to proteases such as trypsin so that the difference in chromatin condensation is detected as the difference of Giemsa staining (Table 23.1).

According to the latest International system for Human Cytogenomic Nomenclature (ISCN2016) [6], idiograms (schematic diagrams of normal karyotypes by G-banding) are expressed in 300, 400, 550, 700, and 850 bands per haploid set. In the report of the result of chromosome analysis, it must be specified, which band level of the test is performed. Chromosome analysis for the prenatal diagnosis requires a minimum of 400 bands for advanced maternal age and positive screening cases and a minimum of 500 bands for fetal morphological abnormalities.

When XX cells were found to be mixed in XY cells, the analysis should be performed on XY cells, considering that XX cells were caused by maternal tissue contamination. However, karyotype analysis of a small number of cells is required for XX cells for confirmation purposes. The attending physician consults with the laboratory staff and considers whether or not maternal tissue contamination was detected at the time of cell culture. If XY/XX cells were detected in CVS, additional tests using amniotic fluid cells should be considered. If XY/XX cells were detected in amniotic fluid cells, it is necessary to confirm the fetal genitalia by ultrasonography.

Table 23.1 Features of G-banding

Official name	Principal reagent	Staining pattern	Structural features	Features of the nonhistone protein
G-bands by trypsin using Giemsa (GTG)	Trypsin, Giemsa	G-dark band	Heterochromatic region, A-T rich, late S-phase replication	Tightly condensed region, rich in protein disulfide cross-links hydrophobic regions that have a high affinity with eosin and thiazine.
		G-light band	Euchromatic region, G-C rich, early S-phase replication	Relatively loose structure, rich in protein sulfur as sulfhydryls less hydrophobic region that does not have a affinity with eosin and thiazine.

In addition to routine G-banding, various banding techniques such as Q-, R-, C-, and N-banding and Alu I-digested C-like banding are used to identify specific chromosome variants and/or abnormalities (Table 23.2), [6]. Based on the results of the G-banding, other banding techniques and FISH are added as necessary. Interpretation and cytogenetic diagnoses are made based on the results of those obtained.

Table 23.2 Features and applications of various banding techniques

Banding (idiom)	Official name	Principal reagent(s)	Features/application/target
Q-	Q-bands by fluorescence using quinacrine (QFQ)	Quinacrine mustard	Specific staining of A-T bases pairs, similar pattern as G-banding Yq12, satellites, centromeric heterochromatin
R-	R-bands by BrdU using Giemsa (RBG) R-bands by BrdU using acridine orange (RBA)	5-Bromodeoxyuridine (BrdU), Hoechst 33258, Giemsa, Acridine orange	The addition of BrdU before harvest to incorporate BrdU into late-replication region. R-bands (inversion of the G-bands) appears by the sequential staining with Giemsa or acridine orange after staining with Hoechst 33258, which has a strong affinity to BrdU.
N-	—	Silver nitrate, Giemsa	Silver staining to the region of satellite stalk of acrocentric chromosomes correspond to Nucleolus Organizing Region (NOR)
C-	C-bands by barium-Hydroxide using Giemsa (CBG)	Barium hydroxide, Giemsa	Specific staining of heterochromatin brocks (1q12, 9q12, 16q11.2, Yq12)
Alu I digested C-like-	—	Restriction enzyme Alu I, Giemsa	Frequent digestion of euchromatin with the enzyme brings staining of heterochromatin brocks (1q12, 9q12, 16q11.2, Yq12)
Sister chromatid exchange (SCE)		BrdU, Hoechst 33258, Giemsa	The addition of BrdU to incorporate for two cell cycles to bring identification of each chromatid. It allows detecting sister chromatid exchange. Diagnostic testing for Bloom syndrome.
High resolution	—	Ethidium Bromide	The addition of ethidium bromide to inhibit chromosome condensation brings harvesting the cells at prophase to prometaphase stage. Thymidine synchronization of cell division frequently used together. It used for the detection or identification of the breakpoints of rearrangement.

23.3 Precise Investigation of Mosaicism and Points of That Interpretation

Anaphase lags frequently occur at the very early stage of embryogenesis so that fetal chromosomal mosaicism becomes not rare [7]. On the other hand, growth factors are fundamentally added to the culture medium used for cell culture of fetal tissue, which enhances cell proliferation while increasing the possibility of generating aneuploidies that do not exist in the original cells (artifacts). Therefore, additional workup needs to be carefully and rationally performed on the mosaic detected in the prenatal chromosome testing, to determine whether the mosaic is a true or a pseudo mosaic.

Mosaics detected by the in situ culture method are classified as follows, and the level 3 mosaic is determined to be a true mosaic.

- Level 1 mosaic: detected in only one cell in one colony or only in a part of one colony
- Level 2 mosaic: detected in all cells in one colony
- Level 3 mosaic: commonly detected in multiple colonies in multiple cultureware

Workups proposed by Hsu and Benn are widely used in the additional mosaic analysis for cultured amniotic fluid cells and chorionic villus cells [8].

Report of the test result should mention what level of the mosaic is determined as a result of the additional workups. The attending physician would be expected to interpret the results appropriately and explain it precisely to the couple.

In the culture of chorionic villus cells, mosaic confined to placental tissue is observed to be about 2%. Depending on the developmental stage of the mosaic that was arisen, trophoblast cells and villous stromal fibroblasts may have different detection patterns and classified into the following types of confined placental mosaicism (CPM).

Type I CPM:

Limited to trophoblast cells. Detected by the direct method (short-term culture), but not detected in fibroblasts derived from the villous stroma (with long-term culture).

Type 2 CPM:

Limited to fibroblasts derived from the villous stroma, not detected in trophoblast cells.

Type 3 CPM:

Detected in both trophoblast cells and fibroblasts derived from the villous stroma.

Since CPM cannot be definite at the step of villus cell examination alone, when mosaicism is detected in villous cells, it is necessary to confirm it with the examination of amniotic fluid cells.

23.4 Points to Care in the Interpretation of Chromosomal Aberrations

When mosaic aneuploidy is detected, it is necessary to examine the fetal structural abnormalities by ultrasonographic examination precisely. Even if a Level 3 mosaic is detected in the culture of chorionic villi or amniotic fluid cells, it might not be detected in the somatic cells of the fetus. Depending on what chromosome is detected as mosaic, the empirical risk of true mosaicism on the fetal somatic cells and the presence of disease complications might have varying degrees, so that the reexamination by invasive sampling should be carefully considered.

Benn carefully reviewed the pregnancy outcomes, and the results of confirmatory testing of the aneuploid mosaic are detected in the amniotic fluid cells [4]. About autosomal aneuploidy mosaic: In CVS, the mosaic containing chromosomes 2, 3, and 7 is common, but is very unlikely to be confirmed by amniocentesis. Mosaics containing chromosomes 8, 9, 18, and 21 are infrequent but are often confirmed by amniocentesis. In Amniotic fluid cells, it is recommended to take into account empirical risks. Mosaic trisomies 2, 4, 9, and 16 have very high risk (>60%) of abnormal consequences; mosaic trisomies 5, 13, 14, 15, 18, and 21 have high risk (40–59%); mosaic trisomies 6, 7, 12, and 17 have moderately high risk (20–39%). Except for mosaic trisomies 8, 9, 13, 18, and 21, additional confirmation by PUBS is not recommended. If a mosaic of chromosomes with imprinting effects (chromosome 6, 7, 11, 14, 15, and 20) is detected, genetic testing of uniparental disomy (UPD) by DNA polymorphism analysis with parental samples is recommended. About sex chromosome aneuploidy mosaic: Mosaic of sex chromosomal aneuploidy is detected at a higher rate than autosomal abnormalities, and almost no abnormalities are observed at birth. For 45, X/46, XY mosaics, it is necessary to confirm the sex of the fetus by ultrasonography and to examine the presence or absence of internal genitals at birth. Long-term prognosis is unknown in many prenatally diagnosed cases.

Caution should be exercised when Robertson translocation is detected during prenatal testing. One-third of the Robertson translocation detected through prenatal testing is known as de novo origin, but when Robertson translocation of the nonhomologous chromosome is detected, the risk with UPD is estimated at 0.6% even if it is de novo or not. The risk with UPD of Robertson translocation of the homologous chromosome (isochromosome) is estimated at 66% [9]. It is necessary to consider the examination of diagnostic testing of UPD when the Robertson translocation involves chromosome 14 or 15 [10].

When a structural chromosome abnormality is detected, whether it is a balanced type or not becomes a problem, and it is necessary to identify breakpoints as precise as possible. However, it is not easy to identify the breakpoints precisely by the proband's G-banding alone. So it is crucial to obtain results in a short period by adding a chromosome analysis of the parents and/or FISH analysis by using appropriate DNA probe such as subtelomeric clones. Sometimes, a confusion might occur in the case identified with de novo morphologically/or apparently balanced structural rearrangement. Additional CMA testing will consider clarifying whether the rearrangement accompanied a genomic deletion or not. Prenatal detection of small supernumerary marker chromosomes (sSMCs) is occasionally detected [11]. sSMC is often derived from acrocentric chromosomes, especially chromosome 15, and a stepwise workup is needed to perform in consideration of the parental origin, which also has the possibility that intact homologous chromosomes 14 and 15 might be UPD [12].

The additional workups consist of chromosome analysis of the parents, FISH, CMA, and UPD tests that need to use DNA extracted from not only fetal tissue but also the parents [13]. It is necessary to proceed while confirming the turnaround time of this testing strictly.

23.5 Normal Chromosome Variants

Normal chromosome variants are morphological abnormalities that are manifested by the chromosome banding and do not affect phenotype or reproduction. It is divided into heteromorphism (Table 23.3) and euchromatic variant [14]. These variants are inherited from one of the parents in principle.

Heteromorphism is the size diversity and pericentric inversion of highly condensed constitutive heterochromatin. The most frequently observed one is inv(9)(p12q13) that is detected in about 2% of the general population (Fig. 23.2). Euchromatin variant is an inversion, deletion, or duplication of euchromatin.

Except for inv(9)(p12q13), in many cases, it is difficult to identify heteromorphism or euchromatic variant by G-banding alone so that we need to identify them by adding various chromosome banding techniques properly. Parental chromosome analysis should also be used to identify the carrier status for these normal variants.

Table 23.3 The representative normal chromosomal variation

Variant	Chromosome	Locus/karyotype
Heteromorphism		
Length or size	1, 9, and 16	Constitutive heterochromatin (1q12, 9q12, and 16q11.2)
	Acrocentric-	Short arm, satellite stalk, satellite
	Y	Yq12
Pericentric-inversion	Y	inv(Y)(p11.2q11.23)
	1	inv(1)(p11q12), inv(1)(p13q21)
	3	inv(3)(p11.2q12)
	9	inv(9)(p12q13)
	16	inv(16)(p11.2q12.1)
Euchromatin		
Pericentric-inversion	2	inv(2)(p11.2q13)
	10	inv(10)(p11.2q21.2)

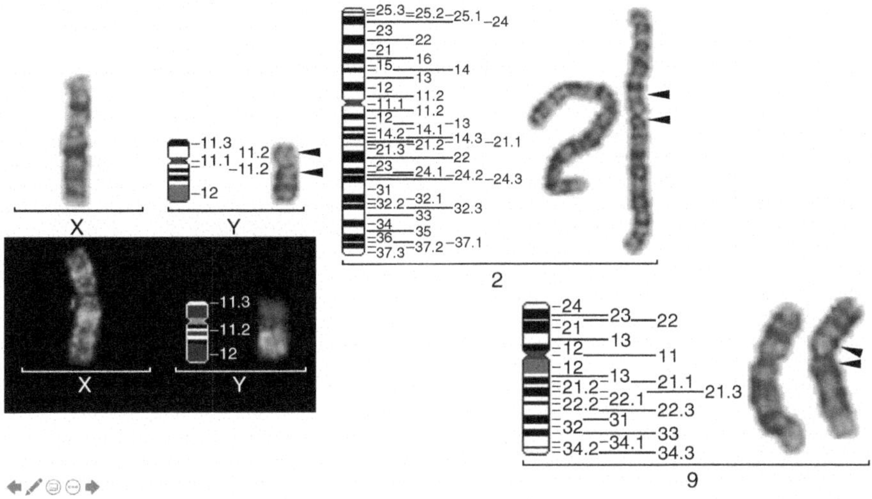

Fig. 23.2 Partial karyotypes of the carriers of pericentric inversion polymorphisms. (From left to right) Chromosome X and inv(Y)(p11.2q11.2), inv(2)(p11.2q13), and inv(9)(p12q13). The inverted chromosome is on the right side of the homologous chromosome, and arrowheads indicate breakpoints of the inversion. The lower part on the left side (with the dark background) is a Q-banded partial karyotype, and the others are G-banded partial karyotypes

23.6 Conclusion

Although the chromosome analysis by using the banding technique is classic genetic testing with a half-century of history, it is still essential clinical testing for a definitive diagnosis of chromosomal abnormalities. Various genetic and genomic analysis technologies are being applied to the medical field. Karyotyping of G-banded cells is having critical advantages of the ability to detect intercellular heterogeneity by a cell-by-cell basis analysis and easily detect balanced chromosome rearrangements. Most chromosome analyses are performed in reference laboratories. All of the testing laboratories are expected to report the results accurately and in an easy-to-understand way when they identified the rare chromosome abnormalities. On the other hand, healthcare professionals such as physicians need the skills to choose additional testing appropriately and to interpret them accurately based on clinical information. Rapid and accurate communication between the two professional parties is required, and collaboration with specialists in clinical cytogenetics is also needed.

References

1. Committee on genetics and society for maternal-fetal medicine. Microarrays and next-generation sequencing technology: the use of advanced genetic diagnostic tools in obstetrics and gynecology. The American College of Obstetricians and Gynecologists Committee Opinion Number 682, December 2016. https://www.acog.org/-/media/project/acog/acogorg/clinical/files/committee-opinion/articles/2016/12/microarrays-and-next-generation-sequencing-technology-the-use-of-advanced-genetic-diagnostic-toolsin-obstetrics-and-gynecology. pdf Accessed 6 Oct 2020.

2. Odibo AO. Amniocentesis, chorionic villus sampling, and fetal blood sampling. In: Milunski A, Milunski M, editors. Genetic disorders and the fetus. 7th ed: Wiley; 2016. p. 68–97.
3. Van Dyke DL, Milunski A. Amniotic fluid constituents, cell culture, and neural tube defects. In: Milunski A, Milunski M, editors. Genetic disorders and the fetus. 7th ed: Wiley; 2016. p. 98–177.
4. Benn PA. Prenatal diagnosis of chromosomal abnormalities through chorionic villus sampling and amniocentesis. In: Milunski A, Milunski M, editors. Genetic disorders and the fetus. 7th ed: Wiley; 2016. p. 178–266.
5. American College of Medical Genetics and Genomics (ACMG). Standard and guidelines for clinical genetics laboratories 2018 Edition, Revised January 2018 E: Clinical Cytogenetics. https://www.acmg.net/PDFLibrary/Standards-Guidelines-Cytogenetics. pdf Accessed 6 Oct 2020.
6. McGowan-Jordan J, Simons A, Schmid M, editors. Normal chromosomes. In: An international system for human cytogenomic nomenclature: Karger; 2016. p. 7–14.
7. Mantikou E, Wong KM, Repping S, Mastenbroek S. Molecular origin of meiotic aneuploidies in preimplantation embryos. Biochim Biophys Acta. 2012;1822:1921–30. https://doi.org/10.1016/j.bbadis.2012.06.013.
8. Hsu LY, Benn PA. Revised guidelines for the diagnosis of mosaicism in amniocytes. Prenat Diagn. 1999;19:1081–2.
9. Berends SA, Horwitz J, McCaskill C, Shaffer LG. Identification of uniparental disomy following prenatal detection of Robertsonian translocations and isochromosomes. Am J Hum Genet. 2000;66:1787–93.
10. Del Gaudio D, Shinawi M, Astbury C, Tayeh MK, Deak KL, Raca G; ACMG Laboratory Quality Assurance Committee. Diagnostic testing for uniparental disomy: a points to consider statement from the American College of Medical Genetics and Genomics (ACMG). Genet Med. 2020;22:1133–41.
11. Liehr T, Weise A. Frequency of small supernumerary marker chromosomes in prenatal, newborn, developmentally retarded and infertility diagnostics. Int J Mol Med. 2007;19:719–31.
12. Schwartz S. Molecular cytogenetics and prenatal diagnosis. In: Milunski A, Milunski M, editors. Genetic disorders and the fetus. 7th ed: Wiley; 2016. p. 313–49.
13. Marle N, Martinet D, Aboura A, Joly-Helas G, Andrieux J, Flori E, et al. Molecular characterization of 39 de novo sSMC: contribution to prognosis and genetic counseling, a prospective study. Clin Genet. 2014;85:233–44.
14. RJM G, Amor DJ, editors. Normal chromosomal variation. In: chromosome abnormalities and genetic counseling. 5th ed: Oxford University Press; 2018. p. 369–86.

Chapter 24
FISH

Kaoru Suzumori

Abstract The establishment of fluorescence in situ hybridization (FISH) techniques has enabled the detection of DNA copy number changes for the mapping of target DNA sequences [Hopman et al. (Molecular neuroanatomy. Elsevier, 1988)]. This technique has a wide range of applications, such as for gene mapping and the ordering of DNA sequences on chromosomes and as an adjunct to conventional cytogenetics for characterizing chromosomal aberrations [Ferguson-Smith and Yates (Am J Hum Genet 48:178, 1991)]. Probes for FISH analysis may consist of DNA segments, such as α-satellite DNA from the centromeric regions, other repetitive DNA sequences, and unique DNA sequences of chromosomes. Widely used chromosome-specific probes are classified as 'repetitive' (centromeric regions) probes [Cremer et al. (Hum Genet 74:346, 1986)], 'painting' probes, and 'locus-specific' probes according to their complementary location on the chromosome. The use of fluorescence microscopy allows the detection of multiple probes, each labeled with a different color. The advancement of this technology now allows combinational fluorescence with 24 different colors that can be visualized on the same metaphase spread, thereby highlighting each chromosome pair [Schröck et al. (Science 273:494, 1996), Speicher et al. (Nat Genet 12:368, 1996)].

This chapter focuses on FISH analysis for fetal aneuploidies, meiotic segregation modes in men with constitutional chromosomal abnormalities, and the prenatal diagnosis of carriers of a complex constitutional chromosome abnormality using spectral karyotyping.

Keywords FISH · Robertsonian translocation · Reciprocal translocation · Meiotic segregation · Spectral karyotyping

K. Suzumori (✉)
Fetal Life Science Center Ltd., Nagoya City University Graduate School of Medical Science, Nagoya, Japan
e-mail: k.suzumori@flsc.jp

H. Masuzaki (ed.), *Fetal Morph Functional Diagnosis*, Comprehensive Gynecology and Obstetrics, https://doi.org/10.1007/978-981-15-8171-7_24

24.1 Rapid Prenatal Diagnosis of Aneuploidies by FISH

The frequency of chromosomal abnormalities has been estimated to be 0.65–0.84% in surveys of newborn babies [1–4], and approximately 80–95% of these abnormalities are common aneuploidies in chromosomes 13, 18, 21, X, or Y [5, 6]. Of note, the risk of these common aneuploidies is correlated with maternal age, and the total frequency of these aneuploidies was 2.26% among pregnancies with a maternal age of over 35 years [7]. Since the 1980s, indications for a prenatal diagnosis of pregnancies at risk of common aneuploidies have included advanced maternal age, abnormal maternal serum screening results, abnormal ultrasound findings in the fetus, and a family history of chromosomal abnormalities. For the past 50 years, G-banding chromosome analysis using cultured amniotic fluid cells has been a key procedure for prenatal diagnosis. Prenatal cytogenetic diagnosis has improved due to the use of metaphase harvesting and a significant reduction in test turnaround times, and final test results can now be obtained within 10–12 days. When cytogenetic results indicate a serious chromosomal abnormality, even a short wait for results can increase the emotional burden on the patient and/or physician.

Rapid detection for aneuploidy in chromosomes 13, 18, 21, X, and Y from interphase amniotic fluid cells is possible with the use of directly labeled, multicolored, commercially available DNA probes. The probes comprise two sets: one set contains 13 unique sequences at 13q14.2 (green), the region 21q22.13 (orange), and the second set contains α-satellite centromere probes for chromosomes X (green), Y (orange), and 18 (blue). Such commercially available probe kits include Cytocell (Oxford Gene Technology, Cambridge, UK) and AneuVysion (AbbotT/Vysis, Downers Grove, IL), among others. Figure 24.1 shows FISH results from four pregnant women with normal female fetus (a), trisomy 21 male (b), trisomy 13 male (c), and trisomy 18 female (d). With probe set 1 (left cell), a normal cell should show two green and two orange (2G, 2O), and with probe set 2 (right cell), a female cell should show two green and two blue signals (2G, 2B) (Fig. 24.1a). While male cells with trisomy 21 should show two green and three orange signals (2G, 3O) with probe set 1, and one green, one orange, and two blue signals with probe set 2 (1G, 1O, 2B) (Fig. 24.1b). With probe sets 1 and 2, male cells with trisomy 13 should show three green and two orange signals (3G, 2O) and two blue, one green, and one orange signals (2B, 1G, 1O) (Fig. 24.1c). However, cells having an extra chromosome 18 should show two green and two orange signals (2G, 2O) and two green and three blue signals in female samples (2G, 3B) (Fig. 24.1d).

Standards for evaluating samples need to be instituted and followed. It has been suggested that a minimum of 50 interphase nuclei with defined hybridization signals should be enumerated for each chromosome and that 80% of cells should show two signals to be considered disomic, while 70% of cells should show three signals to be considered trisomic.

The first clinical trial of FISH analysis for the detection of common aneuploidies involving chromosomes 13, 18, 21, X, and Y was reported in 1990 by Klinger et al. [8]. The usefulness of interphase FISH analysis for the rapid prenatal diagnosis of

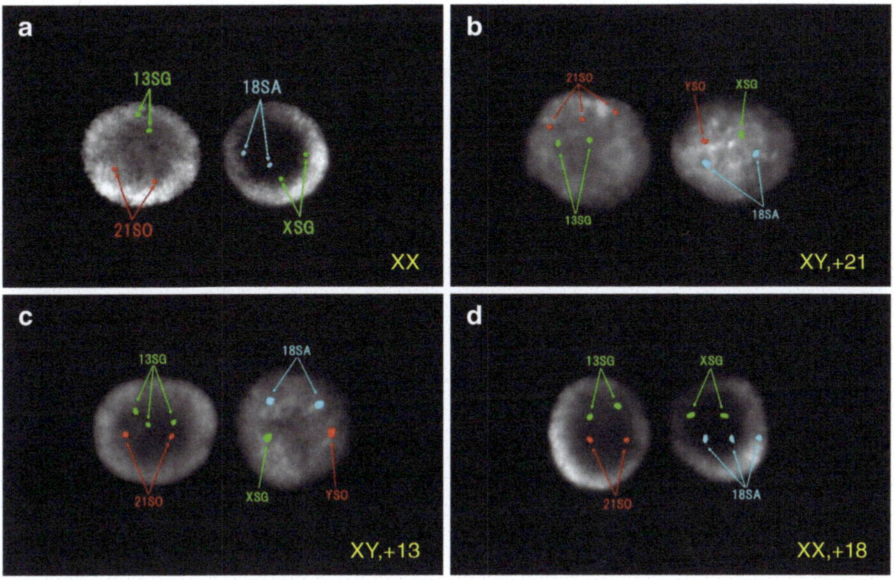

Fig. 24.1 Examples of interphase cell FISH results

aneuploidy has since been confirmed in a number of studies [9–11]. With commercially available FISH prenatal enumeration probe kits, Weremwicz et al. [12] reported an extremely high performance with 94% sensitivity for common aneuploidies and at a 0.1% false positive rate in informative samples. Many papers have demonstrated that inconclusive or informative results are seen in a low percentage of cases, such as those with bloody amniotic fluid or oligohydramnios [13]. In general, this FISH-based procedure cannot detect aneuploidy of nontargeted chromosomes, nor is it currently designed to detect euploid states with other cytogenetic abnormalities, such as translocations, inversions, and marker chromosomes. It has been shown that careful genetic counseling is an important adjunct when ordering FISH testing, and it is essential to explain to patients the limitations of FISH, including its inability to detect all chromosomal abnormalities as well as the possibility of maternal cell contamination, rare technical failures, and uninformative or false negative results in some cases.

Despite its usefulness, care must be taken for the clinical application of FISH assays due to possible pitfalls. The American College of Medical Genetics [14] has issued a policy statement for the clinical application of prenatal interphase FISH assays because of the severe implications of a false positive result. The policy statement called for the reliability, reproducibility, and accuracy of the clinical application of FISH probe sets is to be demonstrated. Prenatal interphase FISH is not a standard procedure and should only be used as an adjunct test with conventional chromosome analysis serving as the primary diagnosis and confirmatory evaluation. Appropriate physician and patient consent should be obtained, and patient management decisions should not be made based on results obtained by FISH alone.

The ACMG recommends the following provisions: (1) Proper informed consent should be obtained following explanations of the purpose, accuracy, potential risks, and limitations of FISH testing; (2) FISH should be used in prenatal interphase cytogenetics only in conjunction with standard cytogenetic analysis; (3) Irreversible therapeutic action should not be initiated on the basis of FISH analysis alone; (4) Providers should confirm the applicability of FISH analysis in prenatal diagnosis after assessing the reproducibility, sensitivity, specificity, and positive and negative predictive values; (5) Appropriate quality assurance/quality control for reagents, as well as techniques in the development of standardized protocols, must be established for FISH analysis.

In conclusion, prenatal FISH detection is valuable for the screening of common aneuploidies, followed by a complete chromosome analysis to confirm anomalies.

24.2 Aneuploidy in Human Spermatozoa: FISH Analysis in Men with Constitutional Chromosomal Abnormalities

Balanced Robertsonian or reciprocal translocations are constitutional chromosomal abnormalities that predispose carriers to the production of chromosomally abnormal gametes. These abnormalities contribute to recurrent abortions of conceptuses with monosomy or trisomy. In general, most autosomal monosomies are eliminated after fertilization, during early pregnancy or in the perinatal period. For this reason, most of them are found in spontaneous abortions [15]. Reproductive failures are closely associated with parental chromosome abnormalities. Male carriers of constitutional chromosome abnormalities may have fertility problems associated with low sperm counts and abnormal sperm morphology. Indeed, among 9207 infertile males reviewed, 0.8% were carriers of a Robertsonian translocation and 0.6% were carriers of a reciprocal translocation [16].

A Robertsonian translocation is a fusion of the long arms of two acrocentric chromosomes 13–15, 21, and 22 after a breakage in the short arms. An individual with what is called a balanced Robertsonian translocation shows only 45 chromosomes, with the translocation chromosomes containing the two complete long arms of the two acrocentric chromosomes involved. The short arm fragments of the translocated chromosomes are lost. Carriers are divided into six groups according to the chromosomes in the translocation: der(13;14), der(14;21), der(13;15), der(14;15), der(13;22), and der(14;22). Logically, during meiosis, pairing and segregation occur through the formation of trivalent in meiosis I. Alternative segregation results in two balanced gametes of either normal chromosomes A and B or derivative der(A;B). The babies with this mode of segregation are usually phenotypically unaffected. In contrast, adjacent segregation modes lead to either sperm nullisomy A or sperm disomy B and produce unbalanced products with monosomy A or trisomy B. The

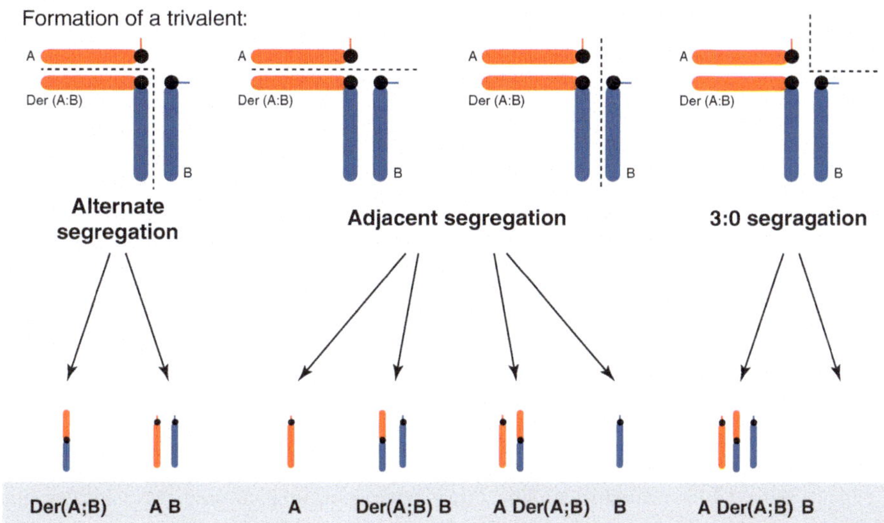

Fig. 24.2 Schematic depiction of trivalent formation and its segregation mode at meiosis in Robertsonian translocation carrier [17]

3:0 mode of segregation leads to sperm double nullisomy or disomy, resulting in unviable monosomy or possibly viable trisomy (Fig. 24.2).

In the late 1980s, investigation of the meiotic segregation of human sperm was made possible by the karyotyping of spermatozoa after the penetration of zona-free golden hamster oocytes [18–20]. However, this test enabled the analysis of only a limited number of spermatozoa. Since the 1990s, FISH has been introduced for the study of the chromosomal content of spermatozoa [21]. Many studies using this technique to estimate meiotic segregation modes in spermatozoa have been published. In the majority of sperm FISH analyses of Robertsonian translocations, dual- or triple-colored FISH approaches have been used, including directly labeled, subtelomeric, locus-specific, centromeric probes for chromosomes involved in the translocation.

There have been several descriptions of meiotic analyses in male Robertsonian translocation carriers. Lamotte et al. [17] reviewed a total aggregated set of 210 patients and analyzed their segregation modes. In the review, spermatozoa from 116 der(13;14), 38 der(14;21), 16 der(13;15), 11 der(14;15), 11 der(14;22), 5 der(13;21), 5 der(13;22), 4 der(21;22), 3 der(15;22), and 1 der(15;21) individuals were described. Dual- and triple-colored FISH analysis using directly labeled subtelomeric and/or locus-specific and/or centromeric probes for chromosomes 13, 14, 15, 21, and 22 was carried out on spermatozoa obtained from translocation carriers. As shown in other literature, the most common Robertsonian translocation is der(13;14), followed by der(14;21). According to the meiotic segregation modes obtained from the compiled Robertsonian translocation carriers, for the alternate segregation mode, it is assumed that translocation carriers have a similar meiotic pattern among the chromosomes involved [22]. This hypothesis is strongly supported by the similarity in the balanced gamete rate among the different Robertsonian translocation carriers. However, Lamotte et al. [17] demonstrated that the alternate segregation mode is predominant in Robertsonian translocation carriers with 73.45% ± 8.05% balanced spermatozoa (min. 50.92%; max. 89.99%). Their results were consistent among the different types of Robertsonian translocations except for der(13;15), which exhibited lower balanced spermatozoa rates when compared to der(13;14), der(14;21), der(13;21), and der(15;22). The proportion of chromosomally normal (balanced) segregation rates commands two over three, whereas the rate of unbalanced segregation (mostly adjacent, but also extremely rare 3:0 segregations) varies, ranging between 10% and 21%. The adjacent segregation modes result in either monosomic or trisomic gametes. Chromosomal monosomy is not identified in conceptuses, while most trisomic conceptuses abort spontaneously, except for those with trisomy 13, 18, and 21, which can remain viable for several hours to several years or more. In a 3:0 segregation, one gamete receives double disomy, resulting in a zygote with 47 chromosomes. The other corresponding gamete receives double nullisomy, resulting in a zygote with 44 chromosomes. The 3:0 segregation mode is quite a rare event (rate of 0.0–5.0%). In the 3:0 segregation mode, one gamete receives three chromosomes, resulting in a double trisomic zygote. The other corresponding gamete receives no chromosome, resulting in a double monosomic zygote. The conceptus resulting from this segregation is not clinically identified.

Reciprocal translocations are the most common structural chromosome rearrangements in humans, with an incidence of 1 per 1175 newborns [23]. A reciprocal translocation does not change the amount of chromosomal material, and it involves the exchange of chromosome segments between arms of two heterologous chromosomes. Carriers of this type of chromosome translocation involving all chromosomes have been described, and ideal empirical data should be available for each translocation. Usually, empirical data exist only for general categories. In general, reciprocal translocations carry an empiric risk of about 10–15% for abnormal offspring [24]. Prenatal counseling would ideally take into account the segregation modes. FISH analysis in sperm samples obtained from reciprocal translocation carriers has been extensively described and reviewed in the literature. During meiosis I in a reciprocal translocation carrier, a quadrivalent is formed between the translocated chromosomes and their normal homologous (Fig. 24.3). This structure may segregate according to five theoretical modes. Alternate and adjacent-1 segregation modes involve a 2:2 disjunction of homologous centromeres to opposite poles. Instead, when any homologous centromeres migrate to the same pole, the possible segregation modes are adjacent-2 (2:2 disjunction), 3:1 or 4:0 disjunction. There is the widespread assumption that 2:2 alternate segregation leads to the formation of normal or balanced gametes, while the other segregation modes produce unbalanced gametes. The other segregation modes, i.e., adjacent-1, adjacent-2, and 3:1 and 4:0 segregations, produce unbalanced gametes. In adjacent-1 segregation, nonhomologous centromeres segregate together and pass to the same gamete. In adjacent-2 segregation, homologous centromeres pass to the same gamete. Both adjacent-1 segregation and adjacent-2 segregation induce partial disomy or nullisomy in the zygote and result in partial trisomy or monosomy in the embryo. In a

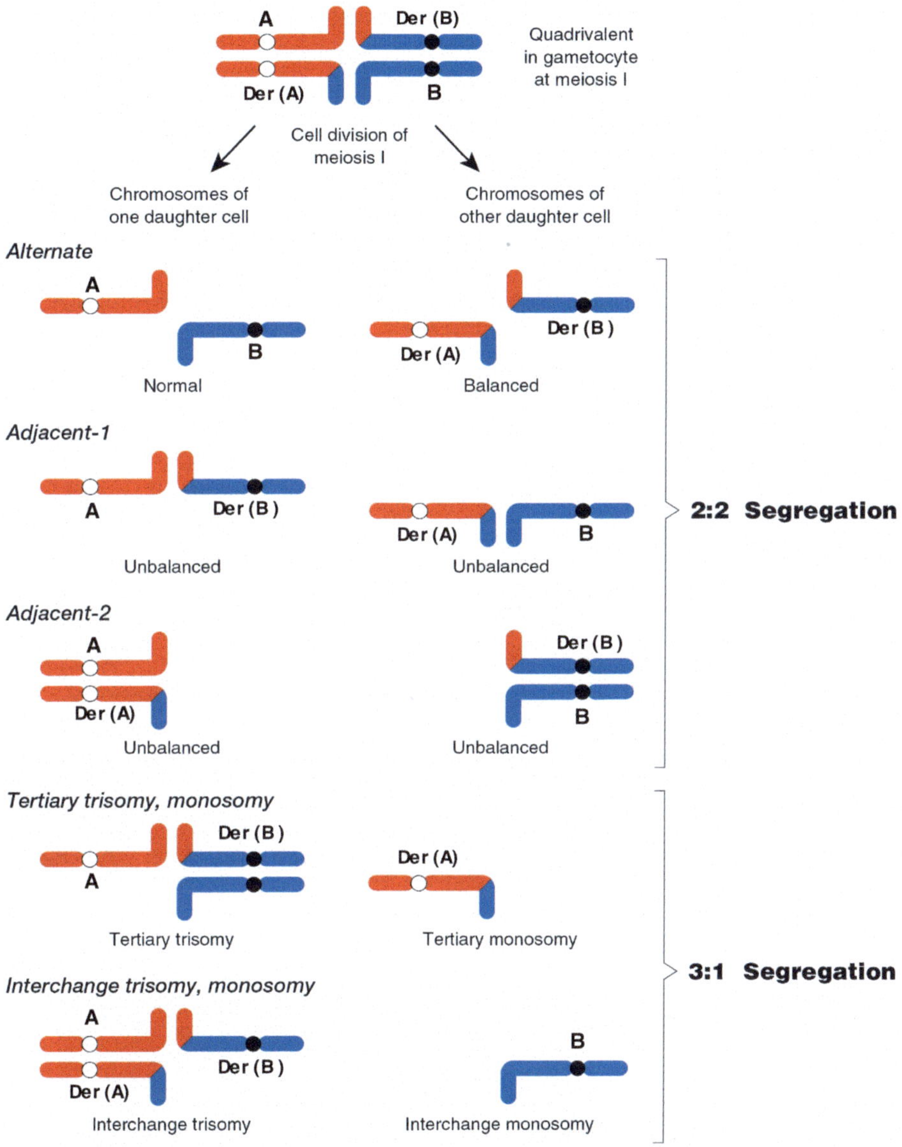

Fig. 24.3 Schematic depiction of quadrivalent formation and its segregation mode at meiosis in reciprocal translocation carrier. A, Chromosome A; B, Chromosome B; der(A), derivative chromosome A; and der(B), derivative B [25]. The 2:2 alternate segregation leads to the formation of normal or balanced gametes, while the 2:2 adjacent-1 or -2 segregations and 3:1 segregation modes produce an unbalanced content

3:1 segregation, one gamete receives two homologous chromosomes (disomy), resulting in a zygote with 47 chromosomes. The other corresponding gamete receives no chromosome (nullisomy), resulting in a zygote with 45 chromosomes. The 4:0 segregation mode produces a gamete with 21 chromosomes and one with 25 chromosomes, but it is quite a rare event.

In meiosis of reciprocal translocation carriers, four chromosomes must pair in reciprocal translocation heterozygotes, and the resulting segregations have a higher frequency of unbalanced chromosomes than Robertsonian translocations. There have been a number of studies on segregation patterns. Zhang et al. [26] summarized numerous previous studies and revealed that alternative segregation was the most frequent mode of segregation (42.71%), followed by adjacent-1, adjacent-2, and 3:1 segregations. Adjacent-1 segregation was observed in 31.13% of spermatozoa, adjacent-2 segregation was observed in 7.87% of spermatozoa, and 3:1 segregation was observed in 4.63% of spermatozoa. In addition, 4:0 and numerical anomalies, presumed to be interchromosomal effects, were observed in 13.66% of spermatozoa. Different studies on meiotic segregation patterns of sperm from reciprocal translocation carriers have revealed variability in the segregation modes, and there is a wide range of unbalanced gamete frequencies, ranging from 18.7% to 91.0%, among patients (Nishikawa et al. 2007) [27–30]. Figure 24.4 shows an

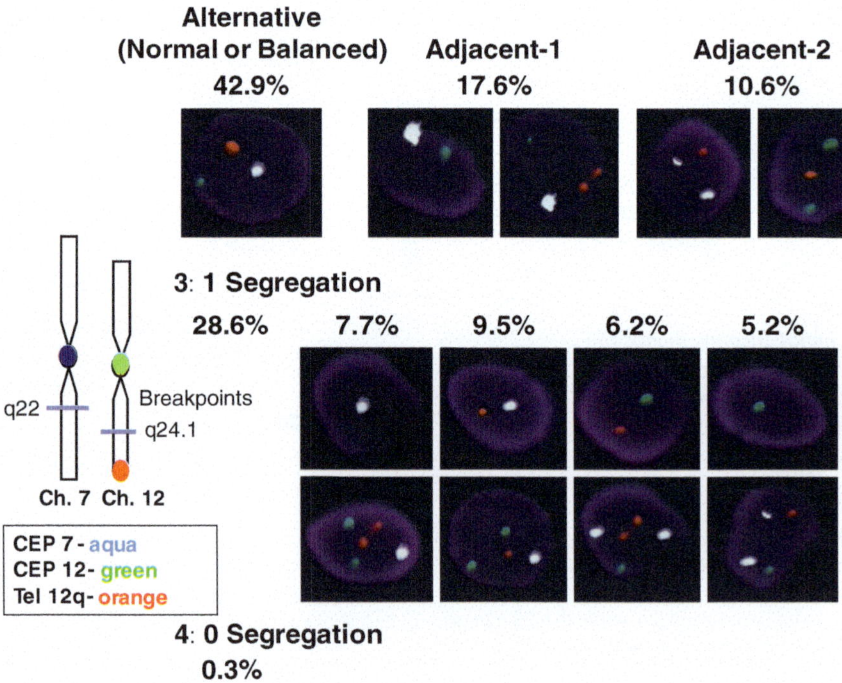

Fig. 24.4 Probes used in the FISH segregation analysis are CEP(centromere) 7 (aqua), CEP 12 (orange), and Tel(telomere) 12q (orange). Pictures show sperm resulting from alternate, adjacent-1, adjacent-2, 3:1, and 4:0 segregations with different signal patterns

example of meiotic segregation analysis on a case with t(7;12)(q22;q24.1) (Nishikawa et al. 2007).

Meiotic segregation patterns can be influenced by many factors. Published data have indicated that patients with shorter centric segments tended to produce higher numbers of adjacent-2 products, whereas those with shorter translocated segments produced more adjacent-1 products [31]. Additionally, 3:1 segregations required the participation of a small chromosome [31]. Studies on spermatozoa from translocation carriers help to broaden the understanding of the mechanisms of meiotic segregation. They should be integrated into the investigations of infertile men to provide a personalized risk assessment of unbalanced spermatozoa, especially since a correlation was found recently between the percentage of abnormal spermatozoa and that of abnormal embryos [32]. Meiotic segregation analysis facilitates the determination of the reproductive prognosis in male balanced translocation carriers and can be used for appropriate genetic counseling.

24.3 Multicolored Spectral Karyotyping for Complex Chromosomal Rearrangements

Complex chromosomal rearrangements (CCRs) are structural chromosome abnormalities that involve three or more breakpoints located on two or more chromosomes, which makes interpretation difficult. Many studies have reported that carriers of a balanced CCR are prone to infertility and recurrent abortions. CCRs with many breakpoints are usually difficult to clarify. In 1996, Schröck et al. [33] developed a novel approach, termed 'spectral karyotyping' or SKY, based on the hybridization of 24 fluorescence-labeled chromosome painting probes, which allows the simultaneous and differential color display of all chromosomes. This approach was used in the case of a pregnant CCR carrier with a previous abnormal child. The first baby, a female, suffered from cardiovascular abnormalities, including a ventral septal defect and patent ductus arteriosus. The karyotype included a 4q 2.3 trisomy, but further details were unknown. Chromosome analysis of the parents revealed that the mother had a complex chromosomal insertion/translocation between three chromosomes with four breakpoints forming der(4)t(4;16)(q22.2;q22.3), der(13)ins(13;4)(q31.2;q22.2q31.3), and der(16)t(4;16)(q31.3;q22.3) detected by G-banding. These findings of the mother's chromosomes were confirmed using SKY (Fig. 24.5). The couple requested prenatal diagnosis for the second pregnancy [34]. Chorionic villus sampling was performed. Cytogenetic analysis by SKY showed a male balanced carrier, the same as the mother.

In recent years, many studies have revealed that carriers of a balanced CCR are at risk of conceptions with various anomalies and reproductive failures owing to unbalanced arrangements due to either the malsegregation of derivative chromosomes or formation of a recombinant chromosome [35]. Many female carriers with CCRs have been identified after having malformed babies or repeated abortions [36]. Most males with CCRs have been shown to be infertile, and there have been

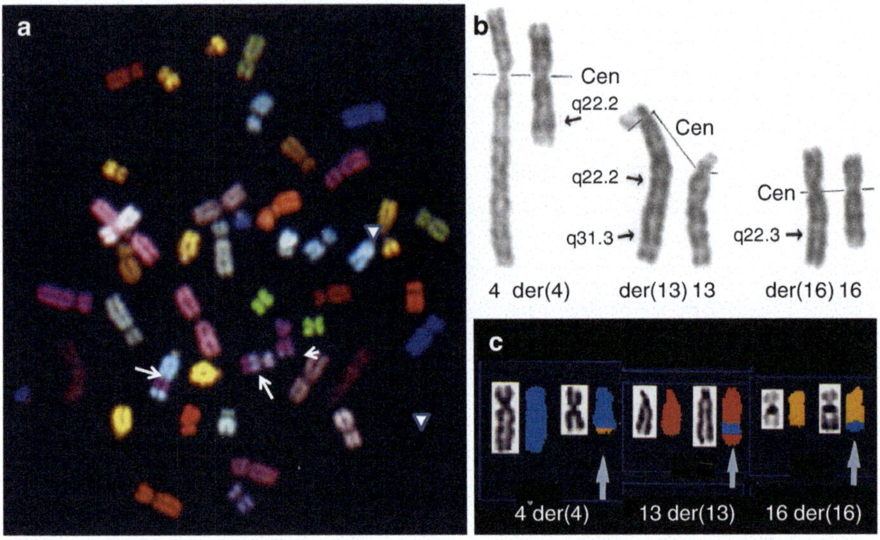

Fig. 24.5 G-banding and spectral karyotyping (SKY) of a case with complex chromosomal rearrangement involving chromosomes 4, 13, and 16. (**a**) Metaphase spread chromosomes stained by SKY (the arrows point to derivative chromosomes), (**b**) G-banded partial karyotypes showing translocation involving chromosomes 4, 13, and 16 and their derivatives (the arrows indicate breakpoints), and (**c**) G-banding and SKY of related chromosomes and their derivatives (the blue arrows indicate translocated chromosomes 4, 13, and 16)

several reports of CCRs in male with oligozoospermia [36–38]. According to the literature, 70–75% of CCRs are de novo in origin. They are found in almost equal proportions among phenotypically normal subjects and individuals with phenotypic abnormalities. The de novo CCRs appear to be mostly of paternal origin. This agrees with the epidemiological finding that most prenatally diagnosed balanced CCRs are maternal in origin (70% maternal versus 30% paternal), while the abnormalities found in newborns are of paternal origin [39].

In conclusion, the complexity of chromosomal rearrangements in patients with CCRs plays a role in male factor infertility and affects the spermatogenetic process rather than the number of chromosomes involved or the location of breakpoints. To corroborate this conclusion, further studies with larger sample sizes and advanced techniques, such as array-based comparative genomic hybridization, are required to characterize the breakpoints in detail [35].

References

1. Hopman AHN, Raap AK, Landegent J, et al. Non-radioactive in situ hybridization. In: Van Leeuwen F, Buijs RM, Pool CW, Pach O, editors. Molecular neuroanatomy. New York: Elsevier Science Publication B.V. (Biomedical Division); 1988. p. 43–68.
2. Ferguson-Smith MA. Putting the genetics back into cytogenetics. Am J Hum Genet. 1991;48:178–82.

3. Cremer T, Landegent J, Bruckner A, School HP, et al. Detection of chromosome aberrations in the human interphase nucleus by visualization of specific target DNAs with radioactive and non-radioactive in situ hybridization techniques: diagnosis of trisomy 18 with probe LI.84. Hum Genet. 1986;74:346–52.
4. Schröck E, du Manoir S, Veldman T, et al. Multicolor spectral karyotyping of human chromosomes. Science. 1996;273:494–7.
5. Speicher MR, Ballard SG, Ward DC. Karyotyping human chromosomes by combinatorial multi-colour FISH. Nat Genet. 1996;12:368–75.
6. Friedrich U, Nielsen J. Chromosome studies in 5,049 consecutive newborn children. Clin Genet. 1973;4(4):333–43.
7. Lubs HA, Ruddle FH. Chromosome abnormalities in the population: estimation of rates based on New Haven newborn study. Science. 1970;169(3944):495–7.
8. Nielsen J, Wohlert M. Chromosome abnormalities found among 34,910 newborn children: results from a 13-year incidence study in Arthus. Hum Genet. 1991;87(1):81–3.
9. Sergovich F, Valentine GH, Chen A, et al. Chromosome aberrations in 2159 consecutive newborn babies. N Engl J Med. 1969;280(16):851–5.
10. Jacobs PA, Melville MM, Ratcliffe SG, Keay AJ, et al. A cytogenetic survey of 11680 newborn infants. Ann Hum Genet. 1974. 1974;37:359–76.
11. Ratcliffe SG, Stewart AL, Melville MM, et al. Chromosome studies on 3500 newborn male infants. Lancet 1970. 1970;1:121–2.
12. Ferguson-Smith MA, Yates JRW. Maternal age specific rates for chromosome aberration and factors influencing them: Report of a collaborative European study of 52965 amniocenteses. Prenat Diagn. 1984;4:5–44.
13. Klinger KW, Dakowski W, et al. Prenatal detection of aneuploidy of 21, 18, 13, X or Y by interphase in situ hybridization. Am J Hum Genet. 1990; Suppl. 47A:224.
14. Baart EB, Martini E, Van Opstal D. Screening for aneuploidies of ten different chromosomes in two rounds of FISH: a short and reliable protocol. Prenat Diagn. 2004;24:955–66.
15. Klinger KW, Landes G, Shook D, Harvey R, Lopez L, et al. Rapid detection of chromosome aneuploidies in uncultured amniocytes by using fluorescence in situ hybridization (FISH). Am J Hum Genet. 1992;51(1):55–65.
16. Ward BE, Gersen SL, Carelli MP, et al. Rapid prenatal diagnosis of chromosomal anueploidies by fluorescene in situ hybridization: clinical experience with 4500 specimens. Am J Hum Genet. 1993;52(5):854–65.
17. Wenemowicz S, Sandstrom DJ, Morten CC, et al. Fluorescence in situ hybridization (FISH) for rapid detection of aneuploidies: experience in 911 prenatal cases. Prenat Diagn. 2001;21:262–9.
18. Winsor EJT, Silver MP, Theve R, et al. Maternal cell contamination in uncultured amniotic fluid. Prenat Diagn. 1996;16:49–54.
19. American College of Medical Genetics. Prenatal interphase fluorescence in situ hybridization (FISH) policy statement. Am J Hum Genet. 1993;53:526–7.
20. Jacobs P, Hassold TJ. The origin of numerical chromosomal abnormalities. Adv Genet. 1995;33:101–3.
21. De Braekeleer M, Dao TN. Cytogenetic studies in human male infertility: a review. Hum Reprod. 1991;6:245–50.
22. Lamotte A, Martinez G, Devillard F, et al. Is sperm FISH analysis still useful for Robertsonina translocation? Meiotic analysis for 23 patients and review of the literature. Basic Clin Androl. 2018;28:2–11.
23. Balkan W, Martin RH. Chromosome segregation into the spermatozoa of two men heterozygous for different reciprocal translocations. Hum Genet. 1983;63:345–8.
24. Martin KH. Analysis of human sperm chromosome complements from a male heterozygous for a reciprocal translocation t(11;22) (q23;q11). Clin Genet. 1984;25:357–61.
25. Rudak F, Jacobs A, Yanagimachi R. Direct analysis of the chromosome constitution of human spermatozoa. Nature. 1978;274:911–3.

26. Perrin A, Morel F, Douet-Guilbert N, et al. A study of meiotic segregation of chromosomes in spermatozoa of translocation carrier using fluorescent in situ hybridization. Andrologia. 2010;42:27–34.
27. Ogur G, Asse EV, Vegetti W, et al. Chromosomal segregation in spermatozoa of 14 Robertsonian translocation carriers. Mol Hum Reprod. 2006;12(3):209–15.
28. De Braekeleer M, Dao TN. Cytogenetic studies in human spontaneous abortions. In: Hafez ESE, editor. Assisted human reproductive technology. New York: Hemisphere Publication Company; 1991. p. 41–5. Google Scholar.
29. Daniel A, Boue A. Prospective risk in reciprocal translocation heterozygotes at amniocentesis as determined by potential chromosome imbalance size. Data of the European Collaborative Prenatal Diagnosis Centres. Prenat Diagn. 1986;6:315–50.
30. Gardner RJM, Sutherland GR. 4. Autosomal reciprocal translocations. In: Chromosome abnormalities and genetic counseling. Oxford Monograph on Medical Genetics No. 46. Oxford: Oxford University Press; 2004. p. 59–97.
31. Zhang S, Lei C, Wu J, et al. Analysis of segregation patterns of quadrivalent structures and the effect on genome stability during meiosis in reciprocal translocation carriers. Hum Reprod. 2018;33(4):757–67.
32. Ko DS, Cho JW, et al. Clinical outcomes of preimplantation genetic diagnosis (PGD) and analysis of meiotic segregation modes in reciprocal translocation carriers. Am J Med Genet A. 2010;152A(6):1428–33.
33. Lim CK, Cho JW, Song IO, et al. Estimation of chromosomal imbalances in preimplantation embryos from preimplantation genetic diagnosis cycles of reciprocal translocations with or without acrocentric chromosomes. Fert Steril. 2008;90:2144–51.
34. Martin RH. Cytogenetic determinations of male fertility. Hum Reprod Update. 2008;14:379–90.
35. Ye Y, Qian Y, Xu C, et al. Meiotic segregation analysis of embryos from reciprocal translocation carriers in PGD cycles. Repro Biomed Online. 2012;24(1):83–90.
36. Nishikawa N, Sato T, Suzumori N, et al. Meiotic segregation analysis male translocation carriers by using fluorescent in situ hybridization. Inter J Androl. 2007;31:60–6.
37. Fraut T, Mermet MA, et al. Cooperation of selection and meiotic mechanisms in the production of imbalances in reciprocal translocation. Cytogenet Cell Genet. 2000;88:15–21.
38. Morel F, Dout-Guilber T, et al. Meiotic segregation of translocations during male gametogenesis. Int J Androl. 2004;27:200–12.
39. Tanemura M, Suzumori K, Nishikawa N, Ishihara Y. Multicolour spectral karyotyping for complex chromosomal rearrangements in repeated abortion or congenital anomalies. Prenat Diagn. 2001;21:1123–8.
40. Kim JW, Chang EM, Song S-H, et al. Complex chromosomal rearrangements in infertile males: complexity of rearrangement affects spermatogenesis. Fertil Steril. 2011;95(1):349–52.
41. Batista DA, Pai GS, Stetten G. Molecular analysis of a complex chromosomal rearrangement and a review of familial case. Am J Med Genet. 1994;53(3):255–63.
42. Coco R, Rahn MI, Estangain PG, Antonioni G, et al. A constitutional complex chromosome rearrangement involving meiotic arrest in a review of familial male: case report. Hum Reprod. 2004;19:2784–90.
43. Kausch K, Haaf T, Khler J, et al. Complex chromosomal rearrangement in a woman with multiple miscarriage. Am J Med Genet. 1988;31:415–20.
44. Pellestor F, Anahory T, Lefort G, et al. Complex chromosomal rearrangements; origin and meiotic behavior. Hum Reprod Update. 2011;178(4):476–94.

Chapter 25
Polymerase Chain Reaction (PCR)

Takahiro Yamada

Abstract Polymerase chain reaction (PCR) is one of the most important techniques for prenatal diagnosis. It can amplify a specific DNA sequence from tiny fetal samples with high efficiency within a few hours. PCR is a cyclic DNA synthesis reaction by DNA polymerase in an automated system that amplifies the target sequence to over 100 million copies in a test tube. This technology is useful not only for invasive prenatal genetic diagnostic testing but also for noninvasive prenatal genetic testing.

Keywords Polymerase chain reaction · PCR · Taq polymerase · DNA · Direct sequencing · Sanger sequencing · Electrophoresis

25.1 The Technical Advantages of Polymerase Chain Reaction in Prenatal Diagnosis

One of the most important molecular technologies for prenatal diagnosis of single gene disorders is polymerase chain reaction (PCR). PCR amplifies a specific DNA sequence against a background of the entire genome. The target DNA sequence of interest is only a small part of the whole genome. When we try to read the sequence of one exon of a single target gene, we need to amplify the genomic region flanking the exon. Assuming that the average size of exons in the human genome is ~300 base pairs, the ratio to the size of whole genome (~3000 Mb) is 1:10,000,000. Moreover, in prenatal diagnosis, we can obtain only a small amount of sample from chorionic villi or amniotic fluid. PCR is able to amplify DNA fragments from such tiny amounts of tissue sample.

T. Yamada (✉)
Department of Medical Ethics and Medical Genetics, Kyoto University School of Public Health, Kyoto, Japan
e-mail: taka0197@kuhp.kyoto-u.ac.jp

H. Masuzaki (ed.), *Fetal Morph Functional Diagnosis*, Comprehensive Gynecology and Obstetrics, https://doi.org/10.1007/978-981-15-8171-7_25

Another indispensable condition of the technique to be useful for prenatal diagnosis is speed to obtain a short turnaround time. PCR is able to complete the amplification of target DNA within a few hours in a test tube. Although clients with affected fetuses may choose the termination of the pregnancy based on the result of prenatal diagnosis, elective abortion is allowed only when the gestational age is less than 22 weeks in Japan. Most countries also have a set limit on gestational weeks for elective abortion. From the point of view, this is important advantage of PCR.

25.2 The PCR Procedure (Fig. 25.1)

First, for prenatal diagnosis using fetal samples from amniocentesis or chorionic villous sampling, DNA must be extracted. The extracted genomic DNA is used as a template for PCR. DNA can be extracted from amniotic fetal cells after cell culture for 2 weeks, whereas DNA can be extracted from chorionic villi just after sampling. Next, we designed and synthesized a pair of unique primers to the sequences upstream and downstream of a region of interest. The primers were oligonucleotides of 20–25 base pairs that are homologous to sequences that flank the DNA segment to be amplified. The length between the primer binding sites is limited by the type of DNA polymerase (e.g., Taq polymerase) and is usually to around 1000 bases or fewer. The primers are designed to bind to opposite strands of the target DNA, which is denatured into single strands by heating to ~95 °C. The primers are allowed to anneal to the opposite genomic strands by cooling to the annealing temperature specific for the primer pairs being used (around 60 °C). Following

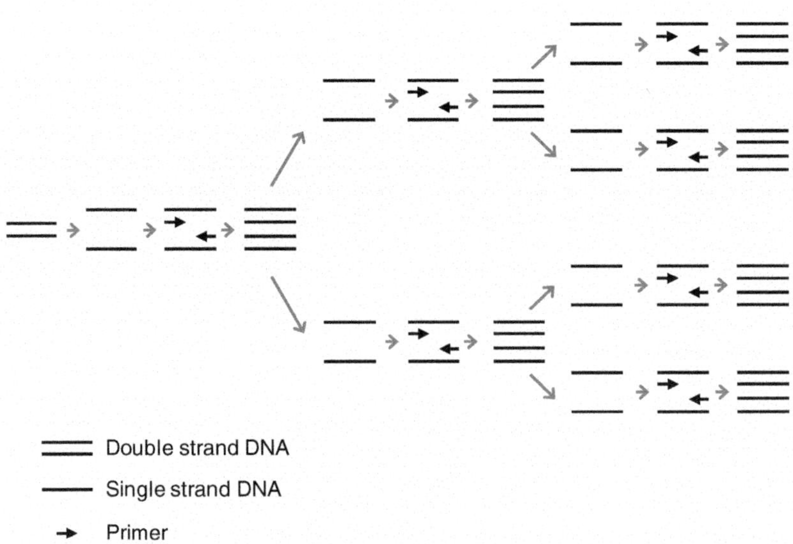

Fig. 25.1 Diagram of polymerase chain reaction

annealing, DNA polymerase (Taq polymerase) directs DNA synthesis during incubation at ~72 °C using four kinds of nucleotides. This produces a pair of hybrid molecules, which are once again separated into single strands by heating. Again, the primers bind and DNA synthesis reactions are allowed to begin. DNA polymerases are derived from bacteria that thrive at high temperatures, allowing the same polymerase to be used in spite of multiple cycles of heating and cooling of the reaction mixture. The process is repeated multiple times, usually 30 or more, using an automated system, which leads to an exponential increase in the target DNA sequence. This results in over 100 million copies of the target sequence in a matter of 2 or 3 h in a test tube.

25.3 Clinical Use of PCR in Prenatal Diagnosis

25.3.1 PCR in Invasive Prenatal Genetic Testing

Prenatal diagnosis of genetic disorders by DNA analysis can be performed either by direct detection of the mutation or by means of closely linked markers. For direct detection of mutations, there are a variety of methods including Southern blotting, PCR, DNA sequencing, and others. Detection of relatively small sized mutation begins with the amplification of the DNA region of interest.

Separation and accurate size estimation of PCR products is the final step for the prenatal diagnosis of single-gene disorder caused by mutation that alters the length of the target sequence (e.g., a triplet repeat). Amplified DNA molecules migrate toward the positive electrode at a different rate depending on its length in a nondenaturing gel. After electrophoresis, DNA is usually visualized by staining the gel with a fluorescent dye, such as ethidium bromide, which binds to DNA.

Detection of each nucleotide change, deletion, or insertion is performed with the use of the Sanger sequencing method. In principle, after denaturing the double stranded amplified target DNA, DNA polymerase is used to synthesize a complimentary strand. During the reaction, different kinds of fluorescently labeled 2′,3′-dideoxynucleotides of adenine, cytosine, guanine, and thymidine (fluorescent dye terminator) are added. When one of the dideoxynucleotides is incorporated, the 3′-end of the reaction is no longer a substrate for chain elongation and the growing DNA chain is terminated. Thus, in the reaction, there are DNA molecules that are fluorescent with different colors according to the type of nucleotide with a common 5′-end, but of varying length because of the incorporation of a specific 3′-end. Next, the reaction product is subjected to electrophoresis in an automated sequencer.

An indirect linkage method by means of closely linked markers also needs PCR. After amplification of the DNA sequence flanking a polymorphic marker, the mutated allele is detected using a restriction fragment length polymorphism, variable number tandem repeat, or other diagnostic feature.

25.3.2 PCR in Noninvasive Prenatal Genetic Testing

PCR plays important roles in noninvasive prenatal genetic testing (NIPT) using cell-free fetal DNA (cfDNA). NIPT for the detection of a fetal chromosomal disease was first applied clinically by massive parallel sequencing using a next-generation sequencer in October 2011 [1]. However, in the early days of NIPT research, the analysis of single-gene disorders by PCR preceded. Lo et al. started with the use of the most obvious difference between maternally and paternally derived genetic material, the Y chromosome [2]. With the use of PCR technology, amplification of a single-gene copy sequence of *DYS14* from the Y chromosome was performed. The detection of this means that the fetus is male. After this research for fetal sex determination, PCR analysis of cfDNA in maternal plasma started to be used for RhD genotyping in RhD-negative pregnant mothers [3] and diagnosis of single-gene disorders in fetuses [4].

References

1. Samura O, Sekizawa A, Suzumori N, et al. Current status of non-invasive prenatal testing in Japan. J Obstet Gynaecol Res. 2017;43:1245–55.
2. Lo YM, Corbetta N, Chamberlain PF, et al. Presence of fetal DNA in maternal plasma and serum. Lancet. 1997;350:485–7.
3. Lo YM, Hjelm NM, Fidler C, et al. Prenatal diagnosis of fetal RhD status by molecular analysis of maternal plasma. N Engl J Med. 1998;339:1734–8.
4. Saito H, Sekizawa A, Morimoto T, et al. Prenatal DNA diagnosis of a single-gene disorder from maternal plasma. Lancet. 2000;356:1170.

Chapter 26
Microarray and Next Generation Sequencing

Hiroki Kurahashi and Takema Kato

Abstract Advance in molecular technologies for genome-wide analysis such as microarray or next generation sequencing (NGS) has provided great improvement in resolution of the analysis and sensitivity of diagnosis. Cytogenetic microarray facilitates the detection of chromosomal copy number gain or loss in undiagnosed cases in the postnatal and prenatal clinical setting. The use of microarray is recommended for a fetus with one or more major structural abnormalities identified on ultrasonographic examination. While NGS has enabled us to perform genome-wide analysis such as whole exome or whole genome sequencing in undiagnosed cases, the quantitative data obtained by NGS also allow us to obtain information of copy number variation, giving us the opportunities for highly sensitive analysis in noninvasive prenatal testing or preimplantation genetic testing. The microarray or NGS often detects a number of benign copy number variants or variants of unknown significance (VUS) frustrating the clinicians. Difficulties are also encountered in handling the secondary findings, identification of variant unrelated to the primary purpose for the testing. Appropriate genetic counseling will be required for such highly sensitive genome-wide analysis in prenatal genetic testing.

Keywords Microarray · Next generation sequencing · Copy number variant
Exome · Variant of unknown significance · Secondary findings

H. Kurahashi (✉)
Division of Molecular Genetics, Institute for Comprehensive Medical Science, Fujita Health University, Toyoake, Japan

Department of Clinical Genetics, Fujita Health University Hospital, Toyoake, Japan
e-mail: kura@fujita-hu.ac.jp

T. Kato
Division of Molecular Genetics, Institute for Comprehensive Medical Science, Fujita Health University, Toyoake, Japan
e-mail: takema@fujita-hu.ac.jp

H. Masuzaki (ed.), *Fetal Morph Functional Diagnosis*, Comprehensive Gynecology and Obstetrics, https://doi.org/10.1007/978-981-15-8171-7_26

26.1 Introduction

In the past three decades, maternal age at childbirth in many high-income countries has been significantly increased. The pregnancy in advanced maternal age is a critical risk factor for fetal chromosomal numerical abnormalities, aneuploidy. Increasing rate of fetal aneuploidy is a significant public health issue due to its adverse impacts on pregnancy outcomes. Prenatal chromosomal testing for fetal cell samples is one of the options for high risk pregnancies. On the other hand, screening by ultrasound examination is the powerful tool for fetal health care. Routine use of ultrasound examination facilitates the detection of structural abnormalities of the fetus during pregnancy, which occasionally requires further analysis to rule out the fetal chromosomal disorders. Karyotyping by G-staining is the conventional cytogenetic technique that has been generally used for standard chromosomal analysis of fetal samples obtained by amniocentesis or chorionic villi sampling. However, the information obtained by microscopic examination is limited to 5–10 Mb resolution. Fluorescence in situ hybridization (FISH) using disease-specific probe improved the sensitivity of the detection of submicroscopic deletions/duplications. However, FISH can be used only for diagnosis of aneuploidy or recognizable microdeletion/microduplication syndromes. Advances in microarray technology open the door for a new era of molecular cytogenetics, cytogenomics. Microarray enabled us to perform the highly sensitive genome-wide analysis for microdeletion/microduplication syndromes. Now, the use of microarray is recommended for a fetus with one or more major structural abnormalities identified on ultrasonographic examination [1].

The second wave of paradigm shift from cytogenetics to cytogenomics was brought by invention of NGS. For the genetic diagnosis for single gene disorders, PCR followed by Sanger sequencing has been the standard laboratory technique. However, NGS enabled us to perform genome-wide analysis such as exome analysis, and it facilitates the diagnosis of undiagnostic cases. Notably, the NGS technique provides not only the sequence information to identify the disease-causing variant at the nucleotide resolution but also the quantitative information at the exon levels [2]. Regarding the undiagnosed patients, the exome analysis is now about to replace the microarray and is the first-tier option for diagnostic procedure for genetic diseases. Further, the quantitative analysis of the whole genome sequencing was applied to noninvasive prenatal genetic testing (NIPT) or preimplantation genetic testing for aneuploidy (PGT-A) (Fig. 26.1). In this chapter, we will learn the concept of recently advanced genome-wide genetic analysis using microarray or NGS.

26.2 Microarray

A cytogenetic microarray is a laboratory tool used for detecting the microdeletions/duplications at the genome-wide loci. A microarray is microscope slides that are printed with thousands of tiny spots at defined positions, with each spot containing

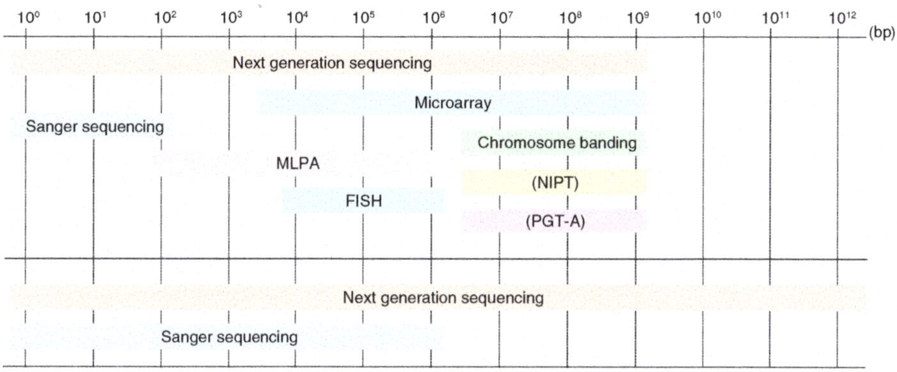

Fig. 26.1 Comparison of methodologies for analysis for disease-causing genomic variant. Upper panel shows the resolution of each method. The data for NIPT and PGT-A are obtained by standard NGS-based method. Lower panel shows the cumulative output per day

a oligonucleotide with known DNA sequence at the certain genome position. The DNA molecules attached to each slide act as probes to measure the signal intensity giving us the information of copy number variation (CNV), which corresponds to the term known as the deletions/duplications by conventional cytogenetic technique. Genomic DNA of test sample is labeled with fluorescent compound, and CNV detection is performed by quantitative analysis of hybridization signal. In general, test sample and reference sample are labeled with different fluorescent compounds and hybridized to microarray competitively. This technique, called comparative genomic hybridization (CGH), is now a standard laboratory test for detection of CNV (Fig. 26.2a).

Microarray-based CGH is generally used for detection of pathogenic CNV in clinically undiagnosed cases often in pediatric clinics. Although diagnosis for clinically recognizable microdeletion/microduplication syndromes can be generally conducted by FISH with region-specific probes, we cannot select the specific FISH probes for others. When we use microarray to find pathogenic CNV in undiagnosed cases, it is often difficult to determine the CNV responsible for the patient's phenotype, since any individuals carry tens of CNVs, most of which are benign and do not affect the phenotype. Since most of the pathogenic CNV is larger than 500 kb, most protocol sets the detection threshold at >400–500 kb [3]. We can refer to the database of CNV in normal population to exclude the benign CNV and also see the database for disease patients to see whether the reported individuals who carry the overlapping CNV are reported to carry the similar phenotype or not. Since de novo CNV is often responsible for the de novo phenotype, trio analysis using the proband and the parental samples is recommended. Some of the genes within the pathogenic CNV might be responsible for the patient's phenotype. To identify gene(s) intolerant to the haploinsufficiency, evaluation of pLI score might be useful [4]. For individuals with any developmental disabilities or congenital anomalies, conventional chromosome karyotyping by G-staining can detect pathogenic cytogenetic

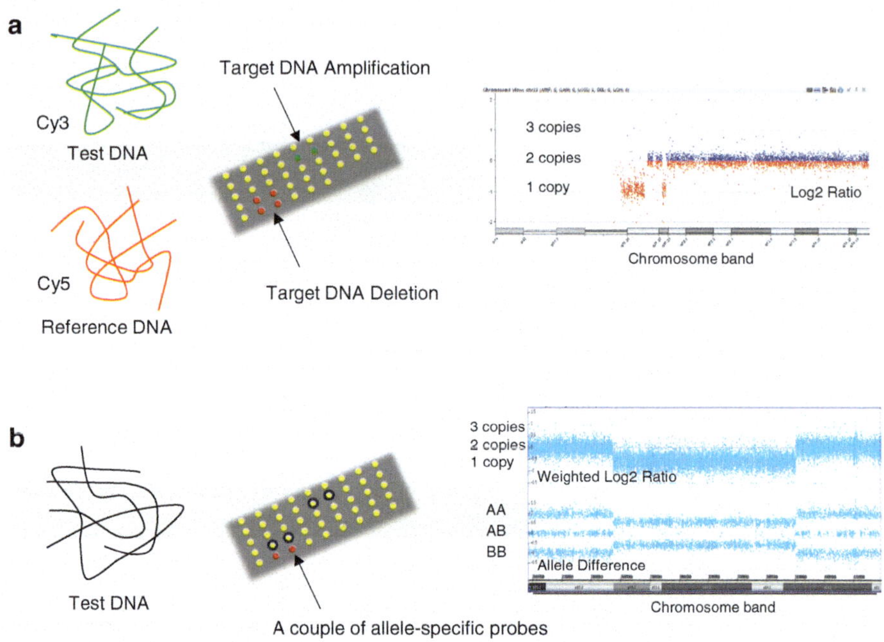

Fig. 26.2 Two types of microarray platforms. (**a**) aCGH. (**b**) SNP microarray

abnormalities in 3–5%. When we use microarray, detection rate of pathogenic CNV increases up to 15–20% [5]. Since microarray was introduced as a diagnostic tool, many new microdeletion/microduplication syndromes have been defined [6].

Cytogenetic microarray is recommended to be the first-tier tool for detecting the pathogenic structural variant in pediatric patients with developmental disabilities or congenital anomalies [5, 7]. It can detect microdeletions/microduplications as well as aneuploidy. As a secondary testing for conventional karyotyping by G-staining, microarray is also useful to identify the origin of small marker chromosome or additional chromosome of unknown origin. Then, can microarray detect all of the cytogenetic abnormalities that can be detected by conventional karyotyping? The answer is no. Although microarray can detect moderate level of CNV mosaicism, low level mosaicism less than 5–10% might be missed. Microarray can detect the unbalanced translocation, but the balanced translocation, whose copy number is neutral, will be missed in microarray analysis. Hence, the microarray has a high potential diagnostic tool for phenotype-based screening, whereas it does not work well in etiological screening of infertility or recurrent pregnancy loss since most of the expected abnormalities are the balanced structural abnormalities such as translocations or inversions.

SNP microarray is the other laboratory tool used for detecting the CNV at the genome-wide loci. On the SNP microarray, there are millions of tiny spots at defined positions, with each spot containing allele-specific oligonucleotide DNA probes at the certain genome position as a couple. Intensity of hybridization signals of the probe couple represents SNP genotype, which allows us to determine the homozygosity or heterozygosity at the loci (Fig. 26.2b). If there is a chromosomal deletion, SNP genotype within the deletion shows long contiguous stretch of homozygosity, i.e., runs of homozygosity or loss of heterozygosity (LOH). Occasionally, long contiguous stretch of copy number neutral LOH can be observed, which indicates uniparental disomy at the loci. SNP microarray is also powerful in detecting polyploidy such as triploidy.

Instead of the high-sensitive nature of genome-wide CNV analysis, it still has a couple of problems. The microarray often detects a number of benign copy number variants or variants of unknown significance (VUS). When the CNV responsible for the phenotype is not found, it is difficult to determine whether the VUS is pathogenic or not. Further, since the evaluation of the CNV is only based on the database information, reanalysis using updated database information might change the VUS to pathogenic or benign CNV. Difficulties are also encountered in handling the secondary findings, identification of variant unrelated to the primary purpose for the testing. Informed consent before the testing will be required including how to report the results.

In the prenatal diagnosis, the use of microarray is recommended for a fetus with phenotypic abnormalities, particularly one or more major congenital structural abnormalities identified on ultrasonographic examination [1]. Accurate diagnosis will provide the information about the prognosis of the fetus and facilitate decision-making of the parents. In the use of microarray for screening of the pregnancy of advanced maternal age, the microarray still has a risk to detect the VUS or secondary findings, which frustrates the clinicians and the parents. Appropriate genetic counseling is necessary before and after the testing, and careful follow-up of the pregnancy is important.

26.3 Next Generation Sequencing

For the diagnosis of recognizable monogenic disease, standard PCR and Sanger sequencing method have been used. Since the Sanger sequencing is based on capillary electrophoresis of the product of each sequencing reaction, sequence output per run is limited to a small number and it is time-consuming. NGS, also known as the massively parallel sequencing technology, is based on taking a photo of a massive number of sequencing reactions on the flow cell using high resolution digital camera, and it enables us to obtain sequencing of 1 million to tens of billion short reads (approximately 100 bases each) per run (Fig. 26.3a). For the whole genome sequencing, sonicated genomic DNA is used for construction of sequencing library. For the exome sequencing, genomic DNAs including certain genes are enriched by hybridization capture-based or amplicon-based approaches before NGS.

Exome sequencing is a powerful tool for diagnosis of monogenic disease in undiagnosed patient. In the case of autosomal recessive polycystic kidney disease, only *PKHD1* is the candidate gene, but it has more than 70 exons and Sanger

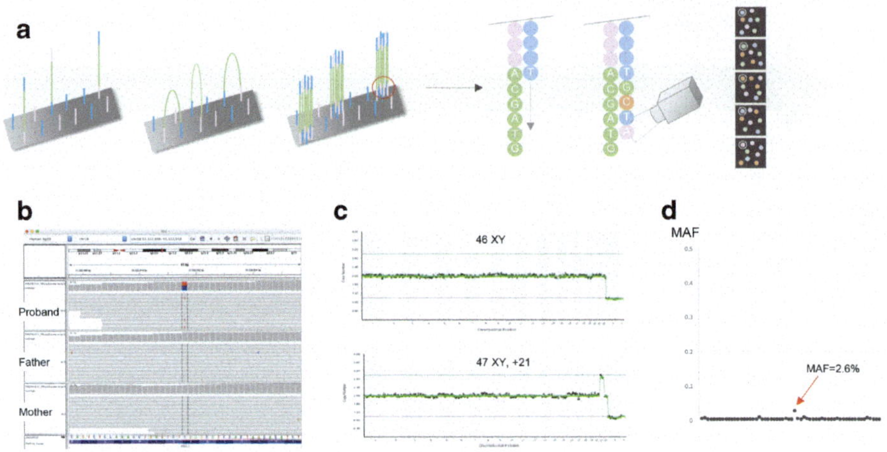

Fig. 26.3 Application of NGS to prenatal diagnosis. (**a**) Principle of NGS short-read sequencer. Massive PCR is performed on the flow cell. Addition of one fluorescent nucleotide in each cycle is monitored by digital camera. (**b**) Exome analysis. Trio analysis using samples of proband and parents indicates de novo mutation. (**c**) Preimplantation genetic diagnosis. Upper panel shows normal embryo, while lower panel shows trisomy 21. (**d**) NIPT for monogenic disease. De novo mutation can be detected by deep sequence of the PCR product by NGS using cell-free DNA from maternal blood as a template

sequencing is impractical. In this instance, exome sequence technique is helpful [8]. Exome sequence technique is also useful for the diseases with genetic heterogeneity. In the case of congenital hearing loss, for which more than 100 genes are known to be responsible, exome sequence technique is helpful to identify the causative variant in a given patient. Generally, tens of candidate variants are identified in the exome analysis. The pathogenicity of the variant should be evaluated by protocol recommended by American Collage of Medical Genetics on the basis of information of population frequency or molecular function and classified into five categories, pathogenic, likely pathogenic, VUS, likely benign, and benign [9].

To identify a new disease gene, whole exome sequencing is a powerful tool. Since de novo variant is often responsible for the de novo phenotype, trio analysis using the proband and the parental samples is recommended for whole exome sequencing (Fig. 26.3b). A considerable number of disease-responsible genes for monogenic disorders have been newly identified in the last few decades. However, the whole exome sequencing can identify only approximately 30% of the undiagnosed cases tested [10]. In the case of undiagnosed cases even when the whole exome sequencing has been used, whole genome sequencing might be the next option for achieving the genetic diagnosis. In the field of cancer genetics, exome sequencing allows us to know the driver mutations to develop the cancer of a given patient when the exome data of the cancer tissue and adjacent normal tissue are compared. It is useful to identify the personalized molecular target therapy.

NGS provides not only qualitative but also quantitative data. Quantitative data depend on the depth of sequence read counts collected on each sample, and it can provide the dosage information of the target genomic region. Quantitative analysis of the whole genome sequence enables us to identify unbalanced structural and numerical chromosomal abnormalities just like microarray analysis. One well-known application is the NIPT. NIPT is a first trimester screening test that can detect the trisomy or other chromosomal copy number abnormalities. Based on the fact that approximately 10% of cell-free DNA (cfDNA) in maternal blood originates from trophoblasts in placenta, cfDNA in maternal blood could be the source of analysis of the fetal genetic or chromosomal diseases. In NIPT, massively parallel sequencing is performed for cfDNA. In the case of pregnancy of trisomy 21, read counts of chromosome 21 should be increased. Due to high negative prediction value, NIPT is now the standard prenatal diagnosis undertaken most frequently. Another application of the quantitative NGS is the PGT-A. PGT-A is a procedure that allows the determination of the chromosomal status in the early embryo. During assisted reproduction technology procedure, a small number of trophoectodermal cells are taken by blastocyst biopsy and subjected to whole genome amplification. Quantitative analysis of the whole genome sequencing of the DNA provides the information regarding the chromosomal contents (Fig. 26.3c). Read depth of x0.01 genome coverage is sufficient to know whether the embryo has the aneuploidy or gross copy number abnormalities or not. Recent application of the cytogenetic NGS is the etiological screening of the recurrent pregnancy loss using the products of concept (POC). So far, the chromosomal analysis for POC was performed by conventional karyotyping using G-staining. However, since it requires cell culture, it is necessary to start the culture immediately after the delivery, but it is occasionally impractical by location or psychological issues. For NGS, POC samples can be stored in freezer, and the cytogenetic test for the subsequent pregnancy can be offered at the teachable moment.

In the prenatal diagnosis, even when using the conventional karyotyping and microarray technique, more than half of the fetuses with structural anomalies remain without a diagnosis. Some of them might be caused by monogenic disorder. Whole exome can identify pathogenic variants in ~20% of fetuses having severe structural anomalies. However, the clinical use of exome for prenatal diagnosis is still controversial since there are many points to consider including interpretation of the results and how to report the VUS or secondary findings [11]. Deep sequence of the target region can provide the information of low level mosaicism. In neonatal diagnosis, deep sequence of the target region for a monogenic disease could identify de novo mutation of the fetus in maternal cfDNA (Fig. 26.3d). This can be applied for identification of de novo *FGFR3* mutation in maternal cfDNA in pregnancy with short-limb bone disease to make an accurate diagnosis of achondroplasia or thanatophoric dysplasia [12].

26.4 Future Perspectives

Conventional karyotyping using G-staining is the simple but genome-wide screening test that can be used in prenatal diagnosis. Whole genome sequencing by NGS has not yet replaced the karyotyping since there are still some sequence gaps in the reference sequence of the human genome. Further, the NGS data cannot differentiate maternal and paternal homologous chromosomes for alignment. Recent advance in long-read NGS technologies allows for the retrieval of 10–100 kb (occasionally >2 Mb) sequence reads as a single DNA molecule, which are much longer than those of standard short-read sequence (approximately 100 bp). This technique might bridge the sequence gap of the human genome reference. Long-read sequencing also enables the phasing of the SNPs to differentiate the two homologues. Further, proximity ligation followed by NGS could also sequence the two homologues separately [13]. Cytogenomics obtained by combination of these comprehensive techniques might replace the conventional microscopic cytogenetics in near future. Then, we can soon see the days when we know all the genomic information of each individual.

However, we have not got ready for genome-wide cytogenomics of the fetus in prenatal diagnosis. In the era of genome-wide prenatal diagnosis using microarray or NGS, to what extent do the parents or medical stuffs want to know? The information contained in the genome is more sensitive because it contains an individual's probabilistic "future diary", and also contains information about an individual's family members [14]. Do they want to know the baby's future? In this chapter, we are discussing only about the simple chromosomal disorders or monogenic diseases. However, most of the common diseases are polygenic diseases and precise information is still lacking for the risk estimation of these diseases. At the same time, concern is also emerging for enhancement application. Accumulation of the evidence as well as establishment of ethical guideline is necessary for the help of the autonomous decision-making of the couple in genome-wide prenatal diagnosis via appropriate genetic counseling.

Acknowledgements We are grateful to Dr. S. Miyai and Dr. F. Suzuki for technical assistances. We also thank the Database Center for Life Science (DBCLS) for providing illustration for the Figures.

References

1. Committee on Genetics and the Society for Maternal-Fetal Medicine. Committee Opinion No.682: Microarrays and next-generation sequencing technology: the use of advanced genetic diagnostic tools in obstetrics and gynecology. Obstet Gynecol. 2016;128(6):e262–8.
2. Fromer M, Moran JL, Chambert K, et al. Discovery and statistical genotyping of copy-number variation from whole-exome sequencing depth. Am J Hum Genet. 2012;91(4):597–607.
3. Cooper GM, Coe BP, Girirajan S, et al. A copy number variation morbidity map of developmental delay. Nat Genet. 2011;43(9):838–46.
4. Lek M, Karczewski KJ, Minikel EV, et al. Exome Aggregation Consortium. Analysis of protein-coding genetic variation in 60,706 humans. Nature. 2016;536(7616):285–91.
5. Miller DT, Adam MP, Aradhya S, et al. Consensus statement: chromosomal microarray is a first-tier clinical diagnostic test for individuals with developmental disabilities or congenital anomalies. Am J Hum Genet. 2010;86(5):749–64.
6. Shaikh TH. Copy number variation disorders. Curr Genet Med Rep. 2017;5(4):183–90.

7. Manning M, Hudgins L, Professional Practice and Guidelines Committee. Array-based technology and recommendations for utilization in medical genetics practice for detection of chromosomal abnormalities. Genet Med. 2010;12(11):742–5.
8. Miyazaki J, Ito M, Nishizawa H, et al. Intragenic duplication in the PKHD1 gene in autosomal recessive polycystic kidney disease. BMC Med Genet. 2015;16:98.
9. Richards S, Aziz N, Bale S, et al. Standards and guidelines for the interpretation of sequence variants: a joint consensus recommendation of the American College of Medical Genetics and Genomics and the Association for Molecular Pathology. Genet Med. 2015;17(5):405–24.
10. Clark MM, Stark Z, Farnaes L, et al. Meta-analysis of the diagnostic and clinical utility of genome and exome sequencing and chromosomal microarray in children with suspected genetic diseases. NPJ Genom Med. 2018;3:16.
11. Monaghan KG, Leach NT, Pekarek D, et al. The use of fetal exome sequencing in prenatal diagnosis: a points to consider document of the American College of Medical Genetics and Genomics (ACMG). Genet Med. 2020; [Epub ahead of print].
12. Terasawa S, Kato A, Nishizawa H, et al. Multiplex PCR in noninvasive prenatal diagnosis for FGFR3-related disorders. Congenit Anom (Kyoto). 2019;59(1):4–10.
13. Selvaraj S, Dixon JR, Bansal V, et al. Whole-genome haplotype reconstruction using proximity-ligation and shotgun sequencing. Nat Biotechnol. 2013;31(12):1111–8.
14. Annas GJ. Privacy rules for DNA databanks. Protecting coded 'future diaries'. JAMA. 1993;270(19):2346–50.

Chapter 27
How to Obtain Certifications and Licenses for Prenatal Diagnosis

Shigehito Yamada and Katsuhiko Naruse

Abstract This chapter describes how medical qualifications related to prenatal diagnosis are utilized in clinical practice and the status of accreditation in Japan and other countries considering the current state of prenatal diagnosis. In Japan, although licenses for performing tests for prenatal diagnosis are not fixed, several credentials for genetic medicine are established and certified by academic societies. The need for genetic medicine specialists is increasing due to advances in genetic medicine. Establishing a system that can effectively solve the concerns of pregnant women and their families while making effective use of qualified personnel is desirable.

Keywords License · Certification · Clinical geneticist · Genetic counselor Prenatal diagnosis

27.1 How to Qualify for Prenatal Diagnosis in Japan

27.1.1 Qualifications

In Japan, there are several qualifications related to perinatal genetic medicine. Here, we introduce the qualifications and explain the types of qualifications, such as licenses, credentials, and certificates. The expert "license" is what the government grants. This means that the government ensures that licensees meet the minimum eligibility criteria and that public health, safety, and welfare are reasonably protected [1]. In Japan, a doctor's license is the sole "license" with regard to clinical

S. Yamada (✉)
Congenital Anomaly Research Center, Kyoto University Graduate School of Medicine, Kyoto, Japan
e-mail: shyamada@cac.med.kyoto-u.ac.jp

K. Naruse
Department of Obstetrics and Gynecology, Nara Medical University, Kashihara, Japan
e-mail: naruse@naramed-u.ac.jp

H. Masuzaki (ed.), *Fetal Morph Functional Diagnosis*, Comprehensive Gynecology and Obstetrics, https://doi.org/10.1007/978-981-15-8171-7_27

genetics. Meanwhile, the term "certification" may be authorized by the government or private specialty associations or boards, and no government-certified "certification" exists for genetic medicine in Japan. However, to become a genetic counselor in Japan, it is necessary to complete a government-approved master's program before taking the qualification test. In that regard, the qualification of the genetic counselor might be the closest to obtaining a "license" or "certification" approved by the government among the qualifications related to genetic medicine listed below. The term "credential" is also used; it is not generally defined in statute but is widely used by professionals, the public, regulators, and legislators as evidence (public or private) of a person's qualifications [1].

In Japan, the medical staff has several "certifications" or "credentials." Since 1987, the Japan Society of Obstetrics and Gynecology has authorized the certification of board-certified medical doctors. To obtain this certification, it is necessary to have 5 years of experience as a medical doctor, including 3 years of senior residency as an obstetrician–gynecologist followed by exams and interviews. Almost all obstetrician–gynecologists in Japan tend to obtain this certification after residency. Once an obstetrician–gynecologist has obtained this certification, the following four related qualifications can be acquired in the field of perinatal diagnosis:

1. The Japan Society of Perinatal and Neonatal Medicine (since 2009)—Certification (Mother and Fetus)

This certification certifies that the specialist has advanced medical experience in the field of general perinatal medicine. However, it is not indicated in genetic medicine [2].

2. The Japan Society of Ultrasonics in Medicine (since 1990)—Certification (Obstetrics and Gynecology)

In addition to basic knowledge of medical ultrasound engineering and clinical ultrasound medicine, this course certifies that the specialist has the knowledge and skills in each specialty (in this case, obstetrics and gynecology), but it is not indicated in genetic medicine [3].

3. Japanese Board of Medical Genetics and Genomics, Clinical Genetics—Clinical Geneticist (since 2002)

This course provides information on clinical genetic medicine that meets the needs of not only patients and their families but also the public. Furthermore, specialists essential for the further development of clinical genetics are trained and accredited by the board. However, it is not specified in prenatal medicine [4].

4. Japan Society of Clinical Genetics in Obstetrics and Gynecology (JSGOG)—Certification (Year certificated, Prenatal Medicine) (since 2019)

This certificate certifies the genetic knowledge and skills necessary for improving the quality of genetic medicine among members in the society to provide appropriate genetic explanation related to obstetric and gynecological care. It comprises three courses: Prenatal Medicine, Gynecological Oncology, and Reproductive

Medicine. The Prenatal Medicine course is limited to prenatal diagnosis and counseling and is intended for physicians engaged in primary care in the field of obstetrics and gynecology [5].

In Japan, nonMD medical staff engaged in prenatal genetic medicine can obtain two certifications: Genetic Counselor and Certified Nurse Specialist.

5. Japanese Nursing Association—Certified Nurse Specialist (Genetic Nursing)

This course aims to identify the genetic problems of clients, assist in decision-making associated with diagnosis, prevention, and treatment, and support lifelong medical treatment to improve the quality of life. However, it is not indicated in prenatal medicine [6].

6. Japanese Board of Genetic Counseling—Genetic Counselor

This course trains and certifies genetic counselors as professionals who work with clinical genetic specialists to provide high-quality clinical genetic care as well as assist clients with genetic problems and protect their rights. The training curriculum is comparable to that of a master's degree; therefore, a bachelor's degree is required for all candidates applying for the genetic counselor courses. However, the curriculum is not indicated in prenatal medicine [7].

27.1.2 History and Present Status

Following the innovation of ultrasonography in obstetrics and gynecology by Professor Ian Donald after World War II [8], the use of ultrasonography in intrauterine diagnosis has expanded and currently includes detection of fetal anomalies, including screening for aneuploidy, by fetal cardiac ultrasound [9] and risk assessment of chromosomal abnormalities in fetuses by measuring the thickness of nuchal fold [10]. Since the last century, transvaginal or transabdominal ultrasound devices have been widely used in clinics across Japan. However, despite the sophisticated technology of ultrasound devices and the improved techniques of medical workers, aneuploidy screening by ultrasound has not been widely introduced in Japan because of disagreements regarding the universal screening of fetal anomalies, similar to maternal serum marker (MSM) tests.

When the first MSM test conducted in the second trimester of pregnancy was introduced in Japan in the mid-1990s [11], the dramatic increase in the number of tests used for screening Down syndrome and aneuploidy-related fetal anomalies was controversial. The ethics regarding prenatal screening based on serum markers was discussed in the context of Japanese law, which does not allow pregnancy termination because of fetal abnormalities [12]. In 1999, the Scientific Council's Expert Committee on Prenatal Diagnosis, which evaluates Japan's advanced medical technology, published the "Overviews on Prenatal Serum Marker Screening" guidelines, which specified that medical workers do not need to provide test-related information to all pregnant women. Subsequently, the number of maternal serum screening tests decreased [13]. In addition, prenatal genetic screening tests such as MSM tests and/or nuchal translucency in ultrasonography were performed as per patient's request rather than as routine procedure because no policy on prenatal screening by the government had been adopted nationwide. Consequently, the rate of prenatal genetic diagnosis performed was relatively low, and the system of care that provides prenatal genetic counseling during routine obstetric care was poorly established in Japan.

Concurrently with this background, noninvasive prenatal testing (NIPT) as a commercial test began to be used in the USA in October 2011. In 2013, NIPT was introduced in Japan as a clinical study and was reportedly performed on more than 30,000 pregnant women over a 3-year period [14]. Since 2016, NIPT has been conducted approximately 14,000 times/year, with no significant change [15].

Meanwhile, the number of amniocentesis cases had been increasing since 1998, when the records were first maintained, but have been decreasing since 2014 [16], possibly because NIPT was introduced in April 2013. From 2000 to 2011, MSM tests were performed 15,000–20,000 times annually, but their use has been steadily increasing since 2012, having been performed approximately 35,900 times in 2016 [16]. This is not unrelated to the fact that NIPT had been extensively reported in Japan as a "new type of prenatal diagnosis" in newspapers and on the internet in Japan in 2012, and the interest about prenatal diagnosis heightened among pregnant women. It is possible that MSM tests were chosen by pregnant women who did not meet the requirements for NIPT.

While the requirements for performing NIPT are strictly defined by the Japanese Association of Medical Sciences [17], a large number of NIPTs are also performed in private clinics aside from obstetrics and gynecology with profit-making intentions [15]. This business is booming because the test can be performed only with blood collection. Unfortunately, pre- and posttest genetic counseling appears to be insufficiently provided to pregnant women and their families. All pregnant women who wish to undergo fetal genetic testing during pregnancy should in principle receive adequate genetic counseling. To achieve this goal, the Ministry of Health, Labour and Welfare and the academic society associated with fetal genetic testing are coordinating to establish a system and develop human resources for prenatal genetic medicine.

27.2 Qualification for Prenatal Diagnosis in Other Countries

27.2.1 Prenatal Testing

In most countries, special credentials in genetic medicine are unnecessary for basic prenatal testing for chromosomal anomalies [18], although fetal aneuploidy screening is incorporated in the core curriculum of geneticist's training in each country [19]. However, low-quality genetic counseling by nongeneticists, including for fetal aneuploidy, had been exposed by a British study at the end of the last century [20].

Thereafter, the training curriculum for general obstetrical practice has incorporated genetic care, at least for prenatal testing for aneuploidy. The basic skills to explain the probability and screening process of congenital anomalies to mothers and family members are incorporated in the senior residential course for obstetricians in the USA [21], the UK [22], and Australia/New Zealand [23]. Clinical geneticists as well as obstetrics consultants in most countries continue to participate in the routine clinical works with prenatal testing, similar to universal screening of fetal aneuploidy.

Credentials for prenatal testing involving fetal ultrasound are managed and certified by several societies. The Fetal Medicine Foundation in the UK [24] and the Nuchal Translucency Quality Review in the US [25] are well-known qualifiers for first-trimester screening ultrasound, and some laboratories that provide combined testing, including nuchal fold thickness, request a valid certificate from these organizations. Other qualifiers, such as the American Registry for Diagnostic Medical Sonography® [26] and the UK National Screening Committee programs [27], provide the certificate or education standards not limited to first-trimester screening (second trimester or fetal heart anomalies) and support sonographers without obstetrics medical licenses, such as radiologists, midwives, obstetrical nurses, and medical technologists. In the UK, the Fetal Anomaly Screening Program recommends that any practitioner, including radiographers, midwives, nurses, and doctors, who performs a fetal anomaly ultrasound scan on pregnant women for screening and diagnosis should acquire the Certificate/Diploma (as appropriate) in Medical Ultrasound from the College of Radiographers or Postgraduate Certificate in Medical Ultrasound [28]. The screening quality in each district of the country was monitored and reviewed strictly by the National Healthcare System [29].

As mentioned above, for geneticists, adhering to guidelines or official statements from national or professional societies for routine clinical works on general prenatal testing seems to be superior to obtaining professional licensing. Furthermore, the technology and knowledge for prenatal diagnosis are improving steadily; hence, updated guidelines or statements must be utilized. A useful website for recent prenatal screening and diagnosis guidelines or recommendations worldwide is provided by the Geneva Foundation for Medical Education and Research in Switzerland [18].

27.2.2 Genetic Counseling

Nearly 7000 professional genetic counselors are currently working worldwide [30], but the accreditation system for genetic counselors varies among countries [31]. In the USA, the genetic counselor training course was started in New York in 1969 [32], and as of 2018, 22 states provide licenses to conduct genetic counseling [30]. The American Board of Genetic Counseling controls the credentials and training programs via the Accreditation Council for Genetic Counseling (ACGC). The curriculum prior to the training course differs based on the program, but it generally includes a BA degree from an accredited university, a GRE exam, and a prerequisite of some courses, such as genetics, statistics, and psychology. The USA and Canada have 35 ACGC-accredited programs as of 2016 [33].

In the UK, genetic counselors have different origins. Midwives and nurses have been performing genetic counseling following their own education system since 1992 [34], and they formed the Association of Genetic Nurses and Counselors (AGNC) and started training programs in genomic counseling in 2016. As recommended by the AGNC, genetic counselors working in the UK and Ireland should be registered at the Genetic Counselor Registration Board (GCRB). GCRB registers members with a nursing background and an MSc degree in genetic counseling [35]. For countries in the European Union, the European Society of Human Genetics has a registration system for genetic nurses and counselors, which is accredited by the European Board of Medical Genetics. The status of genetic counseling as a profession in other countries, including Japan, as of 2016 was previously reviewed [30]; this study also included other conditions, such as organizations accrediting professional genetic counselors and the estimated number of counselors as of 2018 in major countries, as shown in Table 27.1.

Pre- and posttest counseling for prenatal testing including the screening program is recommended [21] in the USA. However, the number of genetic counselors and

Table 27.1 Organizations credentialing professional genetic counselors worldwide as of 2018 [30]

Country	First training program started	Organization	Estimated number of genetic counselors	
United States of America	1969	National Society of Genetic Counselors (NSGC)	4000	
		American Board of Genetic Counseling (ABGC)		
		Accreditation Council for Genetic Counseling (ACGC)		
		Association of Genetic Counseling Program Directors (AGCPD)		
Cuba	1999	National Medical Genetics Network	900	[36]
Canada	1985	Canadian Association of Genetic Counseling (CAGC)	350	
United Kingdom	1992	Association of Genetic Nurses and Counsellors (AGNC)	310	
		Genetic Counsellor Registration Board (GCRB)		
Japan	2005	Japanese Society of Genetic Counseling (JSGC)	267	(April, 2020)
		Japanese Society of Human Genetics (JSHG)		
		Japanese Board of Genetic Counseling (JBGC)		
Australia/New Zealand	1995	Human Genetics Society of Australasia (HGSA)	220	

medical geneticists is limited. Furthermore, there are attempts by healthcare insurers to restrict certified genetic specialists from conducting genetic testing because of the limited access to prenatal testing in an appropriate period [37], but the American College of Obstetricians and Gynecologists is opposed to this restriction. A recent legislation in some states in the USA states that mothers with fetuses with trisomy 21 should be provided positive information regarding the future of the fetus [38]. This counseling can be performed by genetic counselors or well-trained professionals in the field, but the rapid increase in the needs for genetic counseling as well as prenatal testing coupled with the lack of trained specialists worldwide appears to have created a new problem.

27.3 Summary and Future Considerations

Fetal ultrasonography has become an aspect of genetic medicine, and genetic tests such as NIPT and MSM tests are being performed routinely. In brief, many tests in routine obstetrical practice are related to genetic medicine. Meanwhile, at present, genetic medicine is increasingly needed because of genetic research and technological advances focusing on cancer. The proportion of medical staff specializing in genetic medicine against the increasing demand of genetic medicine is low among all people involved in medical care. As has been confirmed, pretest genetic counseling creates an opportunity for pregnant women to satisfactorily consider prenatal testing and promotes its understanding, and it may effectively facilitate informed decision-making after adequate consideration [39]. Hence, all pregnant women who wish to undergo genetic tests should undergo counseling; however, immediately referring women to medical staff with specialized knowledge, such as clinical geneticists or genetic counselors, is discouraged. A more careful and thorough approach is required for women with positive test results [39], and they should be referred to experts in such cases. Currently, genetic counseling is incorporated in the latest core curriculum of medical students in Japan [40], and young medical staff is expected to provide genetic medicine as routine medical care. Moreover, medical staff should acquire sufficient education on genetic medicine so that those who provide routine medical care in obstetrics can support women and their families with a counseling mind.

Acknowledgment We are deeply grateful to Ms. Chieko Tamura (certified genetic counselor in the USA and Japan) and Dr. Yasushi Nakamura (medical geneticist and qualified specialist by The Fetal Medicine Foundation) from FMC Tokyo Clinic, Japan, for the insightful comments and suggestions about circumstances of genetic medicine and terminology about qualifications in other countries.

References

1. Pew Health Professions Commission, Taskforce on Health Care Workforce Regulation. Reforming health care workforce regulation: policy considerations for the 21st century: report of the Taskforce on Health Care Workforce Regulation, Pew Health Professions Commission. 1995.
2. The Japan Society of Perinatal and Neonatal Medicine. Perinatal specialist system regulations (only in Japanese) [Online]. 2020. https://www.jspnm.com/Senmoni/Doc/kisoku_20200310.pdf. Accessed 23 Apr 2020.
3. The Japan Society of Ultrasonics in Medicine. Ultrasonic Specialist System Committee (only in Japanese) [Online]. https://www.jsum.or.jp/capacity/fjsum/qualifications.html. Accessed 23 Apr 2020.
4. Japanese Board of Medical Genetics and Genomics, Clinical Genetics. About the system of clinical geneticist (only in Japanese) [Online]. http://www.jbmg.jp/index.html. Accessed 23 Apr 2020.
5. Japan Society of Clinical Genetics in Obstetrics and Gynecology. Terms of certification (only in Japanese) [Online]. 2019. http://jsgog.kenkyuukai.jp/images/sys/information/20190705140224-05A42052F596AA3711562B32E4303CBF5A8EEC3C-B2A4C85717845EB40A51E187.pdf. Accessed 23 Apr 2020.
6. Japanese Nursing Association. About Certified Nurse Specialist (only in Japanese) [Online]. 2016. https://nintei.nurse.or.jp/nursing/qualification/cns. Accessed 23 Apr 2020.
7. Japanese Board of Genetic Counseling. About the Japanese Board of Genetic Counseling (only in Japanese) [Online]. 2020. http://plaza.umin.ac.jp/~GC/index.html. Accessed 23 Apr 2020.
8. Donald I, Macvicar J, Brown TG. Investigation of abdominal masses by pulsed ultrasound. Lancet. 1958;1:1188–95.
9. Maulik D, Nanda NC, Maulik D, Vilchez G. A brief history of fetal echocardiography and its impact on the management of congenital heart disease. Echocardiography. 2017;34:1760–7.
10. Nicolaides KH, Azar G, Byrne D, Mansur C, Marks K. Fetal nuchal translucency: ultrasound screening for chromosomal defects in first trimester of pregnancy. BMJ. 1992;304:867–9.
11. Onda T, Kitagawa M, Takeda O, Sago H, Kubonoya K, Iinuma K, Bradley LA, Canick JA, Krasikov NE, Ponting NR, Grier RE. Triple marker screening in native Japanese women. Prenat Diagn. 1996;16:713–7.
12. Sago H, Sekizawa A, Japan NC. Nationwide demonstration project of next-generation sequencing of cell-free DNA in maternal plasma in Japan: 1-year experience. Prenat Diagn. 2015;35:331–6.
13. Sasaki A, Sawai H, Masuzaki H, Hirahara F, Sago H. Low prevalence of genetic prenatal diagnosis in Japan. Prenat Diagn. 2011;31:1007–9.
14. Samura O, Sekizawa A, Suzumori N, Sasaki A, Wada S, Hamanoue H, Hirahara F, Sawai H, Nakamura H, Yamada T, Miura K, Masuzaki H, Nakayama S, Okai T, Kamei Y, Namba A, Murotsuki J, Tanemoto T, Fukushima A, Haino K, Tairaku S, Matsubara K, Maeda K, Kaji T, Ogawa M, Osada H, Nishizawa H, Okamoto Y, Kanagawa T, Kakigano A, Kitagawa M, Ogawa M, Izumi S, Katagiri Y, Takeshita N, Kasai Y, Naruse K, Neki R, Masuyama H, Hyodo M, Kawano Y, Ohba T, Ichizuka K, Kido Y, Fukao T, Miharu N, Nagamatsu T, Watanabe A, Hamajima N, Hirose M, Sanui A, Shirato N, Yotsumoto J, Nishiyama M, Hirose T, Sago H. Current status of non-invasive prenatal testing in Japan. J Obstet Gynaecol Res. 2017;43:1245–55.
15. Sekizawa A. NIPT: noninvasive prenatal testing (conference material, only in Japanese) [Online]. 2019. https://www.mhlw.go.jp/content/11908000/000559098.pdf.
16. Sasaki A, Sago H, Yoshihashi H, Yamada S, Miyake H, Suzumori N, Takada F, Masuzaki H, Hirahara F, Kugu K, Konishi I. Current status of prenatal diagnosis in Japan 1998-2016. J Japan Soc Perinat Neonat Med (in Japanese, only abstract in English). 2018;54:101–7.
17. Japanese Association of Medical Sciences. "Gene, Health, and Society" Review Committee (only in Japanese) [Online]. 2013. http://jams.med.or.jp/rinshobukai_ghs/index.html. Accessed 23 Apr 2020.

18. Geneva Foundation for Medical Education and Research. Obstetrics and gynecology guidelines [Online]. https://www.gfmer.ch/Guidelines/Prenatal_screening/Prenatal_screening_mt.htm. Accessed 23 Mar 2020.
19. Driscoll DA, Gross SJ, Professional Practice Guidelines C. Screening for fetal aneuploidy and neural tube defects. Genet Med. 2009;11:818–21.
20. Harris R, Lane B, Harris H, Williamson P, Dodge J, Modell B, Ponder B, Rodeck C, Alberman E. National Confidential Enquiry into counselling for genetic disorders by non-geneticists: general recommendations and specific standards for improving care. Br J Obstet Gynaecol. 1999;106:658–63.
21. Committee on Practice Bulletins-Obstetrics, Committee on Genetics, The Society for Maternal-Fetal Medicine. Practice Bulletin No. 163: Screening for fetal aneuploidy. Obstet Gynecol. 2016;127:e123–37.
22. Royal College of Obstetricians and Gynaecologists. Full details of the Core Curriculum, updated in August 2019 [Online]. 2020. https://www.rcog.org.uk/en/careers-training/specialty-training-curriculum/core-curriculum/. Accessed 23 Mar 2020.
23. The Royal Australian and New Zealand College of Obstetricians and Gynaecologists (RANZCOG). NT eLearning [Online]. https://elearning.nuchaltrans.edu.au/. Accessed 23 Mar 2020.
24. The Fetal Medicine Foundation. https://fetalmedicine.org/. Accessed 23 Mar 2020.
25. Perinatal Quality Foundation. Nuchal Translucency Quality Review [Online]. https://www.ntqr.org/wfAboutUs.aspx. Accessed 23 Mar 2020.
26. American Registry for Diagnostic Medical Sonography (ARDMS). Fetal Echocardiography (FE) [Online]. https://www.ardms.org/get-certified/rdms/fetal-echocardiography/. Accessed 30 Mar 2020.
27. National Institute for Health and Care Excellence (NICE). Quality statement 10: Screening – national fetal anomaly screening programmes [Online]. https://www.nice.org.uk/guidance/qs22/chapter/Quality-statement-10-Screening-national-fetal-anomaly-screening-programmes. Accessed 23 Mar 2020.
28. Public Health England. Fetal anomaly screening: ultrasound practitioners handbook [Online]. https://www.gov.uk/government/publications/fetal-anomaly-screening-ultrasound-practitioners-handbook. Accessed 23 Mar 2020.
29. Public Health England. Antenatal and newborn screening: programme specific operating model for quality assurance [Online]. 2017. https://www.gov.uk/government/publications/antenatal-and-newborn-screening-quality-assurance-procedures. Accessed 23 Apr 2020.
30. Abacan M, Alsubaie L, Barlow-Stewart K, Caanen B, Cordier C, Courtney E, Davoine E, Edwards J, Elackatt NJ, Gardiner K, Guan Y, Huang LH, Malmgren CI, Kejriwal S, Kim HJ, Lambert D, Lantigua-Cruz PA, Lee JMH, Lodahl M, Lunde A, Macaulay S, Macciocca I, Margarit S, Middleton A, Moldovan R, Ngeow J, Obregon-Tito AJ, Ormond KE, Paneque M, Powell K, Sanghavi K, Scotcher D, Scott J, Juhe CS, Shkedi-Rafid S, Wessels TM, Yoon SY, Wicklund C. The global state of the genetic counseling profession. Eur J Hum Genet. 2019;27:183–97.
31. Transnational Alliance for Genetic Counseling. International Committee on Genetic Counselor Credentialing [Online]. http://tagc.med.sc.edu/international_credentialing.asp. Accessed 23 Mar 2020.
32. Davidson RG, Childs B. Perspectives in the teaching of human genetics. In: Harris H, editor. Advances in human genetics: Springer; 1987.
33. International Genetic Counselling Credentialing: A Working Group of the TAGC. Template for comparing credentialing/registration (United States) [Online]. http://tagc.med.sc.edu/documents/credentialing/USACredentialing.pdf.
34. Skirton H, Kerzin-Storrar L, Barnes C, Hall G, Longmuir M, Patch C, Scott G, Walford-Moore J. Building the genetic counsellor profession in the United Kingdom: two decades of growth and development. J Genet Couns. 2013;22:902–6.
35. International Genetic Counselling Credentialing: A Working Group of the TAGC. 2016. Template for comparing credentialing/registration [Online]. http://tagc.med.sc.edu/documents/credentialing/UKCredentialing_2016.pdf. Accessed 23 Apr 2020.

36. Cruz AL. An overview of genetic counseling in Cuba. J Genet Couns. 2013;22:849–53.
37. American College of Obstetricians and Gynecologists (ACOG). Access to genetic testing [Online]. 2018. https://www.acog.org/clinical-information/policy-and-position-statements/position-statements/2018/access-to-genetic-testing. Accessed 23 Apr 2020.
38. Caplan AL. Chloe's Law: a powerful legislative movement challenging a core ethical norm of genetic testing. PLoS Biol. 2015;13:e1002219.
39. Yotsumoto J, Sekizawa A, Suzumori N, Yamada T, Samura O, Nishiyama M, Miura K, Sawai H, Murotsuki J, Kitagawa M, Kamei Y, Masuzaki H, Hirahara F, Endo T, Fukushima A, Namba A, Osada H, Kasai Y, Watanabe A, Katagiri Y, Takeshita N, Ogawa M, Okai T, Izumi S, Hamanoue H, Inuzuka M, Haino K, Hamajima N, Nishizawa H, Okamoto Y, Nakamura H, Kanegawa T, Yoshimatsu J, Tairaku S, Naruse K, Masuyama H, Hyodo M, Kaji T, Maeda K, Matsubara K, Ogawa M, Yoshizato T, Ohba T, Kawano Y, Sago H, Japan NIPT Consortium. A survey on awareness of genetic counseling for non-invasive prenatal testing: the first year experience in Japan. J Hum Genet. 2016;61:995–1001.
40. Ministry of Education, Culture, Sports, Science and Technology. Announcement of Medical Education Model Core Curriculum (2016 revised edition) and Dental Education Model Core Curriculum (2016 revised edition) [Online]. 2017. https://www.mext.go.jp/b_menu/shingi/chousa/koutou/033-2/toushin/1383962.htm. Accessed 23 Apr 2020.

Correction to: Fetal MRI

Keiko Segawa

Correction to:
Chapter 3 in: H. Masuzaki (ed.), *Fetal Morph Functional Diagnosis*, Comprehensive Gynecology and Obstetrics, https://doi.org/10.1007/978-981-15-8171-7_3

We inadvertently published the figures "3.1, 3.3, 3.4, 3.5, 3.6" without the arrow marks. This has been rectified in this version.

The updated version of this chapter can be found at https://doi.org/10.1007/978-981-15-8171-7_3

H. Masuzaki (ed.), *Fetal Morph Functional Diagnosis*, Comprehensive Gynecology and Obstetrics, https://doi.org/10.1007/978-981-15-8171-7_28

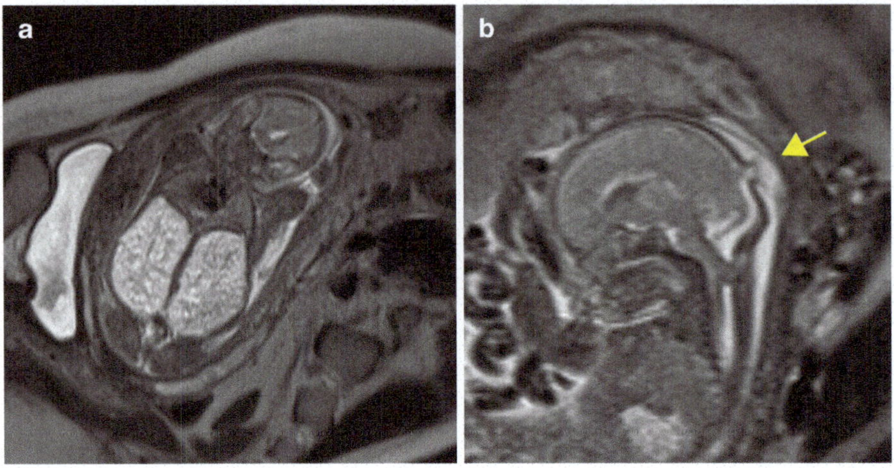

Fig. 3.1 (**a**) Coronal MRI of the fetus at 20 weeks shows severe oligohydramnios. The kidneys are grossly enlarged with abnormal hyperintense parenchyma. (**b**) Sagittal MRI of the brain in the same fetus shows an occipital calvarial defect and posterior encephalocele (arrow). These findings are classic features in Meckel-Gruber syndrome

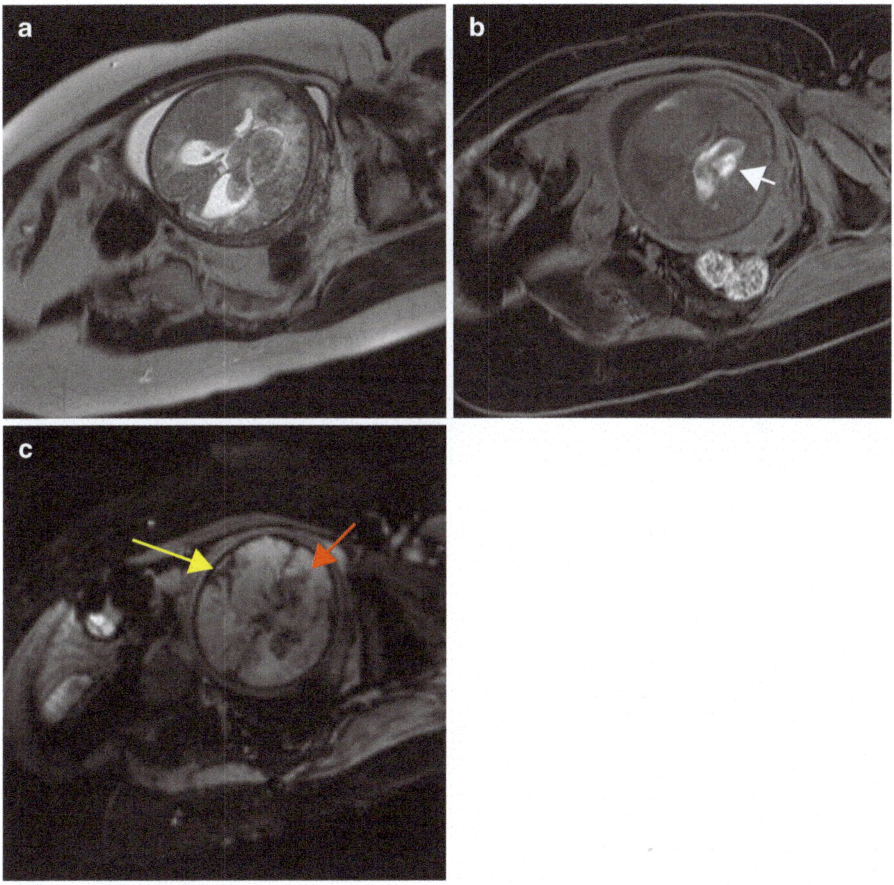

Fig. 3.3 Axial MRI of different sequences of the fetus at 37 weeks with ventriculomegaly and intraventricular hemorrhage. (**a**) T2-weighted image. (**b**) T1-weighted image. (**c**) Echoplanar imaging. Left caudate nucleus shows swelling with ventricular hematoma showing T2-hypointensity/T1-hyperintensity (white arrow). On EP imaging, right Sylvian fissure subarachnoid hemorrhage (yellow arrow) and parenchymal hemorrhage in the left frontal lobe (red arrow) are clear

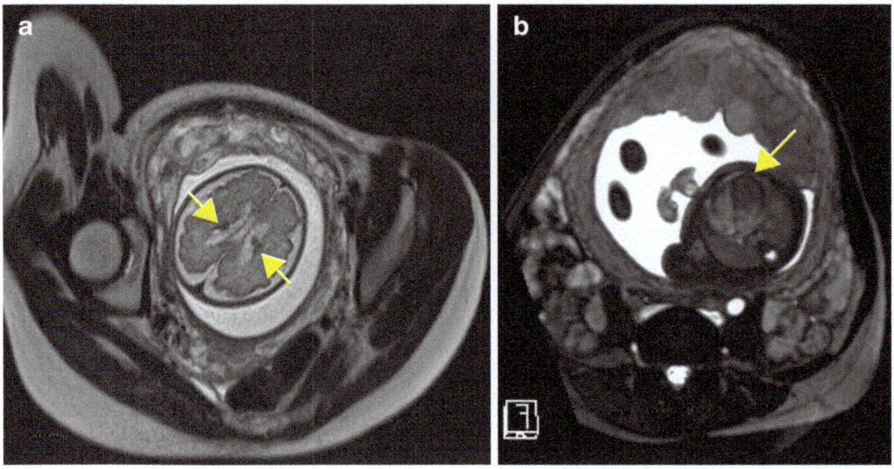

Fig. 3.4 Rhabdomyomas and tuberous sclerosis complex. MRI of the fetus at 29 weeks. (**a**) Axial T2-weighted image shows subependymal nodules (arrows). (**b**) SSFP sequences demonstrate cardiac rhabdomyomas as hypointense area (arrow)

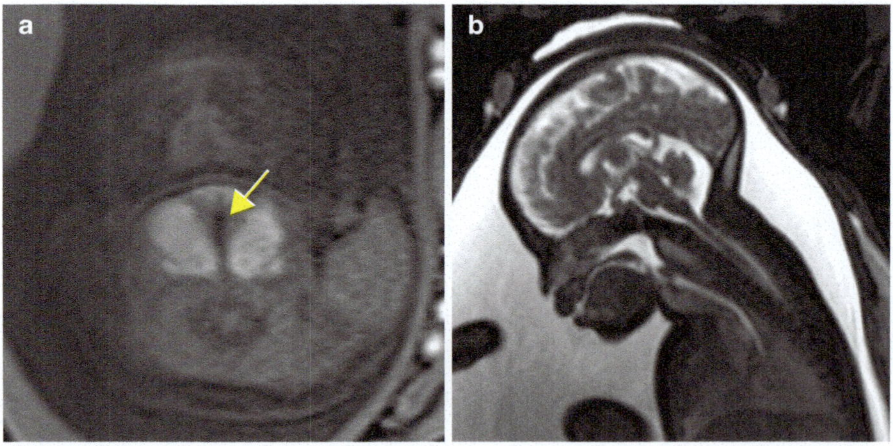

Fig. 3.5 MRI of the fetus at 35 weeks with large goiter. (**a**) On axial T1-weighted image, the large goiter showed hyperintensity and the trachea running in the center was narrowing (arrow). (**b**) Fetal airway patency was assessed with 3D dataset for reconstruction

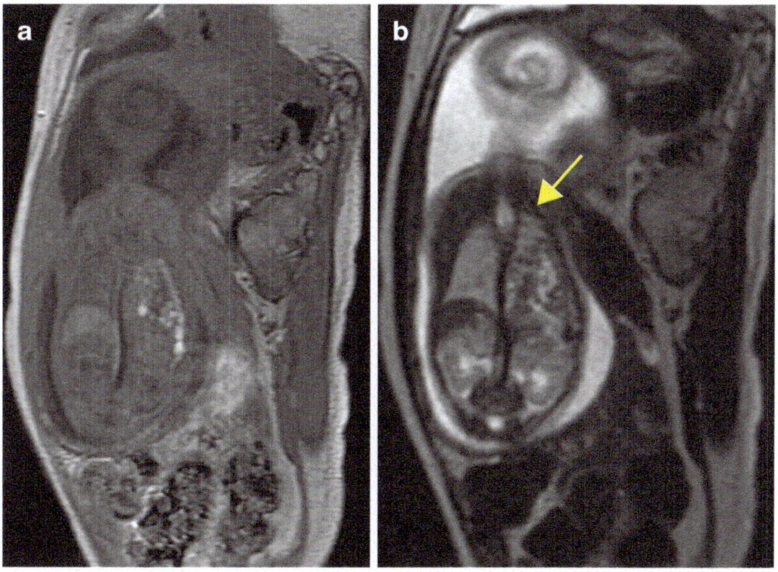

Fig. 3.6 Coronal MRI of the fetus at 28 weeks with congenital diaphragmatic hernia. (**a**) T1-weighted sequence reveal the presence of meconium-filled bowel within the thoracic cavity. (**b**) T2-weighted sequences reveal a tiny left lung at the top of thoracic cavity (arrow)

The manufacturer's authorised representative in the EU is Springer Nature Customer Service Centre GmbH, Europaplatz 3, 69115 Heidelberg, Germany. If you have any concerns regarding our products, please contact ProductSafety@springernature.com

Printed and bound by CPI Group (UK) Ltd, Croydon, CR0 4YY
27/07/2026
02177375-0003